Clinical Nutrition and Inflammatory Bowel Disease

Clinical Nutrition and Inflammatory Bowel Disease

Edited by Jack Marlow

hayle medical

New York

Hayle Medical,
750 Third Avenue, 9th Floor,
New York, NY 10017, USA

Visit us on the World Wide Web at:
www.haylemedical.com

ISBN: 978-1-64647-537-7

Cataloging-in-Publication Data

Clinical nutrition and inflammatory bowel disease / edited by Jack Marlow.
p. cm.
Includes bibliographical references and index.
ISBN 978-1-64647-537-7
1. Inflammatory bowel diseases. 2. Inflammatory bowel diseases--Nutritional aspects.
3. Inflammatory bowel diseases--Diet therapy. 4. Diet therapy. I. Marlow, Jack.
RC862.I53 C55 2023
616.344--dc23

Table of Contents

Preface

Inflammatory bowel disease (IBD) is an umbrella term used to describe intestinal disorders that cause prolonged inflammation (pain and swelling) of the digestive tract. IBD can be divided into two types which include Crohn's disease and ulcerative colitis. Signs and symptoms of IBD include reduced appetite, unintended weight loss, mucus or blood in stool, and upset stomach. IBD can be prevented by certain dietary and lifestyle changes. A patient suffering from IBD is recommended to reduce the intake of foods that irritate the intestines such as fibrous, spicy, greasy, or milk-based products. Vitamin D deficiency is highly prevalent in IBD patients. Exclusive enteral nutrition (EEN) that includes amino acids, sugars, fats, vitamins and minerals is the only established diet for IBD patients. This book investigates the effect of nutrition and diet on inflammatory bowel disease. With state-of-the-art inputs by acclaimed experts of gastroenterology, it targets medical students and professionals.

The researches compiled throughout the book are authentic and of high quality, combining several disciplines and from very diverse regions from around the world. Drawing on the contributions of many researchers from diverse countries, the book's objective is to provide the readers with the latest achievements in the area of research. This book will surely be a source of knowledge to all interested and researching the field.

In the end, I would like to express my deep sense of gratitude to all the authors for meeting the set deadlines in completing and submitting their research chapters. I would also like to thank the publisher for the support offered to us throughout the course of the book. Finally, I extend my sincere thanks to my family for being a constant source of inspiration and encouragement.

Editor

1

Associations between Folate and Vitamin B12 Levels and Inflammatory Bowel Disease

Yun Pan [1], Ya Liu [1], Haizhuo Guo [2], Majid Sakhi Jabir [3], Xuanchen Liu [1], Weiwei Cui [1,*] and Dong Li [4,5,*]

1 Department of Nutrition and Food Hygiene, School of Public Health, Jilin University, 1163 Xinmin Avenue, Changchun 130021, China; yunpan14@mails.jlu.edu.cn (Y.P.); liuya@jlu.edu.cn (Y.L.); liuxc15@mails.jlu.edu.cn (X.L.)
2 Department of Radiology, The Second Part of the First Hospital, Jilin University, Changchun 130031, China; doyouknow_0330@163.com
3 Department of Biotechnology, University of Technology, Baghdad 00964, Iraq; msj_iraq@yahoo.com
4 Department of Immunology, College of Basic Medical Sciences, Jilin University, 126 Xinmin Avenue, Changchun 130021, China
5 Department of Hepatology, The First Hospital, Jilin University, Changchun 130021, China
* Correspondence: cuiweiwei@jlu.edu.cn (W.C.); lidong1@jlu.edu.cn (D.L.)

Abstract: Background: Inflammatory bowel disease (IBD) patients may be at risk of vitamin B12 and folate insufficiencies, as these micronutrients are absorbed in the small intestine, which is affected by IBD. However, a consensus has not been reached on the association between IBD and serum folate and vitamin B12 concentrations. Methods: In this study, a comprehensive search of multiple databases was performed to identify studies focused on the association between IBD and serum folate and vitamin B12 concentrations. Studies that compared serum folate and vitamin B12 concentrations between IBD and control patients were selected for inclusion in the meta-analysis. Results: The main outcome was the mean difference in serum folate and vitamin B12 concentrations between IBD and control patients. Our findings indicated that the average serum folate concentration in IBD patients was significantly lower than that in control patients, whereas the mean serum vitamin B12 concentration did not differ between IBD patients and controls. In addition, the average serum folate concentration in patients with ulcerative colitis (UC) but not Crohn's disease (CD) was significantly lower than that in controls. This meta-analysis identified a significant relationship between low serum folate concentration and IBD. Conclusions: Our findings suggest IBD may be linked with folate deficiency, although the results do not indicate causation. Thus, providing supplements of folate and vitamin B12 to IBD patients may improve their nutritional status and prevent other diseases.

Keywords: folate; vitamin B12; inflammatory bowel disease; meta-analysis; nutrition

1. Introduction

Inflammatory bowel disease (IBD) is characterized by chronic and typically recurrent intestinal inflammation, and it includes Crohn's disease (CD) and ulcerative colitis (UC). Although the exact aetiology and pathogenesis of IBD is still largely unknown, it is considered to be related to individual immunity, an inherited predisposition, environmental factors and the interactions between the mucosal immune system and intestinal antigenic material (e.g., commensal bacteria) [1]. Abnormal immune responses are believed to be the direct cause of intestinal damage [2]. IBD can lead to many clinical symptoms, including impaired nutrient absorption, which can influence the absorption of folate and vitamin B12. Furthermore, many studies have indicated that serum folate and vitamin B12 concentrations influence the development of IBD. Folate is involved in the methylation of DNA and may produce epigenetic changes that affect the interaction between the gut microbiota and systemic immune responses [3]. The gut microbiota [4] and epigenetic changes [5] may be involved in the pathogenesis of IBD. Vitamin B12 acts as a coenzyme in various biochemical reactions, including DNA synthesis and folate metabolism [6]. Deficiencies in vitamin B12 and folate can lead to macrocytic anaemia, hyperhomocysteinemia, and neurologic and psychiatric disorders [7–9]. Compared with healthy subjects, IBD patients are at increased risk of hyperhomocysteinemia [10], and folic acid and vitamin B12 may play pivotal roles in homocysteine metabolic reactions [11]. Moreover, folate and vitamin B12 deficiencies may cause increased homocysteine levels, a risk factor for thrombosis [8,12–14].

Many studies have reported that serum folic and vitamin B12 concentrations differ between IBD patients and healthy individuals. However, the results are not consistent, and differences have been observed between patients with CD and UC. Whether serum folic acid and vitamin B12 concentrations are lower in IBD patients than in non-IBD patients is still largely unknown. Thus, a more comprehensive evaluation of the association between IBD and serum folic acid and vitamin B12 concentrations is needed. In this study, we conducted a meta-analysis to analyse the relationships between the serum concentrations of folic acid and vitamin B12 in IBD patients and healthy controls to provide additional insights into treating and rehabilitating IBD and maintaining a healthy nutritional status.

2. Materials and Methods

2.1. Sources and Methods of Data Retrieval

We performed a comprehensive literature search that included studies from 1970 to December 2016; the electronic databases included PubMed, Medline, Web of Science, and Google Scholar. The searches were conducted to identify all published studies that reported data on the mean differences and standard deviations of serum folate and vitamin B12 concentrations in IBD patients and healthy controls. The following terms were used for the literature search: folic acid, vitamin B9, vitamin M, folvite, folate, vitamin B12, cyanocobalamin, cobalamins, inflammatory bowel disease, Crohn's disease, ulcerative colitis. The term 'OR' was used as the set operator to combine different sets of results. The serum concentrations of folate and vitamin B12 and IBD were determined and used in a meta-analysis to understand how serum folate and vitamin B12 concentrations differ in IBD patients relative to healthy controls. Age, location, detection methods and other confounding factors were also considered.

2.2. Inclusion Criteria

The articles that were included in this meta-analysis matched the following five criteria: (1) inflammatory bowel disease patients were clinically diagnosed; (2) studies included a case group and a control group; (3) the folate and vitamin B12 values were presented as the mean $\pm$ standard deviation (SD); and (4) the patients and controls had not previously received folate and vitamin B12 supplementation; and (5) we excluded studies that did not provide initial data, animal studies, in vitro studies, reviews and conference papers. Three investigators independently reviewed and extracted all of the potentially eligible studies and discussed the inconsistencies until a consensus was reached (Figure 1). Additionally, the Newcastle-Ottawa Scale was used for assessing the quality of studies included in this meta-analysis (Table 1).

2.3. Data Abstraction

We reviewed all of the relevant studies and extracted the following data: (1) lead author, publication year, sample size, mean age of the patients and controls, and gender of the patients and controls; (2) serum folate and vitamin B12 concentrations of the patients and controls; (3) folate and vitamin B12 detection methods; and (4) the diagnosis of the patients and the number of patients and controls.

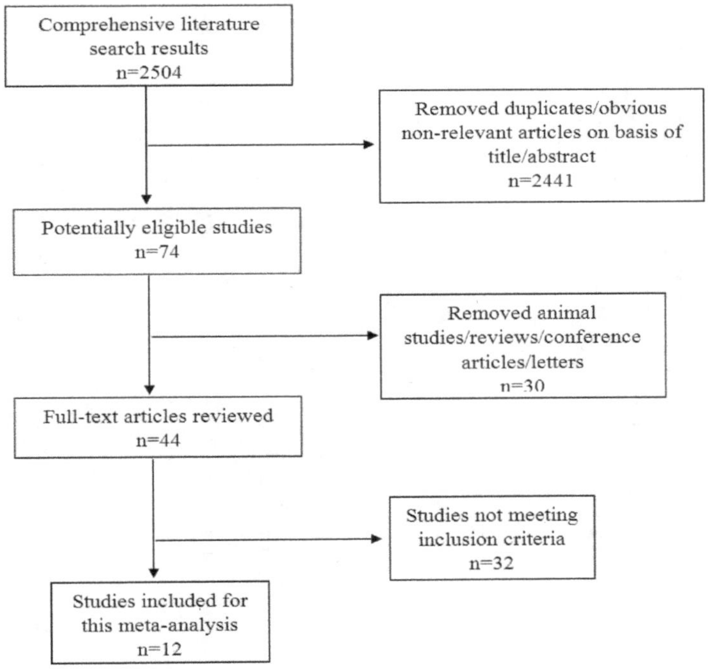

Figure 1. Flow diagram of the literature search.

2.4. Statistical Analysis

All statistical analysis was conducted using the statistical software Stata (version 12.0, StataCorp LLC, College Station, TX, USA). The mean difference, standard deviation and standard error of the serum folate and vitamin B12 concentrations in the IBD and control group were used for the meta-analysis. Units that were not unified were transformed into unified units. We combined the standardized mean difference (SMD) for studies that reported mean and standard deviation values for serum folate and vitamin B12 concentrations in IBD patients and controls. An inverse variance weighted random effect model was used to determine the SMD and 95% confidence intervals (CIs) and measure the different concentrations of folate and vitamin B12 in the patients and controls, and the results were used to evaluate the differences in serum concentrations of folate and vitamin B12 between the IBD patients and normal controls. In order to avoid double counting, both controls in two studies that included both UC and CD patients [15,16] were split approximately evenly into 2 control groups with the means and standard deviations left unchanged before entered into the meta-analysis [17,18].

We used Cochran's Q statistic and the I^2 statistic to assess the statistical heterogeneity in the meta-analysis [19]. If the data were homogeneous ($p > 0.05$), a fixed effect model meta-analysis was performed; if the data were heterogeneous ($p \leq 0.05$), a random effects model meta-analysis was performed. Heterogeneity was considered significant at $p < 0.05$ in the Q test, and the I^2 value was used to evaluate the degree of heterogeneity. We defined low, medium and high heterogeneity at I^2 values of 25%, 50%, and 75%, respectively [20]. Sensitivity analysis was used for analyzing heterogeneity. Subgroup analyses were performed for the type of disease, region of study, and method of detecting the vitamins. In addition, we performed a meta-regression analysis based on the folate and vitamin B12 measurement methods, the year of publication, the sample size, the quality of the study and the average age of the patients. We used a funnel plot to detect publication bias concerning this meta-analysis, with the symmetry of the funnel plot used to determine whether publication bias occurred. Furthermore, a formal statistical assessment of the funnel plot asymmetry was performed with Egger's regression asymmetry test [21].

Table 1. Studies showing the serum folate and vitamin B12 concentrations in IBD patients and controls.

Author	Region	Score	Year	*n*		Assay Method	Age	Gender (Male/Female)		IBD/CD/UC (Mean ± SD)		Controls (Mean ± SD)		*p*	
				IBD/CD/UC	C		IBD/CD/UC/C	IBD/CD/UC	C	FA (ng/mL)	B12 (pg/mL)	FA (ng/mL)	B12 (pg/mL)	FA	B12
Jiang et al. [22]	China	8	2010	252	654	chemiluminescence	-/-/45 ± 14/46 ± 17	147/105	279/374	4.97 ± 2.73 *	437.53 ± 174.12 *	6.74 ± 3.41	572.77 ± 175.33	<0.001	<0.001
Lambert et al. [23]	France	6	1996	21	20	radioimmunoassay	-	11/10	8/12	2.8 ± 2.8 #	190 ± 146 #	4.55 ± 3.26	207 ± 75	NS	NS
Kuroki et al. [24]	Japan	8	1993	24	24	radioimmunoassay	-/26.4 ± 12.4/-/27.0 ± 4.2	17/7	14/10		641 ± 186 #		682 ± 488	<0.001	
Fernández-Miranda et al. [25]	Spain	7	2005	52	186	radioimmunoassay	41.7 ± 11.9/-/-/ 41.9 ± 10.1	23/29	71/115	7.6 ± 4.1	499 ± 287	8.9 ± 3.7	603 ± 231	<0.05	<0.05
Erzin et al. [26]	Turkey	7	2008	105	85	ELISA	38.69 ± 12.13/-/-/ 37.61 ± 10.05	-	-	3.72 ± 1.44	600.14 ± 145.30	4.96 ± 1.19	700.32 ± 141.58	<0.001	
Alkhouri et al. [27]	U.S.	8	2013	61	61	-	12.3 ± 3.9/12.1 ± 4.1/12.3 ± 3.5/12.1 ± 3.6	40/21	30/31	20.1 ± 6.5 20.3 ± 7 # 20.9 ± 5.9 *	775 ± 441 781 ± 372 # 906 ± 669 *	20.4 ± 5.5	727 ± 346		
Yakut et al. [15]	Turkey	6	2010	138	53	chemiluminescence	-	64/74	19/34	7.7 ± 5.3 # 8.6 ± 8.3 *	281 ± 166 # 348 ± 218 *	9.9 ± 3.3	342 ± 179	NS	NS
Akbulut et al. [28]	Turkey	9	2010	55	45	chemiluminescence	-/-/47.4 ± 13.80/ 46.4 ± 13.89	38/17	31/14	5.1 ± 2.19 *	250.4 ± 82.49 *	6.3 ± 0.87	327 ± 73.9	<0.001	<0.001
Kallel et al. [29]	Tunisia	6	2011	89	103	specific immunochemical methods	35.3 ± 12.6/-/-/ 36.5 ± 9.26	47/42	50/53	8.54 ± 3.04	295 ± 180	8.1 ± 3.11	378 ± 170	NS	<0.001
Geerling et al. [30]	Netherlands	7	2000	69	69	radioimmunoassay	-/30.1 ± 10.2/37.8 ± 14.7/35.4 ± 13.7	33/36	23/46	4.72 ± 4.02 #	304.96 ± 82.27 #	5.47 ± 2.47 *	357.82 ± 121.58 *	NS	0.05
										5.03 ± 3.80 *	364.59 ± 119.14 *	5.78 ± 2.96 #	365.95 ± 119.54 #		
Chen et al. [31]	China	6	2011	112	110	ELISA	-/-/39.4 ± 11.7/ 40.3 ± 10.8	58/54	56/54	3.37 ± 0.86 *	147.25 ± 43.67 *	4.03 ± 0.54	152.67 ± 45.17	0.005	0.004
Koutroubakis et al. [16]	Greece	6	2000	108	74	IMx assay	-	66/42	-	6.34 ± 3.05 # 7.02 ± 3.13 *	666.5 ± 366.8 # 478.8 ± 257.7 *	8.78 ± 3.07	377.5 ± 155.6	<0.05	<0.05

* Folate and Vitamin B12 levels reported in ulcerative colitis. # Folate and Vitamin B12 levels reported in Crohn's disease. - Not applicable. P: patients vs. controls; IBD: Inflammatory Bowel Disease; CD: Crohn's Disease; UC: Ulcerative Colitis; C: Controls; FA: Folate Acid; B12: Vitamin B12. SD: standard deviation. IMx assay: a multi-functional immune assay system developed by Abbott Diagnostics, Abbott Park, IL.

3. Results

Our search identified 2504 related references; however, only 12 papers met our inclusion criteria. The 12 studies included 2570 individuals in total, with 1086 IBD patients and 1484 controls [15,16,22–31]. The detailed results are expressed in Table 1. Among the 12 studies, the folate concentration in the study by Kuroki et al. [24] was excluded because it was detected in red blood cells. Folate and vitamin B12 were detected via chemiluminescence immunoassays in three studies [15,22,28], radioimmunoassays in four studies [23–25,30], ELISA in two studies [26,31], a specific immunochemical method in one study [29], and the IMx assay in one study [16]. Three studies did not include the mean age of patients and controls [15,16,23], and one study included the median age of patients and controls [23]. Of the 12 included studies, six studies were conducted in Asia [15,22,24,26,28,31], four in Europe [16,23,25,30], one in America [27], and one in Africa [29]. Seven studies investigated the association between UC and serum folate and vitamin B12 concentrations [15,16,22,27,28,30,31]; six studies investigated the association between CD and serum folate and vitamin B12 [15,16,23,27,29,30]; and two studies investigated IBD patients who were not classified by the type of disease [25,26]. The patients' basic characteristics are presented in Table 1. The participants in one study [27] were children, and those in the other studies were adults. The data included in this analysis was defined as continuous variables.

We conducted a meta-analysis of the serum folic acid and vitamin B12 concentrations in 1086 IBD patients and 1484 controls. The average serum folate concentration in the IBD patients was 0.46 nmol/L lower than that in the controls (SMD = −0.46 ng/mL, 95% CI = −0.64, −0.27 ng/mL, $I^2 = 74.7\%$, $p = 0.000$; Figure 2). An analysis of the results of these studies indicated that IBD patients did not have significantly lower serum vitamin B12 concentrations than the healthy controls (SMD = −0.20 ng/mL, 95% CI = −0.46, 0.05 ng/mL, $I^2 = 87.6\%$, $p = 0.123$; Figure 3). Because of the heterogeneity of the results, we applied a random effects model. In addition, publication bias was not observed in the serum folate concentrations (Egger's test: coefficient = 0.70, $p = 0.627$). However, publication bias was observed in the serum vitamin B12 concentration (Egger's test: coefficient = 4.09, $p = 0.021$). A sensitivity analysis revealed that the studies by Koutroubakis et al. [16] influenced the results; however, when we excluded the study by Koutroubakis et al. on vitamin B12, our final results indicated that the serum vitamin B12 concentrations for IBD patients were 0.35 ng/mL lower than the controls (overall effect size = −0.35 ng/mL, 95% CI = −0.56, −0.13, $I^2 = 79.3\%$, $p = 0.001$).

Significant heterogeneity was observed for the studies (folate: $I^2 = 74.7\%$, $p < 0.001$; vitamin B12: $I^2 = 87.6\%$, $p < 0.001$).

The included articles were divided into three groups by the type of disease as follows: only patients with UC (UC group) [15,16,22,27,28,30,31], only patients with CD (CD group) [15,16,23,27,29,30] and patients from studies [25,26] that did not indicate the type of IBD (IBD group). For the UC group (680 UC patients, 1151 controls), the average serum folate concentration was 0.50 ng/mL lower than that of the controls (SMD = −0.50 ng/mL, 95% CI = −0.71, −0.28 ng/mL, $I^2 = 63.0\%$, $p = 0.000$). For the CD group (247 CD patients, 367 controls), the average serum folate concentration was not statistically significant differences with the controls (SMD = −0.30 ng/mL, 95% CI = −0.63, 0.04 ng/mL, $I^2 = 69.0\%$, $p = 0.080$). For the IBD group, statistically significant differences with the controls were observed (SMD = −0.64 ng/mL, 95% CI = −1.21, −0.06 ng/mL, $I^2 = 85.9\%$, $p = 0.030$) (Figure 4).

The meta-analysis of 12 studies that included the mean serum vitamin B12 concentrations showed an overall non-significant summary effect between the UC patients (SMD = −0.17 pg/mL, 95% CI = −0.59, 0.24 pg/mL, $I^2 = 90.3\%$, $p = 0.406$) and CD patients (SMD = −0.05 pg/mL, 95% CI = −0.46, 0.37 pg/mL, $I^2 = 82.7\%$, $p = 0.829$). However, IBD patients had significantly lower concentrations than healthy controls (SMD = −0.57 pg/mL, 95% CI = −0.83, −0.30 pg/mL, $I^2 = 35.5\%$, $p = 0.000$) (Figure 5).

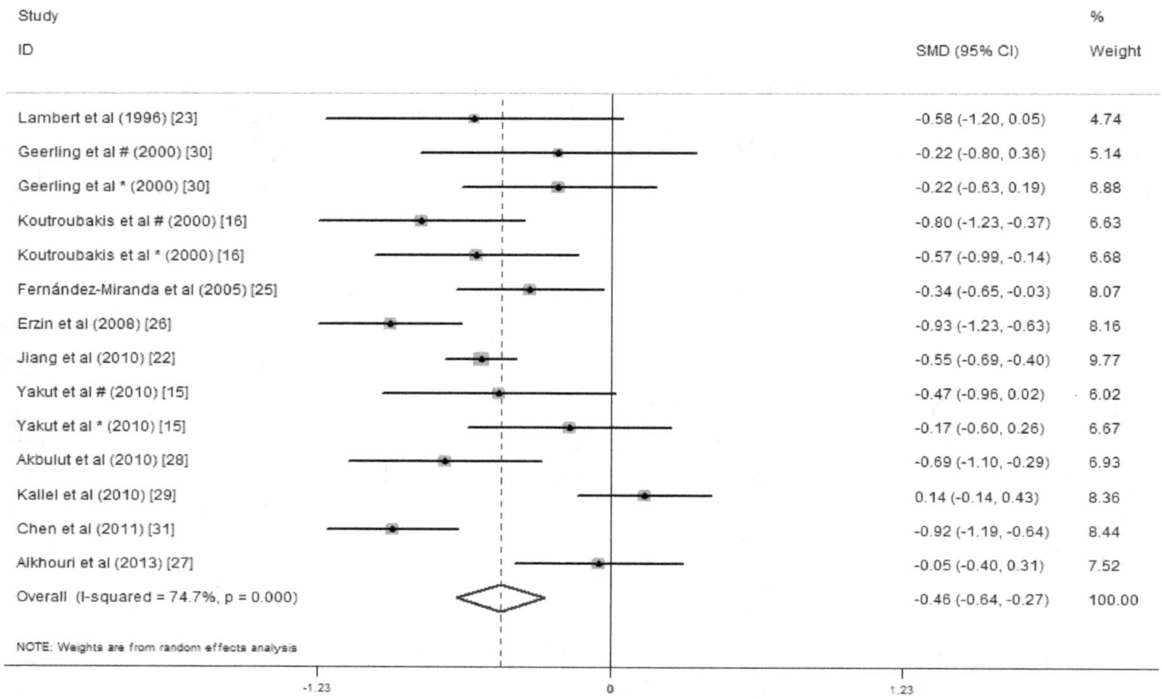

Figure 2. Forest plot of the serum folate concentrations in the inflammatory bowel disease (IBD) patients vs. controls; standardized mean differences with the 95% confidence interval and weight percentage are shown. * Reported in ulcerative colitis; # reported in Crohn's disease.

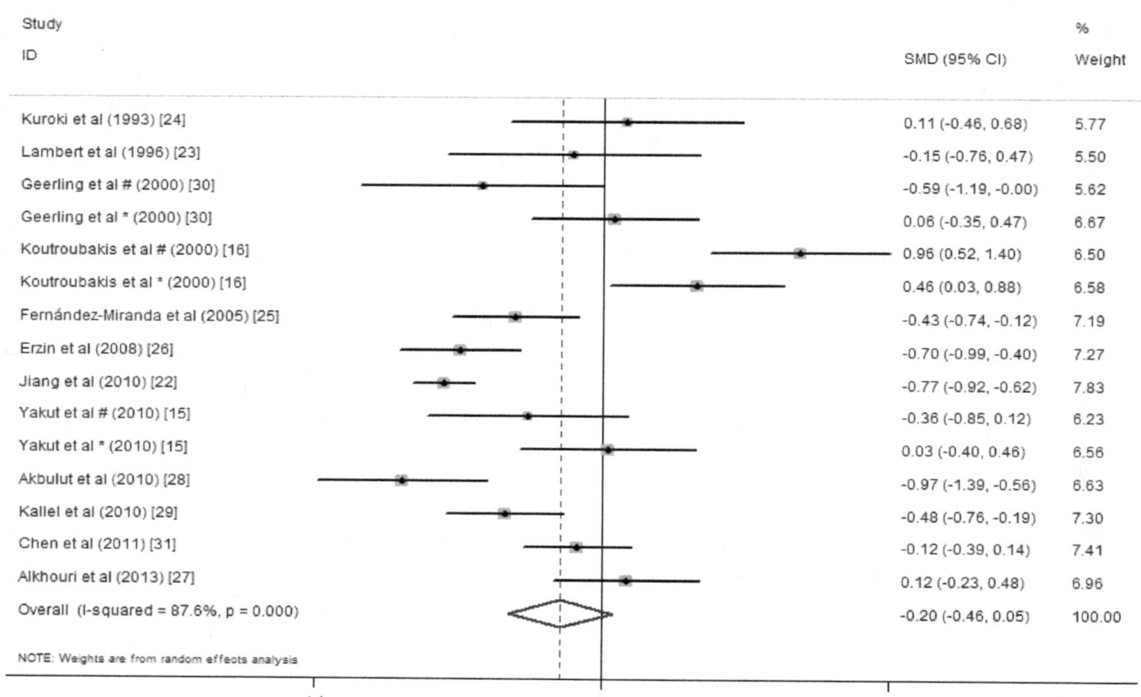

Figure 3. Forest plot of the serum concentrations of vitamin B12 in the IBD patients vs. controls; standardized mean differences with the 95% confidence interval and weight percentage are shown. * Reported in ulcerative colitis; # reported in Crohn's disease.

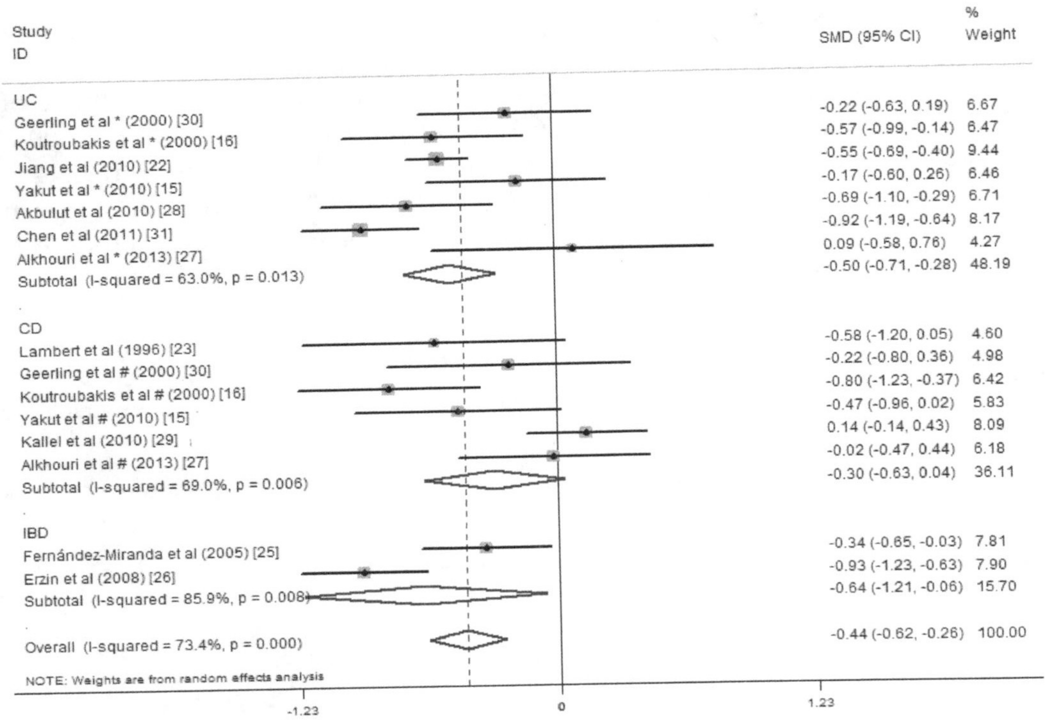

Figure 4. Forest plot of the serum concentrations of folate in the ulcerative colitis (UC), Crohn's disease (CD) and IBD patients vs. controls; standardized mean differences with the 95% confidence interval and weight percentage are shown. Subtotals are for the UC, CD and IBD patients.

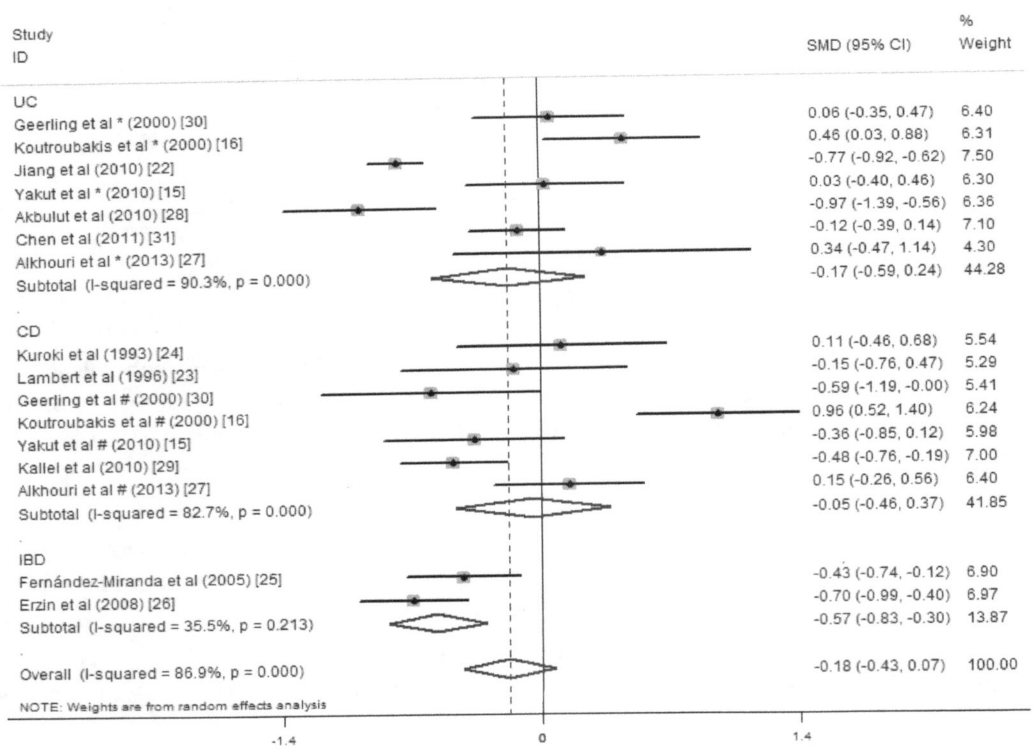

Figure 5. Forest plot of the serum concentrations of vitamin B12 in the UC, CD and IBD patients vs. controls; standardized mean differences with the 95% confidence interval and weight percentage are shown. Subtotals are for the UC, CD and IBD patients.

A subgroup analysis was performed according to the study area, and the studies were divided into three areas: Asia, Europe, and other (America and Africa). The studies in Asia showed that the serum folate concentrations of the IBD patients were significantly lower than those of the healthy controls (SMD = −0.65 ng/mL, 95% CI = −0.86, −0.44 ng/mL, I^2 = 64.3%, p = 0.000). The studies in Europe showed that the serum folate concentrations in the IBD patients were 0.44 ng/mL lower than those of the healthy controls (SMD = −0.44 ng/mL, 95% CI = −0.62, −0.26 ng/mL, I^2 = 3.1%, p = 0.000). The studies in the other areas did not show differences in the serum folate concentrations between the IBD patients and the controls (Figure 6).

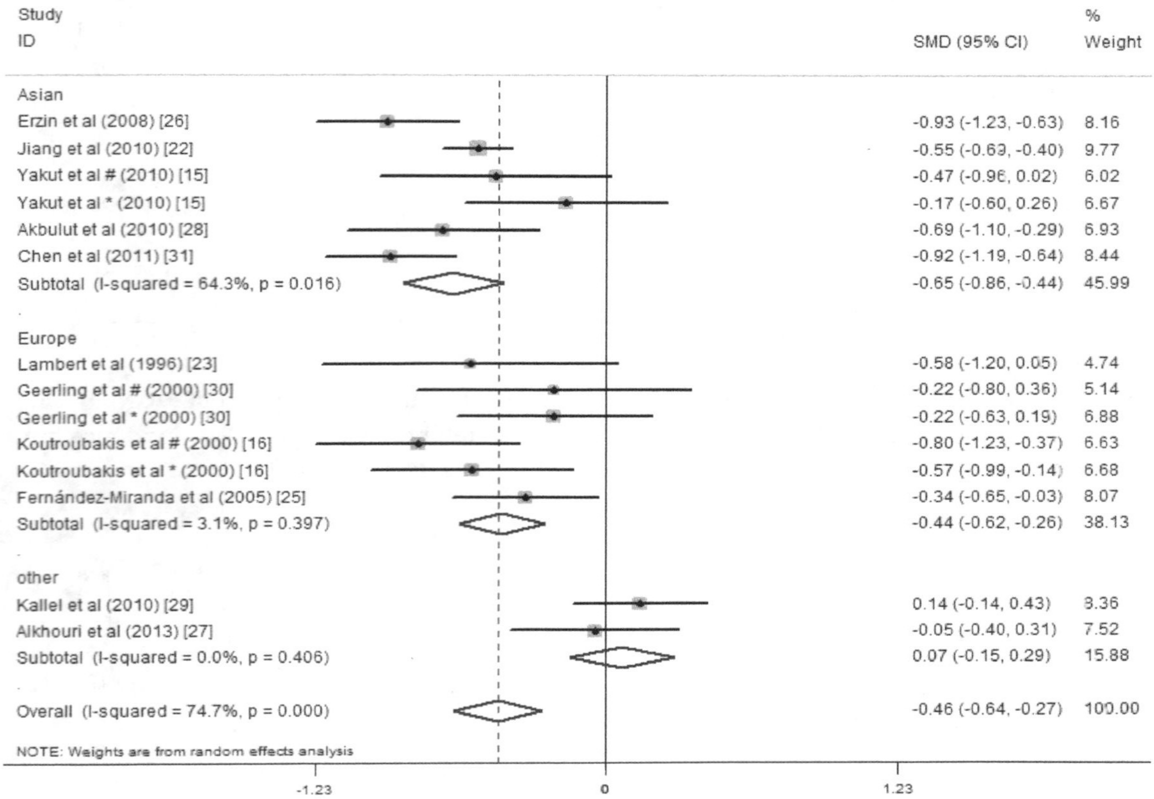

Figure 6. Forest plot of the serum concentrations of folate in the IBD patients vs. controls; standardized mean differences with the 95% confidence interval and weight percentage are shown. Subtotals are for the studies from Asia, Europe, and others. * Reported in ulcerative colitis; # reported in Crohn's disease.

In the subgroup meta-analysis on the mean serum vitamin B12 concentrations, the studies in Asia showed a significant summary effect, and the serum vitamin B12 concentrations of the IBD patients vere 0.43 pg/mL lower than that of the controls (SMD = −0.43 ng/mL, 95% CI = −0.73, −0.13 ng/mL, = 83.4%, p = 0.005). However, significant differences in serum vitamin B12 concentrations were not etected between the IBD patients and controls in the studies from Europe or the other areas (Figure 7).

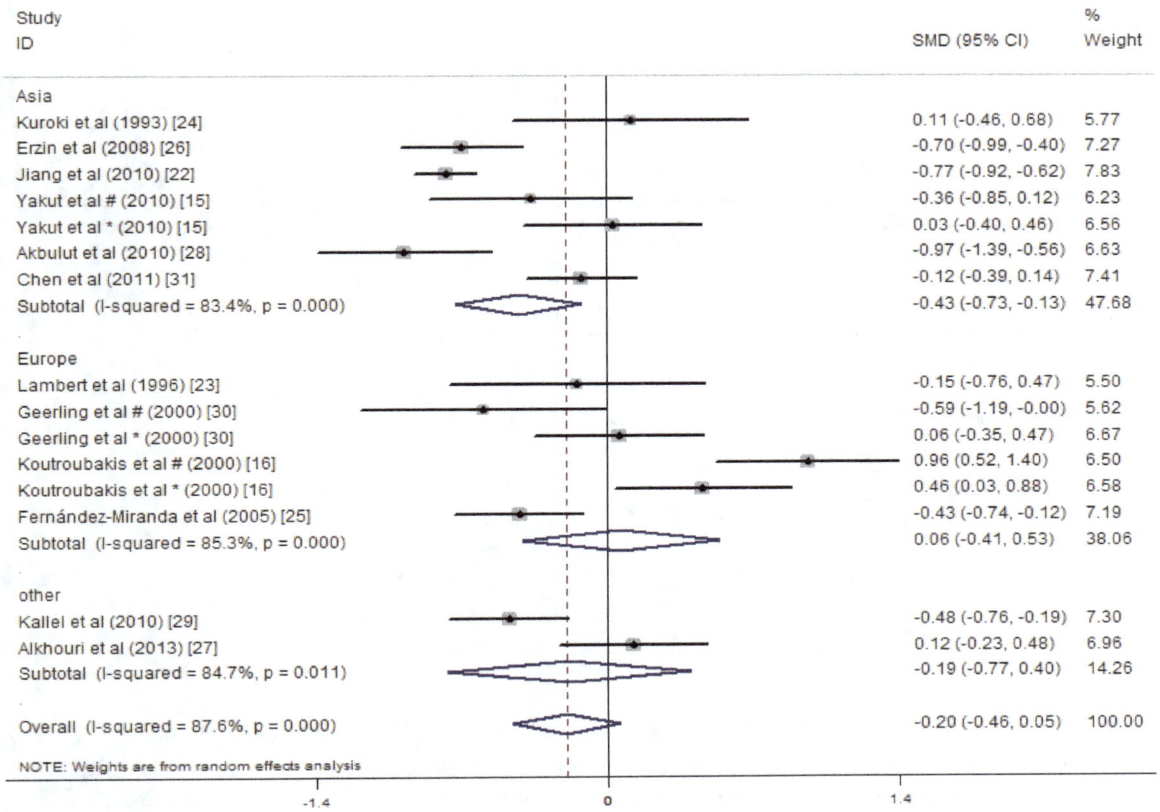

Figure 7. Forest plot of the serum concentrations of vitamin B12 in the IBD patients vs. controls; standardized mean differences with the 95% confidence interval and weight percentage are shown. Subtotals are for the studies from Asia, Europe, and others. * Reported in ulcerative colitis; # reported in Crohn's disease.

The main methods of detecting folic acid and vitamin B12 in the included studies were chemiluminescence immunoassays, radioimmunoassays and ELISA. Alkhouri et al. did not specify the detection method. Kallel et al.'s study used specific immunochemical methods [29], and Koutroubakis et al.'s study used the IMx assay [16]. We performed subgroup analysis according to the three main methods of detecting folate, and the results indicated that the heterogeneity among the three groups was reduced, and the subtotal I^2 values of the chemiluminescence immunoassay, radioimmunoassay and ELISA methods were 11.3%, 0% and 0%, respectively. Studies that applied these three detection methods showed lower average serum folate concentrations in the IBD patients relative to the controls (Figure 8). Thus, the detection methods may introduce heterogeneity into the serum folate concentration results in the different studies. A similar subgroup analysis was performed for the serum vitamin B12 concentrations. Significant differences were only observed among the studies that used chemiluminescence immunoassays, and they indicated that the serum vitamin B12 concentrations of the IBD patients were 0.54 pg/mL lower than that of the controls (SMD = -0.54 pg/mL, 95% CI = -0.94, -0.15 pg/mL, $I^2 = 80.6\%$, $p = 0.010$). However, in studies that detected serum vitamin B12 concentrations via radioimmunoassays and ELISA, statistically significant differences were not observed between the IBD patients and the controls (Figure 9).

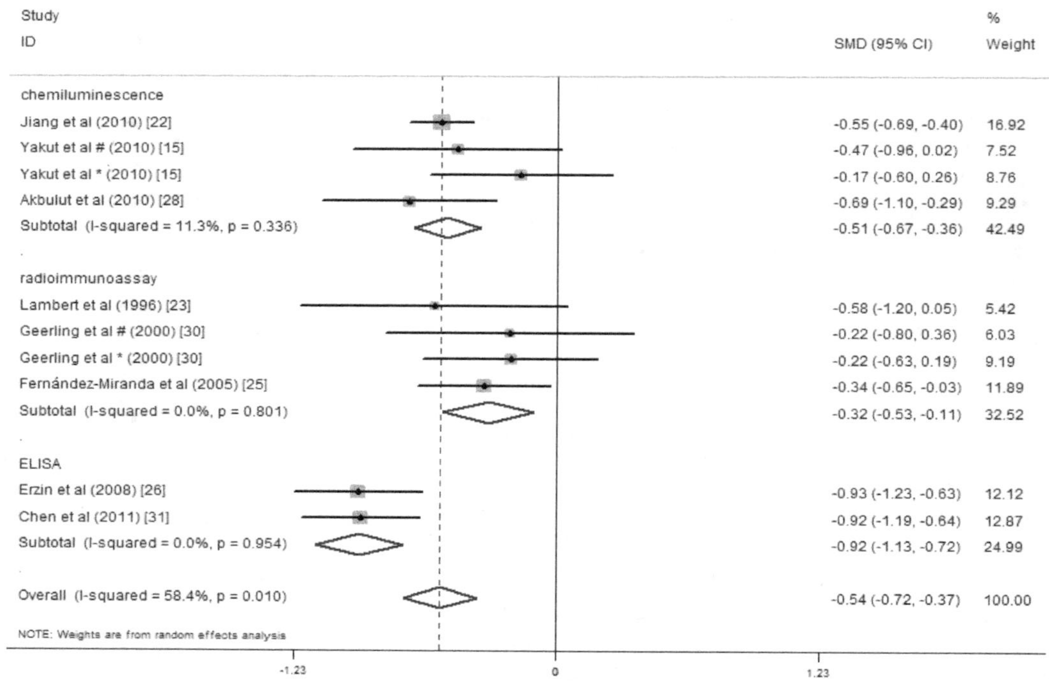

Figure 8. Forest plot of the serum concentrations of folate in the IBD patients vs. controls; standardized mean differences with a 95% confidence interval and weight percentage are shown. Subtotals are for the three detection methods. * Reported in ulcerative colitis; # reported in Crohn's disease.

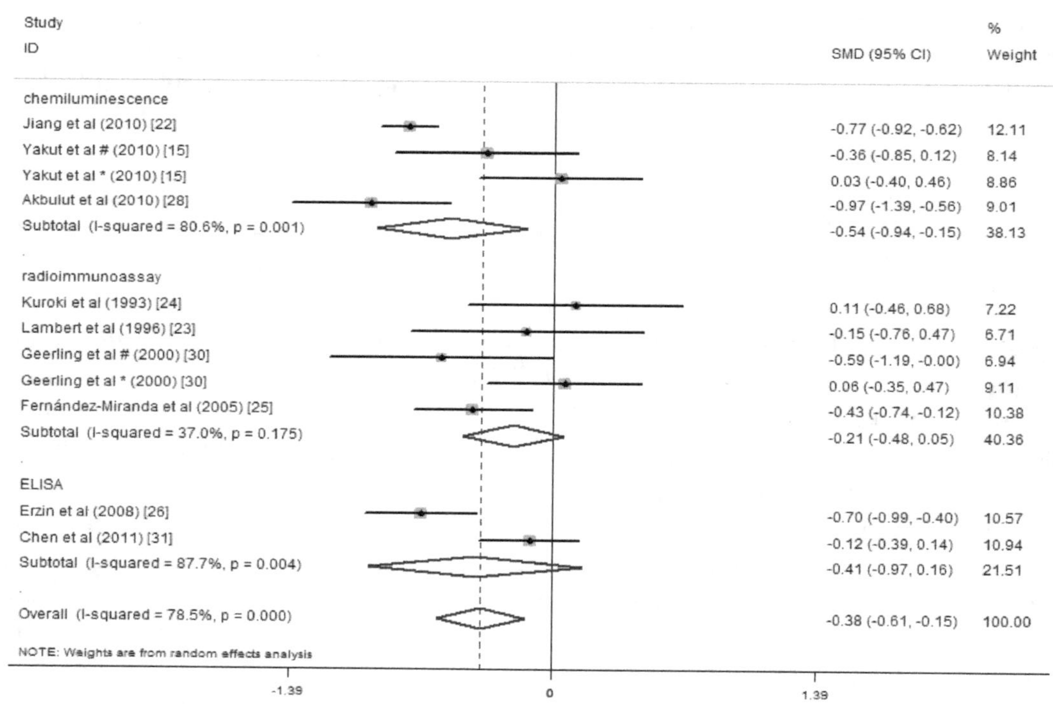

Figure 9. Forest plot of the serum concentrations of vitamin B12 in IBD patients vs. controls; standardized mean differences with a 95% confidence interval and weight percentage are shown. Subtotals are for the three detection methods. * Reported in ulcerative colitis; # reported in Crohn's disease.

A meta-regression analysis was performed because of the significant heterogeneity observed between studies. The meta-regression analysis evaluated the folate and vitamin B12 detection methods, the year of publication, the size of the samples, the quality of the study and the average age of the patients. The results showed that the detection methods impacted the serum folic acid concentrations and the total effect size ($p < 0.05$; Table 2). For serum vitamin B12 concentrations, the mean age of the IBD patients was the source of heterogeneity, and the difference in the results was statistically significant ($p < 0.05$; Table 3). The meta-regression analysis based on the size of the sample and the quality of study could not explain the between-study heterogeneity (Tables 2 and 3).

Table 2. Results of the folate regression analysis.

Variables	n	I^2	Adj R^2	exp(b)	Std. Err.	t	p	95% CI
				0.81	0.10	−1.60	0.154 *	0.61, 1.10
Testing method	10	0.00%	100.00%	0.55	0.08	−4.00	0.005 #	0.38, 0.78
				0.73	0.08	−2.95	0.021 &	0.56, 0.94
Year of publication	14	76.64%	−8.34%	1.007	0.02	0.35	0.729	0.97, 1.05
Sample size	14	76.12%	−11.49%	1.00	0.00	−0.35	0.729	0.99, 1.00
Quality of studies	14	76.51%	−10.63%	0.99	0.10	−0.05	0.959	0.79, 1.25
Average age of patients	9	80.56%	18.27%	0.98	0.01	−1.58	0.159	0.95, 1.01

n: number; I^2: percentage of total variation across studies; Adj R^2: adjusted R^2, the proportion of between-study variance; exp(b): the exponentiation of the B coefficient; Std. Err: standard error; t: t statistic, the coefficient divided by its standard error; p: an independent variable would be significant (<0.05) or not significant (≥0.05) in the model; CI: confidence interval; * chemiluminescence; # radioassay; & ELISA.

Table 3. Results of the vitamin B12 regression analysis.

Variables	n	I^2	Adj R^2	exp(b)	Std. Err.	t	p	95% CI
				0.86	0.27	−0.47	0.654 *	0.43, 1.76
Testing method	11	73.32%	−1.84%	1.22	0.37	0.66	0.530 #	0.60, 2.47
				0.67	0.16	−1.64	0.139 &	0.38, 1.18
Year of publication	15	84.87%	16.62%	0.96	0.02	−1.74	0.105	0.92, 1.01
Sample size	15	81.47%	12.78%	1.00	0.00	−1.58	0.139	0.99, 1.00
Quality of studies	15	82.38%	20.13%	0.78	0.10	−1.92	0.078	0.60, 1.03
Average age of patients	10	65.85%	55.42%	0.97	0.01	−2.73	0.026	0.95, 1.00

n: number; I^2: percentage of total variation across studies; Adj R^2: adjusted R^2, the proportion of between-study variance; exp(b): the exponentiation of the B coefficient; Std. Err: standard error; t: t statistic, the coefficient divided by its standard error; p: an independent variable would be significant (<0.05) or not significant (≥0.05) in the model; CI: confidence interval; * chemiluminescence; # radioassay; & ELISA.

4. Discussion

The results from this meta-analysis showed that the serum folate concentrations of patients with IBD were lower than that in normal controls, and the difference was significant. However, significant differences in serum vitamin B12 concentrations were not observed between the IBD patients and healthy controls. Serum folate concentrations may be reduced because of inadequate dietary intake [32], increased utilization, or drug effects, mainly salicylazosulfapyridine (SASP) [14]. Moreover, Burr et al. [33] showed that folic acid can be used as a supplement for the prevention of colorectal cancer in IBD patients. Considering the results of this study, IBD patients should be supplemented with folic acid. Research has shown that folate deficiency is more common than vitamin B12 deficiency [34]. Folate and vitamin B12 are important water-soluble vitamins for humans. Folate mainly assimilates in the duodenum and the proximal jejunum and is found in a variety of foods. Vitamin B12 is a component of coenzymes, and it is essential for cell biosynthesis and metabolism in vivo. Vitamin B12 is mainly absorbed in the terminal ileum, and the main source of vitamin B12 for humans is animal products. IBD may involve the small intestine; thus, the serum concentrations of folate and vitamin B12 may be lower in patients with IBD despite their presence in a wide range of foods.

Although our findings indicated that the serum concentrations of vitamin B12 were not significantly different between IBD patients and controls, studies have shown that a resection of more than 50–60 cm of the ileum frequently produces vitamin B12 malabsorption [35]. The reason for this difference might be due to 50 patients among 1086 patients included in this meta-analysis underwent surgery, which is less than 5 percent. In CD patients, prior intestinal surgery was an independent risk factor for low serum concentrations of vitamin B12 [15]. A meta-analysis by Battat et al. on vitamin B12 deficiency in IBD patients indicated that the only factor that predisposed CD patients to vitamin B12 deficiency was ileal resections greater than 20 cm [36]. Therefore, IBD patients, especially patients who have had ileal surgery, are recommended to take vitamin B12 supplements.

In the subgroup analysis based on the types of diseases, the serum folate concentrations in UC patients but not CD patients were lower than those in the healthy controls. However, serum folate concentrations in patients with unspecified IBD were lower than that in controls. The subgroup analysis by area showed lower serum concentrations of folate and vitamin B12 in the Asian study populations, which may be related to the typical Asian diet, which mostly includes plant-based foods and less meat than is typical in European diets, because vitamin B12 widely occurs in animal-based food products. Therefore, we suggest these patients may require moderate vitamin B12 supplements.

When we combined the results of all of the studies, a large degree of heterogeneity was observed, so we performed analysis to identify the source of heterogeneity. Firstly, the subgroup analysis of the detection methods showed that the serum folate concentrations were lower in the IBD patients than in the healthy control patients, regardless of the techniques that were used (chemiluminescence immunoassay, radioimmunoassay or ELISA), and the heterogeneity was lower when grouping by detection methods compare to by disease types. Therefore, we concluded that different test methods for folic acid may be one of the sources of heterogeneity in the associated studies. Secondly, the results of the sensitivity analysis showed that the studies by Koutroubakis et al. introduced a large amount of heterogeneity [16]. This might be due to inclusion of three control groups (healthy blood donors, visitors to the gynaecology/obstetrics and orthopaedics wards and normal hospital personnel) by investigators (Koutroubakis et al. [16]), which might have introduced a number of uncontrollable confounding factors. Thirdly, the results of meta-regression analysis showed that the method of detection explained the heterogeneity among the studies that examined serum folate concentrations; the average age of the patient was a heterogeneous factor among the studies that examined the serum vitamin B12 concentrations. Moreover, IBD patients often present morphological and functional disorders of the liver [23], and patients with hepatic dysfunction may have normal or high serum concentrations of vitamin B12 rather than increased body stores of vitamin B12 [37]. We did not analyse the disease severity because of the different ratings criteria for severity. In addition, certain studies did not specify or excluded severe patients, which led to incomplete data; also, disease severity may be not associated with lower serum vitamin concentrations [24].

We still need to acknowledge that this review has several limitations, which means that our results should be interpreted with caution. We only included studies that fit our inclusion criteria described in Section 2.2. Several important studies were excluded due to variety of reasons. These include: Ward et al. only reported the prevalence of vitamin B12 deficiency, but did not show the mean or standard deviation of serum concentrations of vitamin B12 [38]. We excluded this study based on our inclusion criteria (3). Jayaprakash et al. reported their data without a healthy control group, and some of the patients they included had been receiving vitamin B12 supplementation [39]. We excluded this study based on our inclusion criteria (2) and (4). The data included in the analysis were from observational studies; thus, potentially confounding factors may have been included in the baseline characteristics of the selected population. The serum concentrations of folate and vitamin B12 could be affected by ethnicity, gender and complications. Moreover, case-controlled studies and cross-sectional studies lack sufficient proof of the causal link between serum concentrations of folic acid and vitamin B12 and IBD status. Also, observational studies alone to prove cause–effect relationship between certain nutrition factors and certain diseases are very difficult unless the study is as large as the China–Cornell–Oxford Project in the late 20th century [40]. Future prospective studies are needed to identify the causal factors linking serum folate and vitamin B12 concentrations and IBD.

5. Conclusions

In conclusion, the serum folate concentrations in patients with IBD were lower than those in healthy controls, and low serum concentrations of folic acid may be an important risk factor for IBD patients. In addition, the serum vitamin B12 concentrations were lower in Asian patients. We recommend routine screening of patients with IBD for vitamin B12 and folate deficiency to determine whether supplements of folic acid or vitamin B12 should be administered to ensure the nutritional status of IBD patients and to improve the health of patients.

Acknowledgments: This work was supported by the National Natural Science Foundation of China (No. 81501423) and the Norman Bethune Program of Jilin University (No. 2015223).

Author Contributions: W.C., Y.P. and D.L. contributed to the data collection, analysis and manuscript preparation; H.G., M.S.J. and X.L. contributed to the data collection and analysis; and W.C., Y.L. and D.L. developed the study protocol, secured funds, supervised the study and guided the manuscript preparation.

References

1. Leone, V.; Chang, E.B.; Devkota, S. Diet, microbes, and host genetics: The perfect storm in inflammatory bowel diseases. *J. Gastroenterol.* **2013**, *48*, 315–321. [CrossRef] [PubMed]
2. Kaser, A.; Zeissig, S.; Blumberg, R.S. Inflammatory bowel disease. *Annu. Rev. Immunol.* **2010**, *28*, 573–621. [CrossRef] [PubMed]
3. Leddin, D.; Tamim, H.; Levy, A.R. Is folate involved in the pathogenesis of inflammatory bowel disease? *Med. Hypotheses* **2013**, *81*, 940–941. [CrossRef] [PubMed]
4. Shanahan, F. The microbiota in inflammatory bowel disease: Friend, bystander, and sometime-villain. *Nutr. Rev.* **2012**, *70* (Suppl. 1), S31–S37. [CrossRef] [PubMed]
5. Kellermayer, R. Epigenetics and the developmental origins of inflammatory bowel diseases. *Can. J. Gastroenterol.* **2012**, *26*, 909–915. [CrossRef] [PubMed]
6. Bermejo, F.; Algaba, A.; Guerra, I.; Chaparro, M.; De-La-Poza, G.; Valer, P.; Piqueras, B.; Bermejo, A.; Garcia-Alonso, J.; Perez, M.J.; et al. Should we monitor vitamin b12 and folate levels in crohn's disease patients? *Scand. J. Gastroenterol.* **2013**, *48*, 1272–1277. [CrossRef] [PubMed]
7. Owczarek, D.; Rodacki, T.; Domagala-Rodacka, R.; Cibor, D.; Mach, T. Diet and nutritional factors in inflammatory bowel diseases. *World J. Gastroenterol.* **2016**, *22*, 895–905. [CrossRef] [PubMed]
8. Lachner, C.; Steinle, N.I.; Regenold, W.T. The neuropsychiatry of vitamin B12 deficiency in elderly patients. *J. Neuropsychiatry Clin. Neurosci.* **2012**, *24*, 5–15. [CrossRef] [PubMed]
9. Cario, H.; Smith, D.E.; Blom, H.; Blau, N.; Bode, H.; Holzmann, K.; Pannicke, U.; Hopfner, K.P.; Rump, E.M.; Ayric, Z.; et al. Dihydrofolate reductase deficiency due to a homozygous DHFR mutation causes megaloblastic anemia and cerebral folate deficiency leading to severe neurologic disease. *Am. J. Hum. Genet.* **2011**, *88*, 226–231. [CrossRef] [PubMed]
10. Oussalah, A.; Gueant, J.L.; Peyrin-Biroulet, L. Meta-analysis: Hyperhomocysteinaemia in inflammatory bowel diseases. *Aliment. Pharmacol. Ther.* **2011**, *34*, 1173–1184. [CrossRef] [PubMed]
11. Stipanuk, M.H. Sulfur amino acid metabolism: Pathways for production and removal of homocysteine and cysteine. *Annu. Rev. Nutr.* **2004**, *24*, 539–577. [CrossRef] [PubMed]
12. Hoffbrand, V.; Provan, D. Abc of clinical haematology. Macrocytic anaemias. *Br. Med. J.* **1997**, *314*, 430–433. [CrossRef]
13. Vasilopoulos, S.; Saiean, K.; Emmons, J.; Berger, W.L.; Abu-Hajir, M.; Seetharam, B.; Binion, D.G. Terminal ileum resection is associated with higher plasma homocysteine levels in crohn's disease. *J. Clin. Gastroenterol.* **2001**, *33*, 132–136. [CrossRef] [PubMed]
14. Chowers, Y.; Sela, B.A.; Holland, R.; Fidder, H.; Simoni, F.B.; Bar-Meir, S. Increased levels of homocysteine in patients with Crohn's disease are related to folate levels. *Am. J. Gastroenterol.* **2000**, *95*, 3498–3502. [CrossRef] [PubMed]
15. Yakut, M.; Ustun, Y.; Kabacam, G.; Soykan, I. Serum vitamin B12 and folate status in patients with inflammatory bowel diseases. *Eur. J. Intern. Med.* **2010**, *21*, 320–323. [CrossRef] [PubMed]
16. Koutroubakis, I.E.; Dilaveraki, E.; Vlachonikolis, I.G.; Vardas, E.; Vrentzos, G.; Ganotakis, E.; Mouzas, I.A.; Gravanis, A.; Emmanouel, D.; Kouroumalis, E.A. Hyperhomocysteinemia in Greek patients with inflammatory bowel disease. *Dig. Dis. Sci.* **2000**, *45*, 2347–2351. [CrossRef] [PubMed]

17. Deeks, J.; Altman, D. Chapter 16: Special topics in statistics. In *Cochrane Handbook for Systematic Reviews of Interventions*; Version 5.1.0; The Cochrane Collaboration: London, UK, 2011.
18. Senn, S. Overstating the evidence: Double counting in meta-analysis and related problems. *BMC Med. Res. Methodol.* **2009**, *9*, 10. [CrossRef] [PubMed]
19. Cochran, W.G. The combination of estimates from different experiments. *Biometrics* **1954**, *10*, 101–129. [CrossRef]
20. Higgins, J.P.; Thompson, S.G.; Deeks, J.J.; Altman, D.G. Measuring inconsistency in meta-analyses. *Br. Med. J.* **2003**, *327*, 557–560. [CrossRef] [PubMed]
21. Egger, M.; Davey Smith, G.; Schneider, M.; Minder, C. Bias in meta-analysis detected by a simple, graphical test. *Br. Med. J.* **1997**, *315*, 629–634. [CrossRef]
22. Jiang, Y.; Zhao, J.; Jiang, T.; Ge, L.; Zhou, F.; Chen, Z.; Lei, Y.; Huang, S.; Xia, B. Genetic polymorphism of methylenetetrahydrofolate reductase g1793a, hyperhomocysteinemia, and folate deficiency correlate with ulcerative colitis in central China. *J. Gastroenterol. Hepatol.* **2010**, *25*, 1157–1161. [CrossRef] [PubMed]
23. Lambert, D.; Benhayoun, S.; Adjalla, C.; Gelot, M.A.; Renkes, P.; Felden, F.; Gerard, P.; Belleville, F.; Gaucher, P.; Gueant, J.L.; et al. Crohn's disease and vitamin B12 metabolism. *Dig. Dis. Sci.* **1996**, *41*, 1417–1422. [CrossRef] [PubMed]
24. Kuroki, F.; Iida, M.; Tominaga, M.; Matsumoto, T.; Hirakawa, K.; Sugiyama, S.; Fujishima, M. Multiple vitamin status in Crohn's disease. Correlation with disease activity. *Dig. Dis. Sci.* **1993**, *38*, 1614–1618. [CrossRef] [PubMed]
25. Fernandez-Miranda, C.; Martinez Prieto, M.; CasisHerce, B.; Sanchez Gomez, F.; Gomez Gonzalez, P.; Martinez Lopez, J.; Saenz-Lopez Perez, S.; Gomez de la Camara, A. Hyperhomocysteinemia and methylenetetrahydrofolate reductase 677c→t and 1298a→c mutations in patients with inflammatory bowel disease. *Rev. Esp. Enferm. Dig.* **2005**, *97*, 497–504. [CrossRef] [PubMed]
26. Erzin, Y.; Uzun, H.; Celik, A.F.; Aydin, S.; Dirican, A.; Uzunismail, H. Hyperhomocysteinemia in inflammatory bowel disease patients without past intestinal resections: Correlations with cobalamin, pyridoxine, folate concentrations, acute phase reactants, disease activity, and prior thromboembolic complications. *J. Clin. Gastroenterol.* **2008**, *42*, 481–486. [CrossRef] [PubMed]
27. Alkhouri, R.H.; Hashmi, H.; Baker, R.D.; Gelfond, D.; Baker, S.S. Vitamin and mineral status in patients with inflammatory bowel disease. *J. Pediatr. Gastroenterol. Nutr.* **2013**, *56*, 89–92. [CrossRef] [PubMed]
28. Akbulut, S.; Altiparmak, E.; Topal, F.; Ozaslan, E.; Kucukazman, M.; Yonem, O. Increased levels of homocysteine in patients with ulcerative colitis. *World J. Gastroenterol.* **2010**, *16*, 2411–2416. [CrossRef] [PubMed]
29. Kallel, L.; Feki, M.; Sekri, W.; Segheir, L.; Fekih, M.; Boubaker, J.; Kaabachi, N.; Filali, A. Prevalence and risk factors of hyperhomocysteinemia in Tunisian patients with Crohn's disease. *J. Crohns Colitis* **2011**, *5*, 110–114. [CrossRef] [PubMed]
30. Geerling, B.J.; Badart-Smook, A.; Stockbrugger, R.W.; Brummer, R.J. Comprehensive nutritional status in recently diagnosed patients with inflammatory bowel disease compared with population controls. *Eur. J. Clin. Nutr.* **2000**, *54*, 514–521. [CrossRef] [PubMed]
31. Chen, M.L.; Mei, Q.; Xu, J.M.; Hu, N.Z.; Lu, C.X.; Fang, H.M. Significance of plasmichomocysteine, folate and vitamin B(12) in ulcerative colitis. *Zhonghua Wei Chang Wai Ke Za Zhi* **2011**, *14*, 185–187. (in Chinese). [PubMed]
32. Zezos, P.; Papaioannou, G.; Nikolaidis, N.; Vasiliadis, T.; Giouleme, O.; Evgenidis, N. Hyperhomocysteinemia in ulcerative colitis is related to folate levels. *World J. Gastroenterol.* **2005**, *11*, 6038–6042. [CrossRef] [PubMed]
33. Burr, N.E.; Hull, M.A.; Subramanian, V. Folic acid supplementation may reduce colorectal cancer risk in patients with inflammatory bowel disease: A systematic review and meta-analysis. *J. Clin. Gastroenterol.* **2017**, *51*, 247–253. [CrossRef] [PubMed]
34. Hwang, C.; Ross, V.; Mahadevan, U. Micronutrient deficiencies in inflammatory bowel disease: From A to zinc. *Inflamm. Bowel Dis.* **2012**, *18*, 1961–1981. [CrossRef] [PubMed]
35. Bermejo, F.; Algaba, A.; Gisbert, J.P.; Nogueiras, A.R.; Poza, G.; Chaparro, M.; Valer, P.; Piqueras, B.M.; Villa, J.C.; Bermejo, A. Prospective controlled analysis of vitamin B12 and folate deficiency in Crohn's disease. *Gastroenterology* **2011**, *140*, S-434.
36. Battat, R.; Kopylov, U.; Szilagyi, A.; Saxena, A.; Rosenblatt, D.S.; Warner, M.; Bessissow, T.; Seidman, E.; Bitton, A. Vitamin B12 deficiency in inflammatory bowel disease: Prevalence, risk factors, evaluation, and management. *Inflamm. Bowel Dis.* **2014**, *20*, 1120–1128. [CrossRef] [PubMed]

37. Jacobson, S. Serum concentration of cobalamines during total parenteral nutrition in Crohn's disease. *JPEN J. Parenter. Enter. Nutr.* **1986**, *10*, 223–226. [CrossRef] [PubMed]
38. Ward, M.; Kariyawasam, V.; Mogan, S.; Patel, K.; Pantelidou, M.; Sobczyńska-Malefora, A.; Porté, F.; Griffin, N.; Anderson, S.; Sanderson, J.; et al. Prevalence and Risk Factors for Functional Vitamin B12 Deficiency in Patients with Crohn's Disease. *Inflamm. Bowel Dis.* **2015**, *21*, 2839–2847. [CrossRef] [PubMed]
39. Jayaprakash, A.; Creed, T.; Stewart, L.; Colton, B.; Mountford, R.; Standen, G.; Probert, C. Should we monitor vitamin B12 levels in patients who have had end-ileostomy for inflammatory bowel disease? *Int. J. Colorectal Dis.* **2004**, *19*, 316–318. [CrossRef] [PubMed]
40. Campbell, T.C.; Campbell, T.M. *The China Study*, 1st ed.; BenBella Books: Dallas, TX, USA, 2006.

2

Therapeutic Potential of Amino Acids in Inflammatory Bowel Disease

Yulan Liu [1,*], **Xiuying Wang** [1] **and Chien-An Andy Hu** [1,2,*]

[1] Hubei Collaborative Innovation Center for Animal Nutrition and Feed Safety, Hubei Key Laboratory of Animal Nutrition and Feed Science, Wuhan Polytechnic University, Wuhan 430023, China; xiuyingdk@foxmail.com

[2] Department of Biochemistry and Molecular Biology, University of New Mexico School of Medicine, Albuquerque, NM 87131, USA

* Correspondence: yulanflower@126.com (Y.L.); AHu@salud.unm.edu (C.-A.A.H.)

Abstract: Inflammatory bowel disease (IBD), which includes both ulcerative colitis and Crohn's disease, is a chronic relapsing inflammation of the gastrointestinal tract, and is difficult to treat. The pathophysiology of IBD is multifactorial and not completely understood, but genetic components, dysregulated immune responses, oxidative stress, and inflammatory mediators are known to be involved. Animal models of IBD can be chemically induced, and are used to study etiology and to evaluate potential treatments of IBD. Currently available IBD treatments can decrease the duration of active disease but because of their adverse effects, the search for novel therapeutic strategies that can restore intestinal homeostasis continues. This review summarizes and discusses what is currently known of the effects of amino acids on the reduction of inflammation, oxidative stress, and cell death in the gut when IBD is present. Recent studies in animal models have identified dietary amino acids that improve IBD, but amino acid supplementation may not be adequate to replace conventional therapy. The animal models used in dietary amino acid research in IBD are described.

Keywords: inflammatory bowel disease; animal models; amino acids

---

1. Introduction

Inflammatory bowel disease (IBD) is a chronic, idiopathic and relapsing inflammation of the gastrointestinal tract with characteristics of severe diarrhea, electrolyte loss, bleeding and abdominal pain, and causes significant morbidity [1,2]. IBD also increases the risk of developing colorectal cancer [3]. Crohn's disease and ulcerative colitis, the two types of IBD, have distinct pathological and clinical characteristics: Crohn's disease can involve any part of the gastrointestinal tract, but most commonly affects the terminal ileum and perianal regions [2,4]. Ulcerative colitis usually affects the large intestine and the rectum [2,4]. Transmural inflammation is characteristic of Crohn's disease, but in ulcerative colitis, inflammation is typically limited to the mucosa and caused by white blood cell infiltration [1,4]. Because of its complex etiology and complicated symptoms, IBD is very difficult to treat.

Genetics, environmental and microbial factors, components of the innate and adaptive immune systems, oxidative stress, and inflammatory mediators, are all known to be risk factors of IBD [4,5], but little is known about how they interact with each other in the progression of IBD. Experimental chemical-induced, immune-mediated, spontaneous, genetically engineered, and transgenic mouse and pig models can mimic the progression of IBD [5]. They have been used to study the pathophysiology and etiology of human IBD and for drug discovery and development.

Amino acids are required for intestinal growth and maintenance of mucosal integrity and barrier function. They are used by small intestinal mucosal cells as essential precursors for metabolically active proteins, glutathione (GSH), nitric oxide, polyamines, and other molecules [6]. They are also used as building blocks of macromolecule synthesis for intestinal mucosal wound healing, and energy substrates of enterocytes [7]. The gut bacteria can utilize the amino acid to synthesize proteins and varieties of metabolites [8]. Amino acid metabolism in gut microbiota plays an important role in nutrition and physiology of the host [8]. Some studies, primarily conducted in rodents and pigs, are of interest because they have provided evidence that certain amino acids, particularly glutamine and arginine, may influence the progress of IBD [7]. They may act to reduce inflammation, oxidative stress, and the levels of proinflammatory cytokines. The current use of animal models in IBD research and the potential for use of specific amino acids in IBD treatment are reviewed below.

2. Animal Models of IBD—The Chemical-Induced Models

The complexity of IBD may account for the successful development of several different types of animal models. The chemical-induced models, include dextran sulfate sodium (DSS), trinitrobenzene sulfonic acid (TNBS), or acetic acid-induced models, are widely used experimentally because they are reproducible and easy to work with. In this section, the use of these models to study the pathogenesis of IBD and to test novel amino acid therapies are reviewed (Table 1).

Table 1. Examples of chemical-induced inflammatory bowel disease (IBD) animal models.

Colitis Models	Procedure	Animals	References
DSS	1.5–5% (wt/vol) DSS (molecular weight 36–50 kDa) in the drinking water for 5–7 days	rodent	[9–15]
	1.25 g DSS per kg body weight twice a day for 5 days	piglets	[16]
	Chronic colitis: cyclic treatment with 2% DSS repeated 3 times for 30 days	C57BL/6 mice	[9]
TNBS	2 mg/100 mL of TNBS in 45% ethanol	C57BL/6 mice	[9]
	30 mg TNBS in 0.25 mL 50% ethanol	Wistar rats	[17]
	15 mg TNBS in 0.6 mL 50% ethanol	Sprague-Dawley rats	[18]
	15 mg/kg TNBS in 5 mL 50% ethanol	piglets	[19]
	30-mL of 120 mg/kg TNBS in 50% ethanol	minipigs	[20]
	10 mL of 100% ethanol and 1 g of TNBS in 10 mL of distilled water	adult mongrel dogs	[21]
acetic acid	4% acetic acid for 15 s	rats	[22]
	1 mL of 4% acetic acid in 0.9% NaCl	rats	[23,24]

DSS, dextran sulfate sodium; TNBS, trinitrobenzene sulfonic acid.

2.1. DSS

DSS is a sulfated polymer that alters tight junction proteins, leading to the disruption of the intestinal barrier, and is toxic to epithelial cells. Results obtained in DSS-induced animal IBD models have helped to understand the pathogenesis of IBD and to screen potential therapeutic agents. DSS-induced IBD is simple and reproducible and results in symptoms resembling those of ulcerative colitis. The development of acute, chronic, or relapsing symptoms of IBD is dose-dependent, and the size of the DSS is key not only in the induction of colitis but also the location. A comparative study found that colitis developed in animals treated with 5 kDa and 40 kDa DSS but not 500 kDa, and severe colitis developed in the lower colon following administration of 40 kDa, whereas mild colitis developed in the cecum and upper colon after 5 kDa [25]. Various DSS dosage and duration are used to induce IBD in some animal models (Table 1) [9–16]. Following DSS administration, animals usually develop colitis with weight loss and severe, bloody diarrhea [11,13,16,26,27]. DSS colitis is characterized by mucosal ulceration, leukocyte infiltration, intestinal crypt distortion and epithelial hyperplasia [11,13].

It is believed that DSS colitis results in epithelial cell injury and increases the permeability of the intestinal mucosa to large molecules. DSS colitis is accompanied with dysregulation of the gut microbiota [28,29], and is associated with stimulation of innate and adaptive lymphoid elements and secretion of proinflammatory cytokines and chemokines [30,31]. The percentages of $CD3^+$ T lymphocytes in Peyer's patches, natural killer (NK) and B lymphocytes in mesenteric lymph nodes, and NK $CD8^-$ cells in intraepithelial lymphocytes are elevated in DSS-treated animals [32].

Expression of P-selectin glycoprotein ligand-1, leukocyte function-associated antigen-1, and C-C chemokine receptor type 9 by T helper and cytotoxic T cells also increase after DSS treatment [10]. Tissue cytokine and chemokine levels, including interleukin (IL)-1α, IL-1β, IL-6, IL-17, granulocyte colony-stimulating factor, granulocyte-macrophage colony-stimulating factor, eotaxin-1, monocyte chemoattractant protein 1, macrophage inflammatory protein (MIP)-1α, and MIP-1β also change following exposure to DSS [14]. Redox status is also disturbed as shown by decreased GSH and catalase (CAT) and increased reactive oxygen species (ROS), malondialdehyde (MDA), nitric oxide and myeloperoxidase (MPO) [26,33]. Activation of the nuclear factor-κB (NF-κB) pathway has been linked with the pathogenesis of DSS-induced colitis [11], and DSS induces cell death signaling by modulating B-cell lymphoma (Bcl)-2 and Bcl-2-associated X protein (Bax) apoptosis factors [34,35], and receptor-interacting protein 3, mixed lineage kinase domain-like protein, and caspase-8 necroptosis factors [35–37]. Intestinal inflammation resulting from increased cell death has been reported to occur in IBD [34,36,38].

2.2. TNBS

TNBS elicits dysregulation of the intestinal immune system, and induces both acute and chronic colonic inflammation and ulceration [39]. Animal models that present characteristics similar to those of human IBD, predominantly Crohn's disease, have been developed by injection of TNBS in ethanol. The model advantages include simple induction, rapid establishment, and development of reproducible, long-lasting colon damage accompanied by inflammatory cell infiltration and ulcer formation [40]. In the TNBS model, ethanol facilitates disruption of the intestinal barrier and helps TNBS enter the mucosal layer to induce colitis [41,42]. Various dosage combinations of TNBS and ethanol have been reported to induce IBD in various animal models (Table 1) [9,17–21].

Clinical phenotypes in TNBS/ethanol-induced animal models include diarrhea, weight loss, high mortality, and severe inflammation [9,39,43]. Massive bowel edema, and disruption of epithelial cells by large ulcerations are frequent, severe macroscopic injuries [9]; severe and intense transmural inflammation and/or diffuse necrosis, inflammatory granulomas, and submucosal neutrophil infiltration are also characteristic of this model [39].

Oxidative, inflammatory, and apoptotic damage may be among the causes of TNBS-induced colitis [44,45], leading to increased generation of prostaglandin E_2 (PGE_2) [18], increased MDA [44], NF-κB [44], MPO [46], nitric oxide synthase (iNOS) [18], and caspase-3 [44], increases of IL-1α, IL-1β, IL-4, IL-6, tumor necrosis factor (TNF)-α [17,46], and cyclooxygenase (COX)-2 [18], and decreased GSH in colon tissue [44]. Increased $CD3^+$, $CD4^+$ and $CD8^+$ T lymphocytes in peripheral blood have also been reported in TNBS-induced colitis animal models [43].

2.3. Acetic Acid

Acetic acid-induced colitis is a common experimental IBD model. Animals treated with acetic acid develop many pathological and histopathological characteristics in common with human ulcerative colitis. Rectal application of acetic acid damages the mucosal epithelium and produces ulcerative colitis [47]. The severity of the mucosal lesions that develop in acetic acid-induced colitis depends on the acetic acid concentration and the length of exposure. Injection of 25% acetic acid into the gastric lumen causes larger ulcerative lesions than injection of 5% acetic acid [48]. Different concentrations of acetic acid and different exposure times have been reported to induce IBD in rat model (Table 1) [22–24]. Transmural necrosis in all layers of the bowel wall, severe neutrophil infiltration of the intestinal tissue, goblet cell depletion, edema, and submucosal ulceration are common manifestations of this model [23,49–51]. Bloody diarrhea [52], reduction of the intestinal mucus [51], decreased nucleic acid (DNA and RNA) and total protein content [51], and increased colon weight [23,51] and vascular permeability [50] have also been observed. MPO activity and MDA levels are elevated, and contents of GSH, superoxide dismutase (SOD) and CAT are significantly reduced in acetic acid-induced colitis [53,54]. Serum nitrate [53] and lactate dehydrogenase [50], caspase-3 [54,55], proinflammatory mediators iNOS, COX-2, IL-1β, IL-6, and TNF-α [49–51,55] were all significantly increased in acetic acid-treated animals. Acetic acid-induced colitis is also associated with changes NF-κB, inhibitor of κB (IκB) and IκB kinase expression [49].

The chemically induced IBD models are relatively easy and rapid to develop and can be used with wild-type mice or other normal animals. Thus, these models have been most commonly used to identify potential therapeutic agents [56]. However, the acute models may provide only limited information about the pathogenesis of IBD in humans, as the chemical damage to the intestinal barrier results in self-limiting inflammatory response rather than chronic disease [56]. Hence, these models are more relevant in research about acute inflammation. In fact, the intestinal microbiota signature may be different in animals suffering from chronic colitis [57]. In addition, these models may only partially reflect the human situation, e.g., in terms of genetics, environmental factors, dysbiosis, inflammatory response or disturbed permeability in human IBD [56]. Hence, findings in animal models of IBD may not always be consistent with observations in human IBD.

3. Potential Roles of Amino Acids in IBD

Aminosalicylates, corticosteroids, and thiopurines can decrease the duration of active disease and contribute to the maintenance of IBD remission, but these treatments have adverse effects, especially with long-term use [58]. Novel adjunct therapies are thus needed to overcome the limitations of current pharmacological treatment. Interestingly, serum amino acid levels have been shown to differ in IBD patients and healthy controls, suggesting the existence of a link between amino acid profiles and IBD [12,14,59]. Moreover, malnutrition in IBD patients is common, and nutritional therapy is frequently used to overcome nutrient deficiencies and to alter the inflammatory status [58]. Amino acids, as therapeutic candidates, may ultimately help to maintain intestinal integrity in IBD patients (Table 2 and Figures 1 and 2).

Table 2. Summary of the effect of amino acid supplementation on IBD in animal models.

Amino Acids	Effects	Animal Models	References
Glutamine	↓body weight loss, colon edema, endothelial adhesion molecules, infiltrating Th cells, PSGL-1, LFA-1, CCR9	C57BL/6 mice; DSS	[10]
	↓epithelium injury and loss, mucosal hypoplasia	Sprague-Dawley rats; acetic acid	[60]
	↓disruption of colonic architecture, submucosal and serosal fibrosis, collagen Iα2, collagen III, TGFβ, phosphorylated Smad3, PDGF, CTGF	Wistar rats; TNBS	[17]
	↑HO-1, GSH ↓MDA, caspase-3, NF-κB	Wistar-albino rats; TNBS	[44]
	↑GSH ↓MDA, caspase-3	Wistar-albino rats; TNBS	[61]
	↓histopathological scores, cytosolic concentration of TBARS, hydroperoxide-initiated chemiluminescence, NF-κB, iNOS, COX-2	Wistars rats; acetic acid	[49]
	↓histopathological scores, cytosolic concentration of TBARS, hydroperoxide-initiated chemiluminescence, MPO, iNOS, COX-2, NF-κB, TNF-α, IFN-γ, phosphorylated forms of STAT1, STAT5, Akt	Wistar rats; TNBS	[62]
	↑Th22 and Treg cell expression ↓Th1/Th17-associated cytokine expression	C57BL/6 mice; DSS	[11]
	↓NF-κB, PI3K-Akt	ICR mice; DSS	[12]
	↑HSP25, HSP70 ↓diarrhea	Sprague-Dawley rats; DSS	[15]
	↓oxidative stress, ER stress, apoptosis	Wistar rats; TNBS	[45]
Glutamate	↑PCNA-positive cells, SOD, Bcl-2 ↓MDA, Bax, caspase-3, TNF-α, IL-1β	Sprague-Dawley rats; TNBS	[63]
Arginine	↑iNOS ↓mucosal permeability, number of MPO-positive neutrophils, and expression of pro-inflammatory cytokine and chemokine	$iNOS^{-/-}$ C57BL/6 mice; DSS	[14]
	↑T-SOD ↓Akt, MLCK	ICR mice; DSS	[12]
	↓body weight loss, colon weights, macroscopic and microscopic damage of colonic tissues	Wistar rats; acetic acid	[64]

Table 2. *Cont.*

Amino Acids	Effects	Animal Models	References
Sulphur-containing amino acids	↓colon lesions, cytoskeleton damage, serum amyloid A, TNF-α	BALB/C mice; DSS	[27]
	↑caspase-8 ↓chemokine, neutrophil influx, TNF-α, IL-6, IL-12p40, IL-1β, cFLIP and Bcl-xL	Yorkshire piglets; DSS	[16]
	↑goblet cell number, protein/DNA ratio, claudin-1 ↓IEL number, caspase-3, MPO, MDA, TNF-α	piglets; acetic acid	[54]
	↑GSH, SOD, CAT ↓MPO, MDA	Wistar-albino rats; acetic acid	[65]
	↑PON1,GSH ↓macroscopic colonic damage, histopathologic changes, MPO, ROS, TNF-α, IL-1β	BALB/c mice; DSS	[26]
	↑GSH, SOD ↓MPO, MDA, TNF-α, IL-1β, IL-6	Wistar albino rats; acetic acid	[24]
	↓COX2, PGE_2	Sprague-Dawley rats; TNBS	[18]
	↓chronic ulcerative colitis-associated colorectal adenocarcinoma development	C57BL/6J mice; DSS	[66]
Tryptophan	↓body weight loss, frequency of bloody stools, nitrotyrosine content of the colonic tissues	C57black6 mice; DSS	[67]
	↑caspase-8, Bax ↓gut permeability, TNF-α, IL-6, IFN-γ, IL-12p40, IL-1β, IL-17, IL-8, ICAM-1	Piglets; DSS	[68]
	↑Ahr, IL-22, STAT3 ↓colitis symptoms, IL-6, TNF-α, IL-1β, Ccl2, Cxcl1, Cxcl2	C57BL/6 WT and KO mice; DSS	[69]
Glycine	↓diarrhea, body weight loss, ulceration, MPO, IL-1β, TNF-α, CINC, MIP-2	Wistar rats; TNBS/DSS	[70]
Histidine	↓histologic damage, colon weight, TNF-α, IL-6, NF-κB	$IL-10^{-/-}$ mice	[71]

Ahr, aryl hydrocarbon receptor; Akt, protein kinase B; Bcl, B-cell lymphoma; Bax, Bcl-2-associated X protein; CAT, catalase; CCR9, C-C chemokine receptor type 9; cFLIP, FLICE-like inhibitory protein; CINC, cytokine-induced neutrophil chemoattractant; COX-2, cyclooxygenase-2; CTGF, connective tissue growth factor; DSS, dextran sulfate sodium; ER, endoplasmic reticulum; GSH, glutathione; HO-1, heme oxygenase-1; HSP, heat shock protein; ICAM-1, intracellular adhesion molecule-1; ICR, institute for cancer research; IEL, intraepithelial lymphocyte; IFN, interferon; IL, interleukin; iNOS, inducible nitric oxide synthase; LFA, leukocyte function-associated antigen; MDA, malondialdehyde; MIP-2, macrophage inflammatory protein-2; MLCK, myosin light chain kinase; MPO, myeloperoxidase; NF-κB, nuclear factor-κB; PCNA, proliferating cell nuclear antigen; PDGF, platelet-derived growth factor; PGE_2, prostaglandin E_2; PI3K, phosphoinositide-3-kinases; PON1, paraoxonase 1; PSGL, P-selectin glycoprotein ligand; ROS, reactive oxygen species; SOD, superoxide dismutase; STAT, signal transducers and activators of transcription; TBARS, thiobarbituric acid reactive substances; TGF-β, transforming growth factor-β; Th, T-helper; TNBS, trinitrobenzene sulfonic acid; TNF-α, tumor necrosis factor-α; Treg, T regulatory.

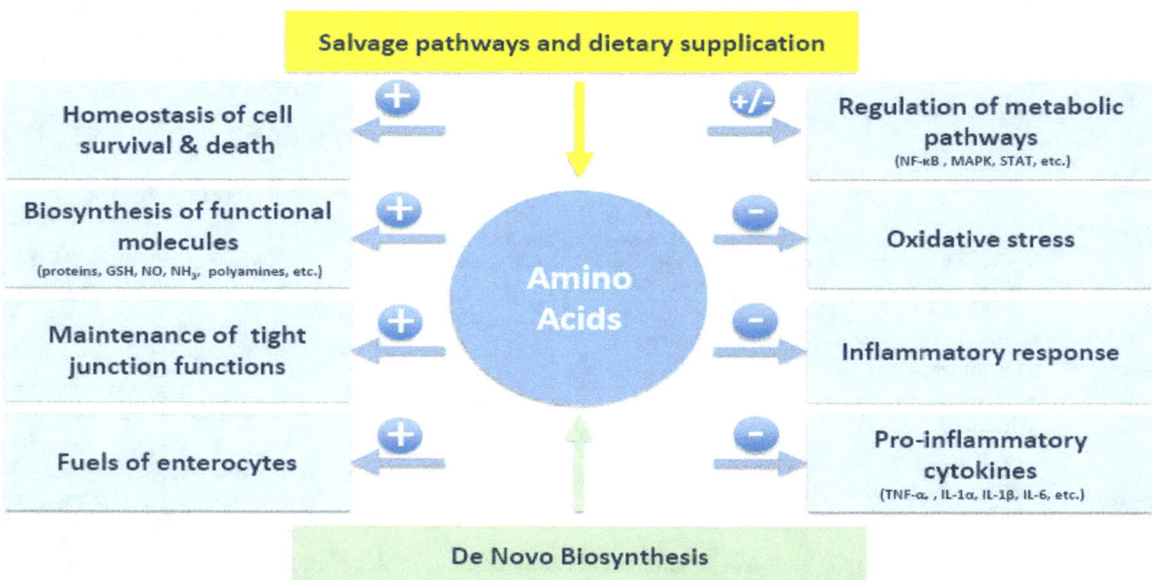

Figure 1. Projected mechanisms by which amino acids exert their beneficial effects on IBD. GSH, glutathione; IL, interleukin; MAPK, mitogen-activated protein; NF-κB, nuclear factor-κB; NO, nitric oxide; STAT, signal transducers and activators of transcription; TNF-α, tumor necrosis factor-α.

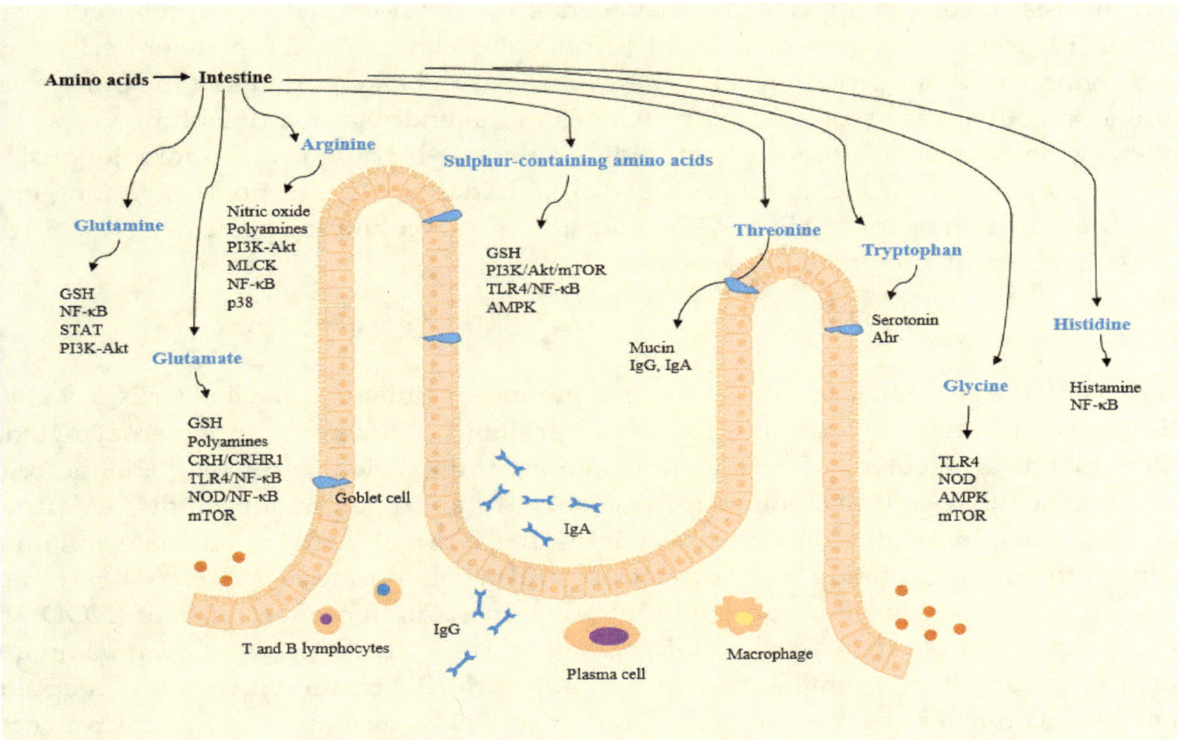

Figure 2. Amino acid-derived metabolites and amino acid-regulated signals. Ahr, aryl hydrocarbon receptor; Akt, protein kinase B; AMPK, AMP-activated protein kinase; CRH, corticotropin-releasing hormone; CRHR, CRH receptor; GSH, glutathione; MLCK, myosin light chain kinase; mTOR, mammalian target of rapamycin; NF-κB, nuclear factor-κB; NOD, nucleotide-binding oligomerization domain protein; PI3K, phosphoinositide-3-kinases; STAT, signal transducers and activators of transcription; TLR, toll like receptor.

3.1. Glutamine

Glutamine is an important gut nutrient, required by enterocytes, and a precursor for biosynthesis of GSH, other amino acids, nucleic acids, and other biologically important molecules [72,73]. Glutamine supplementation is beneficial in improving disease symptoms and intestinal structure and barrier function [72,73]. This amino acid can increase intestinal-friendly microbiota (*Bacteroidetes* and *Actinobacteria*), while decrease pernicious bacteria (*Oscillospira* and *Treponema*) [74]. Its role in IBD is controversial [72,75–78], but the results of most glutamine studies support further evaluation as a potential therapeutic agent. In animal models, glutamine was found to protect against TNBS-, DSS- or acetic acid-induced intestinal damage and preserve gastrointestinal function. Weight loss [10], epithelium injury and loss [60], mucosal hypoplasia [60], submucosal and serosal fibrosis [17], colon edema [10], and disruption of colonic architecture [17] characteristic of chemically induced models were attenuated by glutamine administration. The evidence suggests glutamine may have antioxidant, antiapoptotic, and anti-inflammatory activity in IBD. In IBD models, glutamine has been found to decrease MDA level and caspase-3 activity and increase GSH level and heme oxygenase 1 expression [44,61]. The therapeutic effect of glutamine in experimental colitis results from a decrease in inflammation by modulation of NF-κB [49,62] and signal transducers and activators of transcription (STAT) signaling pathways [62], and from suppression of T cell migration [10,11]. Glutamine supplementation has been shown to regulate NF-κB and phosphoinositide-3-kinases (PI3K)-protein kinase B (Akt) signaling in vivo in a DSS-induced colitis model [12] and to enhance heat shock protein (HSP) expression both in vitro and in vivo in an experimental colitis models [15]. San-Miguel et al. [17] reported that glutamine supplementation prevented fibrosis development in TNBS-treated rats by down-regulating expression of collagen Iα2, collagen III, transforming growth factor-β, phosphorylated Smad3, platelet-derived growth factor, and connective tissue growth factor genes. Crespo et al. [45] reported that the protective effect of glutamine in colitis was associated with changes in the endoplasmic reticulum stress response (cytosine-cytosine-adenosine-adenosine-thymidine enhancer-binding protein homologous protein, binding immunoglobulin protein, and caspase-12), unfolded protein response signaling branches (activating transcription factor (ATF) 4, ATF6, and spliced X-box-binding protein-1), Jun N-terminal kinase, Bcl-2 family proteins, and caspase activation [45].

3.2. *Glutamate*

In most cells, the immediate enzyme-converted product of glutamine metabolism is glutamate [79], which is active as an excitatory neurotransmitter [80], participates in enterocyte oxidative metabolism [81], is a precursor of various polyamines, amino acids, and GSH [82], and regulates oxidative reactions [83] and metabolic pathways [83]. In an inflammation model, we previously demonstrated that glutamate could improve intestinal barrier function, alleviate inflammation and inhibit protein degradation via corticotropin-releasing hormone (CRH)/CRH receptor 1, toll-like receptor (TLR) 4 and nucleotide-binding oligomerization domain protein (NOD)/NF-κB, and mammalian target of rapamycin (mTOR) signaling, respectively [84,85]. Given its unique role in the gastrointestinal tract, glutamate may be an adjuvant IBD treatment with broad application, which has been confirmed by Li et al. [63]. In a rat model of ulcerative colitis, microinjection of glutamate into the hypothalamic paraventricular nucleus (PVN) promoted cell proliferation (increase of proliferating cell nuclear antigen-positive cells) and increased antioxidant levels (reduced MDA content and elevated SOD activity), inhibited apoptosis (upregulation of Bcl-2 protein and downregulation of Bax and caspase-3 protein), and the expression of proinflammatory factors TNF-α and IL-1β [63]. The glutamate mechanism of action may depend on binding to a glutamate receptor on the membrane of PVN neurons.

3.3. *Arginine*

Arginine is a conditionally essential amino acid and a precursor of numerous physiologically active molecules including nitric oxide and polyamines. Dietary arginine induces a shift in the Firmicutes:Bacteroidetes ratio to favor Bacteroidetes in gut [86]. Arginine has important functions in intestinal nutrition and health, is considered as a crucial nutrient for fetuses and neonates, and, especially in the disease states [87]. A study that assessed the expression of arginine transporters and downstream metabolic enzymes, revealed altered arginine metabolism in the gut tissue of IBD patients [88]. Tissue arginine level is also decreased in IBD patients [88], suggesting that dietary arginine supplementation might compensate the arginine deficiency in IBD tissues. Arginine administration has been shown to maintain normal intestinal physiology and to facilitate mucosal healing when the intestine is affected by inflammation [89–91]. Arginine treatment of mice with DSS colitis was shown to reduce mucosal permeability, the number of MPO-positive neutrophils, and expression of proinflammatory cytokines and chemokines and to increase iNOS activity [14]. Other evidence from animal models indicates that dietary arginine may improve clinical and biochemical parameters in DSS colitis via effects on PI3K-Akt and myosin light chain kinase signaling [12]. Histopathological evaluation has revealed alleviation of macroscopic and microscopic damage of colonic tissues induced in an acetic acid IBD model by arginine supplementation [64]. The protective effects were attributed to arginine's nitric oxide donating property and modulation of NF-κB expression [64]. When it was combined with glutamine, arginine had synergistic effects on reduction of major proinflammatory cytokines mediated by the NF-κB and p38 pathways in active Crohn's disease [92]. Oral coadministration of garlic and arginine attenuated the alterations induced by acetic acid, and increased GSH content [53].

3.4. Sulfur-Containing Amino Acids (Methionine and Cysteine)

Methionine is known to improve intestinal antioxidant capacity, villus morphology and development, transepithelial electrical resistance, and abundance of tight junction proteins, and to reduce plasma urea nitrogen [93,94]. Interestingly, reduction in dietary methionine intake has also resulted in improvement of epithelial barrier function [95] and suppression of colonic tumor development [96]. Consistent with this, rats fed with methionine-restricted diet were found to have higher transepithelial electrical resistance and claudin-3 protein expression, and decreased severity of epithelial injury in an ulcerative colitis model induced by DSS [97]. However, methionine-deficient diets can cause enterotoxigenic *Escherichia coli* adhesion, reduce autophagy and accelerate death of intestinal epithelial cells infected with enterotoxigenic *Escherichia coli* [98]. *S*-adenosylmethionine, a GSH precursor and the activated form of methionine, can inhibit lipopolysaccharide-induced TNF-α expression in macrophages [99]. Colon lesions, increased serum amyloid A and TNF-α, and cytoskeleton damage of cells in the intestinal mucosa in DSS-treated mice were reversed when treated with S-adenosylmethionine [27].

Cysteine is a sulfur-containing amino acid, and although high intake of cysteine is extremely toxic in animals [100], dietary cysteine has important anti-inflammatory and antioxidation activities [101]. Kim et al. [16] reported that cysteine attenuated IBD symptoms by restoring gut immune homeostasis and susceptibility of activated immune cells to apoptosis. Cysteine decreased chemokine expression, neutrophil influx, expression of TNF-α, IL-6, IL-12p40, and IL-1β inflammation-related cytokines and FLICE-like inhibitory protein and Bcl-xL prosurvival genes, and increased caspase-8 expression [16].

N-acetylcysteine (NAC), the precursor of cysteine, is rapidly metabolized by the gut to generate GSH [102], and improve intestinal bacteria with an increase in Lactobacillus and Bifidobacterium counts and a decrease in *Escherichia coli* count [103]. NAC is protective of intestinal health, and has beneficial effects in pathological conditions. Supplementation with exogenous GSH or NAC has been shown to attenuate dimethyl fumarate-induced necroptosis of CT26 murine colon adenocarcinoma cells [104]. In a pig model, dietary supplementation with 500 mg/kg NAC increased goblet cell number, and protein/DNA ratio, claudin-1 protein expression, and prevented increase of intraepithelial lymphocytes and caspase-3 protein expression in the colonic mucosa [54]. Cetinkaya et al. [65] demonstrated that intraperitoneal or intrarectal NAC decreased MPO activity and MDA level, elevated GSH level and SOD and CAT activities in an acetic acid-induced rat IBD model. Others have shown that NAC attenuated macroscopic colonic damage and histopathologic changes, decreased colonic MPO activity and ROS, upregulated paraoxonase 1 (an antioxidant enzyme), and scavenged oxygen-derived free radicals in a mouse DSS colitis model [24,26]. In addition to restoring normal levels of antioxidant enzymes, NAC administration also decreased TNF-α, IL-1β, IL-6 proinflammatory cytokines [24,54]. Rectal administration of 13 mg/kg NAC limited TNBS-induced intestinal damage in rats by suppressing COX2 gene expression and PGE_2 level [18]. NAC (0.2%) has the potential to suppress chronic ulcerative colitis-associated colorectal adenocarcinoma development, as shown by inhibition of cellular damage and inflammation-related hyperproliferation [66]. The evidence strongly suggests an NAC benefit in colitis, with alleviation of colitis-induced inflammation, oxidative stress, and tissue damage. The effects of NAC have been reported to be correlated with PI3K/Akt/mTOR, epithelial growth factor receptor, and TLR4/NF-κB signaling, AMP-activated protein kinase (AMPK), and type I interferon [102,105].

3.5. Threonine

Threonine is an essential amino acid necessary for intestinal mucosal protein synthesis, especially mucin, and for intestinal integrity, immune barrier function, and oxidative status [106,107]. Supplementation with 1 or 3 g/kg threonine for 21 days resulted in an increase in intestinal villus height, goblet cell density, mucin-2 expression, and immunoglobulin G, immunoglobulin M and secretory immunoglobulin A concentrations in young broiler chickens [107]. Threonine also decreased *Escherichia coli* and *Salmonella* colonies, and increased the *Lactobacillus* colonies in the cecal contents [107]. The mechanisms of threonine-induced protection of intestinal epithelial cells may involve cytoskeletal stabilization, HSP upregulation and nuclear translocation, and a decrease in apoptosis [108]. Pathological conditions (e.g., ileitis and sepsis) may increase the amount of threonine required by the gastrointestinal tract [106]. In a TNBS-induced minipig ileitis model, Rémond et al. [20] reported that intestinal inflammation increased the gastrointestinal tract requirement for threonine. Indeed, generation of mucosal layer and mucin are often quantitatively and qualitatively impaired in IBD [109] and the increased threonine requirement reflects the increased demand for mucin production during intestinal inflammation. Faure et al. [110] reported that increased feeding of an amino acid cocktail containing threonine promoted mucin production and a healthy microbiota and favor colonic protection and mucosal healing in DSS-treated rats. An adequate threonine supply appears crucial to restoration of intestinal integrity during IBD and therefore to enhance recovery.

3.6. *Tryptophan*

Tryptophan regulates intestinal intracellular protein turnover, expression of tight junction proteins [111] and microbiota diversity [112], and reduces intestinal inflammation [113]. It is a precursor of serotonin (5-hydrotryptamine) [67], which is associated with the pathogenesis of experimental colitis [114]. Decreased serum tryptophan observed in IBD patients was shown to reflect a reduction in availability of tryptophan and its metabolites in gut cells and/or an increase in consumption during the inflammatory process [115]. The effect of low serum tryptophan on serotonin biosynthesis can result in impaired quality of life and depression, and tryptophan deficiency may result in immunodeficiency in the presence of persistent immune activation [116]. Tryptophan seems to have a role in IBD, as tryptophan treatment attenuates the symptoms and severity of DSS-induced colitis. In a mouse IBD model, a tryptophan diet ameliorated body weight loss and frequency of bloody stools [67]. It also improved histological evidence of colitis, and decreased the nitrotyrosine content of colon tissues following DSS treatment [67]. A study of its effects on mucosal inflammation found that tryptophan supplementation reduced gut permeability, expression of proinflammatory cytokines, and increased expression of the apoptosis initiators caspase-8 and Bax [68]. In a study comparing the responses of wild-type and aryl hydrocarbon receptor (Ahr)-deficient mice, Islam et al. [69] found that colitis symptoms and production of intestinal inflammatory cytokines were suppressed by activation of Ahr with a 0.5% tryptophan diet. Ahr is a key transcription factor involved in the regulation of inflammation and immunity. Tryptophan was also associated with increased IL-22 and STAT3 expression and protection of epithelial integrity [69]. Thus, tryptophan could be considered as a promising candidate for the treatment of IBD.

3.7. *Glycine*

Glycine, although can be synthesized from serine, is a nutritionally essential amino acid for neonatal growth and development, and appears to protect against ischemic-reperfusion injury [117], oxidative stress [118], endotoxemia [119], and necrotizing enterocolitis [120]. It has been shown to have anti-inflammatory, immunomodulatory, and direct cytoprotective activity [121–123]. We previously demonstrated that glycine administration increased intestinal protein content, protein/DNA, RNA/DNA, and villus height/crypt depth ratios and the activities of several tricarboxylic acid cycle enzymes (citrate synthase, isocitrate dehydrogenase and the α-ketoglutarate dehydrogenase complex) under inflammatory conditions [122]. Glycine downregulated proinflammatory cytokines and enhanced protein mass via regulation of TLR4, NOD, AMPK and mTOR signaling [122]. The experimental evidence is sufficient to support a hypothesis that glycine can protect against IBD. Tsune et al. [70] confirmed that glycine alleviated diarrhea, body weight loss, ulceration, and inflammatory changes in the colon caused by TNBS and DSS in animal models. TNBS- or DSS-induced increases in colon MPO activity, proinflammatory IL-1β and TNF-α cytokines and cytokine-induced neutrophil chemoattractant and MIP-2 chemokine secretion were largely blunted in animals fed glycine-supplemented diets [70]. These results suggest that glycine might have prophylactic and therapeutic activity against colitis; data on the effect of glycine on IBD is still limited.

3.8. Histidine

Histidine is a conditionally essential amino acid, and is an efficient scavenger of hydroxyl radicals and singlet oxygen [124]. Histidine decarboxylase initiates an immunologically significant pathway for histidine utilization by generating histamine, which can affect acute and chronic inflammation and regulate key events of the immune response [125]. Histidine supplementation can suppress oxidative stress- and TNF-α-induced IL-8 secretion in intestinal epithelial cells [126]. Hasegawa et al. [127] reported that histidine exhibited anti-inflammatory effects in THP-1 human monocytic leukemia cells, and speculated that histidine may also have therapeutic efficacy in IBD. Consistent with this, dietary histidine ameliorated colitis in an IL-10-deficient (IL-10$^{-/-}$) cell transfer model of Crohn's disease, by regulation of NF-κB activation, and subsequent inhibition of proinflammatory cytokine production by macrophages [71]. Other recent results suggest that decreased plasma histidine predicts risk of relapse in patients with ulcerative colitis in remission [128]. The collective evidence suggests that histidine may be an effective agent in treating various immunopathologic conditions.

3.9. Other Amino Acids

Aspartate, asparagine and proline also participate in immune responses [129] that may maintain intestinal health and protect against animal and human diseases. We previously demonstrated that aspartate and asparagine improved intestinal tissue integrity, enhanced mucosal energy status via AMPK signaling, and reduced proinflammatory cytokine expression (via TLR4, NODs and p38) and enterocyte apoptosis (via p38 and extracellular signal-regulated kinase 1/2) in pathological conditions [130–133]. Proline inhibited lipopolysaccharide-induced inflammation in vivo in weaned piglets [134]. Dietary threonine, serine, proline, and cysteine supplementation improved mucin production, restored healthy microbiota, protected gut epithelium and promoted mucosal healing in DSS-treated rats [110].

Experimental studies investigating the efficacy of amino acids such as glutamine and arginine in animal models of IBD are promising. Some clinical studies with oral supplementation of glutamine in IBD patients are disappointing, but new formulations and targeting at the site of mucosal lesions could improve the efficacy of glutamine [135]. The role of arginine in IBD patients still remains controversial [135]. However, the effects of these amino acids in IBD patients have been poorly investigated. The clinical effects of other amino acids should also be investigated in the future.

4. Conclusions

IBD is a complex disease with complex pathogenesis, and no single animal model can fully reflect the entire spectrum of human IBD phenotypes. However, the available models are useful for the study of various aspects and mechanisms of IBD pathogenesis. Amino acids may be necessary for maintaining normal immunocompetence and protecting against human and animal diseases. We predict that these nutrients will likely be used as alternative or ancillary IBD treatments. Additional research is also warranted to add to the understanding of the underlying mechanisms of IBD, and to investigate the clinical effects of these amino acids.

Acknowledgments: This work was supported by the National Natural Science Foundation of China (31372318 and 31422053), State's Key Project of Research and Development Plan (2016YFD0501210) and the Project of the Hubei Provincial Department of Education (T201508).

Author Contributions: Y.L., X.W. and C.A.H. designed and wrote the paper; Y.L. and C.A.H. edited and revised the manuscript. All authors read and approved the final manuscript.

References

1. Shi, X.Z.; Winston, J.H.; Sarna, S.K. Differential immune and genetic responses in rat models of Crohn's colitis and ulcerative colitis. *Am. J. Physiol. Gastrointest. Liver Physiol.* **2011**, *300*, G41–G51. [CrossRef] [PubMed]
2. Randhawa, P.K.; Singh, K.; Singh, N.; Jaggi, A.S. A review on chemical-induced inflammatory bowel disease models in rodents. *Korean J. Physiol. Pharmacol.* **2014**, *18*, 279–288. [CrossRef] [PubMed]
3. Snider, A.J.; Bialkowska, A.B.; Ghaleb, A.M.; Yang, V.W.; Obeid, L.M.; Hannun, Y.A. Murine model for colitis-associated cancer of the colon. *Methods Mol. Biol.* **2016**, *1438*, 245–254. [PubMed]
4. Corridoni, D.; Arseneau, K.O.; Cominelli, F. Inflammatory bowel disease. *Immunol. Lett.* **2014**, *161*, 231–235. [CrossRef] [PubMed]
5. Goyal, N.; Rana, A.; Ahlawat, A.; Bijjem, K.R.; Kumar, P. Animal models of inflammatory bowel disease: A review. *Inflammopharmacology* **2014**, *22*, 219–233. [CrossRef] [PubMed]
6. Wu, G. Intestinal mucosal amino acid catabolism. *J. Nutr.* **1998**, *128*, 1249–1252. [PubMed]
7. Vidal-Lletjós, S.; Beaumont, M.; Tomé, D.; Benamouzig, R.; Blachier, F.; Lan, A. Dietary protein and amino acid supplementation in inflammatory bowel disease course: What impact on the colonic mucosa? *Nutrients* **2017**, *9*, 310. [CrossRef] [PubMed]
8. Dai, Z.; Wu, Z.; Hang, S.; Zhu, W.; Wu, G. Amino acid metabolism in intestinal bacteria and its potential implications for mammalian reproduction. *Mol. Hum. Reprod.* **2015**, *21*, 389–409. [CrossRef] [PubMed]
9. Oh, S.Y.; Cho, K.A.; Kang, J.L.; Kim, K.H.; Woo, S.Y. Comparison of experimental mouse models of inflammatory bowel disease. *Int. J. Mol. Med.* **2014**, *33*, 333–340. [PubMed]
10. Hou, Y.C.; Wu, J.M.; Wang, M.Y.; Wu, M.H.; Chen, K.Y.; Yeh, S.L.; Lin, M.T. Glutamine supplementation attenuates expressions of adhesion molecules and chemokine receptors on T cells in a murine model of acute colitis. *Mediat. Inflamm.* **2014**, *2014*, 837107. [CrossRef] [PubMed]
11. Hsiung, Y.C.; Liu, J.J.; Hou, Y.C.; Yeh, C.L.; Yeh, S.L. Effects of dietary glutamine on the homeostasis of $CD4^+$ T cells in mice with dextran sulfate sodium-induced acute colitis. *PLoS ONE* **2014**, *9*, e84410. [CrossRef] [PubMed]
12. Ren, W.; Yin, J.; Wu, M.; Liu, G.; Yang, G.; Xion, Y.; Su, D.; Wu, L.; Li, T.; Chen, S.; et al. Serum amino acids profile and the beneficial effects of L-arginine or L-glutamine supplementation in dextran sulfate sodium colitis. *PLoS ONE* **2014**, *9*, e88335. [CrossRef] [PubMed]
13. Chu, C.C.; Hou, Y.C.; Pai, M.H.; Chao, C.J.; Yeh, S.L. Pretreatment with alanyl-glutamine suppresses T-helper-cell-associated cytokine expression and reduces inflammatory responses in mice with acute DSS-induced colitis. *J. Nutr. Biochem.* **2012**, *23*, 1092–1099. [CrossRef] [PubMed]
14. Coburn, L.A.; Gong, X.; Singh, K.; Asim, M.; Scull, B.P.; Allaman, M.M.; Williams, C.S.; Rosen, M.J.; Washington, M.K.; Barry, D.P.; et al. L-arginine supplementation improves responses to injury and inflammation in dextran sulfate sodium colitis. *PLoS ONE* **2012**, *7*, e33546. [CrossRef] [PubMed]
15. Xue, H.; Sufit, A.J.; Wischmeyer, P.E. Glutamine therapy improves outcome of in vitro and in vivo experimental colitis models. *JPEN J. Parenter. Enteral Nutr.* **2011**, *35*, 188–197. [CrossRef] [PubMed]
16. Kim, C.J.; Kovacs-Nolan, J.; Yang, C.; Archbold, T.; Fan, M.Z.; Mine, Y. L-cysteine supplementation attenuates local inflammation and restores gut homeostasis in a porcine model of colitis. *Biochim. Biophys. Acta* **2009**, *1790*, 1161–1169. [CrossRef] [PubMed]
17. San-Miguel, B.; Crespo, I.; Kretzmann, N.A.; Mauriz, J.L.; Marroni, N.; Tuñón, M.J.; González-Gallego, J. Glutamine prevents fibrosis development in rats with colitis induced by 2,4,6-trinitrobenzene sulfonic acid. *J. Nutr.* **2010**, *140*, 1065–1071. [CrossRef] [PubMed]
18. Ancha, H.R.; Kurella, R.R.; McKimmey, C.C.; Lightfoot, S.; Harty, R.F. Effects of *N*-acetylcysteine plus mesalamine on prostaglandin synthesis and nitric oxide generation in TNBS-induced colitis in rats. *Dig. Dis. Sci.* **2009**, *54*, 758–766. [CrossRef] [PubMed]
19. Pouillart, P.R.; Dépeint, F.; Abdelnour, A.; Deremaux, L.; Vincent, O.; Mazière, J.C.; Madec, J.Y.; Chatelain, D.; Younes, H.; Wils, D.; et al. Nutriose, a prebiotic low-digestible carbohydrate, stimulates gut mucosal immunity and prevents TNBS-induced colitis in piglets. *Inflamm. Bowel. Dis.* **2010**, *16*, 783–794. [CrossRef] [PubMed]

20. Rémond, D.; Buffière, C.; Godin, J.P.; Mirand, P.P.; Obled, C.; Papet, I.; Dardevet, D.; Williamson, G.; Breuillé, D.; Faure, M. Intestinal inflammation increases gastrointestinal threonine uptake and mucin synthesis in enterally fed minipigs. *J. Nutr.* **2009**, *139*, 720–726. [CrossRef] [PubMed]
21. Shibata, Y.; Taruishi, M.; Ashida, T. Experimental ileitis in dogs and colitis in rats with trinitrobenzene sulfonic acid—Colonoscopic and histopathologic studies. *Gastroenterol. Jpn.* **1993**, *28*, 518–527. [PubMed]
22. Fabia, R.; Willén, R.; Ar'Rajab, A.; Andersson, R.; Ahrén, B.; Bengmark, S. Acetic acid-induced colitis in the rat: A reproducible experimental model for acute ulcerative colitis. *Eur. Surg. Res.* **1992**, *24*, 211–225. [CrossRef] [PubMed]
23. Tahan, G.; Aytac, E.; Aytekin, H.; Gunduz, F.; Dogusoy, G.; Aydin, S.; Tahan, V.; Uzun, H. Vitamin E has a dual effect of anti-inflammatory and antioxidant activities in acetic acid-induced ulcerative colitis in rats. *Can. J. Surg.* **2011**, *54*, 333–338. [CrossRef] [PubMed]
24. Uraz, S.; Tahan, G.; Aytekin, H.; Tahan, V. *N*-acetylcysteine expresses powerful anti-inflammatory and antioxidant activities resulting in complete improvement of acetic acid-induced colitis in rats. *Scand. J. Clin. Lab. Investig.* **2013**, *73*, 61–66. [CrossRef] [PubMed]
25. Kitajima, S.; Takuma, S.; Morimoto, M. Histological analysis of murine colitis induced by dextran sulfate sodium of different molecular weights. *Exp. Anim.* **2000**, *49*, 9–15. [CrossRef] [PubMed]
26. You, Y.; Fu, J.J.; Meng, J.; Huang, G.D.; Liu, Y.H. Effect of *N*-acetylcysteine on the murine model of colitis induced by dextran sodium sulfate through up-regulating PON1 activity. *Dig. Dis. Sci.* **2009**, *54*, 1643–1650. [CrossRef] [PubMed]
27. Oz, H.S.; Chen, T.S.; McClain, C.J.; de Villiers, W.J. Antioxidants as novel therapy in a murine model of colitis. *J. Nutr. Biochem.* **2005**, *16*, 297–304. [CrossRef] [PubMed]
28. Håkansson, Å.; Tormo-Badia, N.; Baridi, A.; Xu, J.; Molin, G.; Hagslätt, M.-L.; Karlsson, C.; Jeppsson, B.; Cilio, C.M.; Ahrné, S. Immunological alteration and changes of gut microbiota after dextran sulfate sodium (DSS) administration in mice. *Clin. Exp. Med.* **2015**, *15*, 107–120. [CrossRef] [PubMed]
29. Munyaka, P.M.; Rabbi, M.F.; Khafipour, E.; Ghia, J.-E. Acute dextran sulfate sodium (DSS)-induced colitis promotes gut microbial dysbiosis in mice. *J. Basic Microbiol.* **2016**, *56*, 986–998. [CrossRef] [PubMed]
30. Perše, M.; Cerar, A. Dextran sodium sulphate colitis mouse model: Traps and tricks. *J. Biomed. Biotechnol.* **2012**, *2012*, 718617. [CrossRef] [PubMed]
31. Kiesler, P.; Fuss, I.J.; Strober, W. Experimental models of inflammatory bowel diseases. *Cell Mol. Gastroenterol. Hepatol.* **2015**, *1*, 154–170. [CrossRef] [PubMed]
32. Vicario, M.; Amat, C.; Rivero, M.; Moretó, M.; Pelegrí, C. Dietary glutamine affects mucosal functions in rats with mild DSS-induced colitis. *J. Nutr.* **2007**, *137*, 1931–1937. [PubMed]
33. Amrouche-Mekkioui, I.; Djerdjouri, B. *N*-acetylcysteine improves redox status, mitochondrial dysfunction, mucin-depleted crypts and epithelial hyperplasia in dextran sulfate sodium-induced oxidative colitis in mice. *Eur. J. Pharmacol.* **2012**, *691*, 209–217. [CrossRef] [PubMed]
34. Dagenais, M.; Douglas, T.; Saleh, M. Role of programmed necrosis and cell death in intestinal inflammation. *Curr. Opin. Gastroenterol.* **2014**, *30*, 566–575. [CrossRef] [PubMed]
35. Qu, C.; Yuan, Z.W.; Yu, X.T.; Huang, Y.F.; Yang, G.H.; Chen, J.N.; Lai, X.P.; Su, Z.R.; Zeng, H.F.; Xie, Y.; et al. Patchouli alcohol ameliorates dextran sodium sulfate-induced experimental colitis and suppresses tryptophan catabolism. *Pharmacol. Res.* **2017**, *121*, 70–82. [CrossRef] [PubMed]
36. Günther, C.; Martini, E.; Wittkopf, N.; Amann, K.; Weigmann, B.; Neumann, H.; Waldner, M.J.; Hedrick, S.M.; Tenzer, S.; Neurath, M.F.; et al. Caspase-8 regulates TNF-α-induced epithelial necroptosis and terminal ileitis. *Nature* **2011**, *477*, 335–339. [CrossRef] [PubMed]
37. Liu, Z.Y.; Wu, B.; Guo, Y.S.; Zhou, Y.H.; Fu, Z.G.; Xu, B.Q.; Li, J.H.; Jing, L.; Jiang, J.L.; Tang, J.; Chen, Z.N. Necrostatin-1 reduces intestinal inflammation and colitis-associated tumorigenesis in mice. *Am. J. Cancer Res.* **2015**, *5*, 3174–3185. [PubMed]
38. Welz, P.S.; Wullaert, A.; Vlantis, K.; Kondylis, V.; Fernández-Majada, V.; Ermolaeva, M.; Kirsch, P.; Sterner-Kock, A.; van Loo, G.; Pasparakis, M. FADD prevents RIP3-mediated epithelial cell necrosis and chronic intestinal inflammation. *Nature* **2011**, *477*, 330–334. [CrossRef] [PubMed]
39. Motavallian-Naeini, A.; Andalib, S.; Rabbani, M.; Mahzouni, P.; Afsharipour, M.; Minaiyan, M. Validation and optimization of experimental colitis induction in rats using 2,4,6-trinitrobenzene sulfonic acid. *Res. Pharm. Sci.* **2012**, *7*, 159–169. [PubMed]

40. Zheng, L.; Gao, Z.Q.; Wang, S.X. A chronic ulcerative colitis model in rats. *World J. Gastroenterol.* **2000**, *6*, 150–152. [CrossRef] [PubMed]
41. Tran, C.D.; Katsikeros, R.; Abimosleh, S.M. Current and Novel Treatments for Ulcerative Colitis. In *Ulcerative Colitis from Genetics to Complications*; InTech: Rijeka, Croatia, 2012.
42. Antoniou, E.; Margonis, G.A.; Angelou, A.; Pikouli, A.; Argiri, P.; Karavokyros, I.; Papalois, A.; Pikoulis, E. The TNBS-induced colitis animal model: An overview. *Ann. Med. Surg.* **2016**, *11*, 9–15. [CrossRef] [PubMed]
43. Wang, J.; Chen, H.; Wang, Y.; Cai, X.; Zou, M.; Xu, T.; Wang, M.; Wang, J.; Xu, D. Therapeutic efficacy of a mutant of keratinocyte growth factor-2 on trinitrobenzene sulfonic acid-induced rat model of Crohn's disease. *Am. J. Transl. Res.* **2016**, *8*, 530–543. [PubMed]
44. Giriş, M.; Erbil, Y.; Doğru-Abbasoğlu, S.; Yanik, B.T.; Aliş, H.; Olgaç, V.; Toker, G.A. The effect of heme oxygenase-1 induction by glutamine on TNBS-induced colitis. The effect of glutamine on TNBS colitis. *Int. J. Colorectal. Dis.* **2007**, *22*, 591–599. [CrossRef] [PubMed]
45. Crespo, I.; San-Miguel, B.; Prause, C.; Marroni, N.; Cuevas, M.J.; González-Gallego, J.; Tuñón, M.J. Glutamine treatment attenuates endoplasmic reticulum stress and apoptosis in TNBS-induced colitis. *PLoS ONE* **2012**, *7*, e50407. [CrossRef] [PubMed]
46. Siddiqui, A.; Ancha, H.; Tedesco, D.; Lightfoot, S.; Stewart, C.A.; Harty, R.F. Antioxidant therapy with *N*-acetylcysteine plus mesalamine accelerates mucosal healing in a rodent model of colitis. *Dig. Dis. Sci.* **2006**, *51*, 698–705. [CrossRef] [PubMed]
47. Low, D.; Nguyen, D.D.; Mizoguchi, E. Animal models of ulcerative colitis and their application in drug research. *Drug Des. Devel. Ther.* **2013**, *7*, 1341–1357. [PubMed]
48. Nakao, K.; Ro, A.; Kibayashi, K. Evaluation of the morphological changes of gastric mucosa induced by a low concentration of acetic acid using a rat model. *J. Forensic Leg. Med.* **2014**, *22*, 99–106. [CrossRef] [PubMed]
49. Fillmann, H.; Kretzmann, N.A.; San-Miguel, B.; Llesuy, S.; Marroni, N.; González-Gallego, J.; Tuñón, M.J. Glutamine inhibits over-expression of pro-inflammatory genes and down-regulates the nuclear factor kappaB pathway in an experimental model of colitis in the rat. *Toxicology* **2007**, *236*, 217–226. [CrossRef] [PubMed]
50. Sakthivel, K.M.; Guruvayoorappan, C. Amentoflavone inhibits iNOS, COX-2 expression and modulates cytokine profile, NF-κB signal transduction pathways in rats with ulcerative colitis. *Int. Immunopharmacol.* **2013**, *17*, 907–916. [CrossRef] [PubMed]
51. Aleisa, A.M.; Al-Rejaie, S.S.; Abuohashish, H.M.; Ola, M.S.; Parmar, M.Y.; Ahmed, M.M. Pretreatment of Gymnema sylvestre revealed the protection against acetic acid-induced ulcerative colitis in rats. *BMC Complement. Altern. Med.* **2014**, *14*, 49. [CrossRef] [PubMed]
52. Niu, X.; Fan, T.; Li, W.; Huang, H.; Zhang, Y.; Xing, W. Protective effect of sanguinarine against acetic acid-induced ulcerative colitis in mice. *Toxicol. Appl. Pharmacol.* **2013**, *267*, 256–265. [CrossRef] [PubMed]
53. Harisa, G.E.; Abo-Salem, O.M.; El-Sayed, S.M.; Taha, E.I.; El-Halawany, N. L-arginine augments the antioxidant effect of garlic against acetic acid-induced ulcerative colitis in rats. *Pak. J. Pharm. Sci.* **2009**, *22*, 373–380. [PubMed]
54. Wang, Q.; Hou, Y.; Yi, D.; Wang, L.; Ding, B.; Chen, X.; Long, M.; Liu, Y.; Wu, G. Protective effects of *N*-acetylcysteine on acetic acid-induced colitis in a porcine model. *BMC Gastroenterol.* **2013**, *13*, 133. [CrossRef] [PubMed]
55. Ali, A.A.; Abd Al Haleem, E.N.; Khaleel, S.A.; Sallam, A.S. Protective effect of cardamonin against acetic acid-induced ulcerative colitis in rats. *Pharmacol. Rep.* **2017**, *69*, 268–275. [CrossRef] [PubMed]
56. Wirtz, S.; Popp, V.; Kindermann, M.; Gerlach, K.; Weigmann, B.; Fichtner-Feigl, S.; Neurath, M.F. Chemically induced mouse models of acute and chronic intestinal inflammation. *Nat. Protoc.* **2017**, *12*, 1295–1309. [CrossRef] [PubMed]
57. Berry, D.; Kuzyk, O.; Rauch, I.; Heider, S.; Schwab, C.; Hainzl, E.; Decker, T.; Müller, M.; Strobl, B.; Schleper, C.; et al. Intestinal microbiota signatures associated with inflammation history in mice experiencing recurring colitis. *Front. Microbiol.* **2015**, *6*, 1408. [CrossRef] [PubMed]
58. Mowat, C.; Cole, A.; Windsor, A.; Ahmad, T.; Arnott, I.; Driscoll, R.; Mitton, S.; Orchard, T.; Rutter, M.; Younge, L.; et al. Guidelines for the management of inflammatory bowel disease in adults. *Gut* **2011**, *60*, 571–607. [CrossRef] [PubMed]
59. Xin, L.; Li, N.; Zhu, W.; Wu, K.; Zhang, L.; Zhai, J.; Wang, Y.; Zhu, J.; Wang, X.; Shi, Y.; et al. An analysis of amino acid metabolic profile and its clinical significance in ulcerative colitis. *Zhonghua Nei Ke Za Zhi* **2015**, *54*, 210–213. [PubMed]

60. Swaid, F.; Sukhotnik, I.; Matter, I.; Berkowitz, D.; Hadjittofi, C.; Pollak, Y.; Lavy, A. Dietary glutamine supplementation prevents mucosal injury and modulates intestinal epithelial restitution following acetic acid induced intestinal injury in rats. *Nutr. Metab.* **2013**, *10*, 53. [CrossRef] [PubMed]
61. Değer, C.; Erbil, Y.; Giriş, M.; Yanik, B.T.; Tunca, F.; Olgaç, V.; Abbasoğlu, S.D.; Oztezcan, S.; Toker, G. The effect of glutamine on pancreatic damage in TNBS-induced colitis. *Dig. Dis. Sci.* **2006**, *51*, 1841–1846. [CrossRef] [PubMed]
62. Kretzmann, N.A.; Fillmann, H.; Mauriz, J.L.; Marroni, C.A.; Marroni, N.; González-Gallego, J.; Tuñón, M.J. Effects of glutamine on proinflammatory gene expression and activation of nuclear factor kappa B and signal transducers and activators of transcription in TNBS-induced colitis. *Inflamm. Bowel Dis.* **2008**, *14*, 1504–1513. [CrossRef] [PubMed]
63. Li, T.T.; Zhang, J.F.; Fei, S.J.; Zhu, S.P.; Zhu, J.Z.; Qiao, X.; Liu, Z.B. Glutamate microinjection into the hypothalamic paraventricular nucleus attenuates ulcerative colitis in rats. *Acta Pharmacol. Sin.* **2014**, *35*, 185–194. [CrossRef] [PubMed]
64. Farghaly, H.S.; Thabit, R.H. L-arginine and aminoguanidine reduce colonic damage of acetic acid-induced colitis in rats: Potential modulation of nuclear factor-κB/p65. *Clin. Exp. Pharmacol. Physiol.* **2014**, *41*, 769–779. [CrossRef] [PubMed]
65. Cetinkaya, A.; Bulbuloglu, E.; Kurutas, E.B.; Ciralik, H.; Kantarceken, B.; Buyukbese, M.A. Beneficial effects of *N*-acetylcysteine on acetic acid-induced colitis in rats. *Tohoku J. Exp. Med.* **2005**, *206*, 131–139. [CrossRef] [PubMed]
66. Seril, D.N.; Liao, J.; Ho, K.L.; Yang, C.S.; Yang, G.Y. Inhibition of chronic ulcerative colitis-associated colorectal adenocarcinoma development in a murine model by *N*-acetylcysteine. *Carcinogenesis* **2002**, *23*, 993–1001. [CrossRef] [PubMed]
67. Shizuma, T.; Mori, H.; Fukuyama, N. Protective effect of tryptophan against dextran sulfate sodium- induced experimental colitis. *Turk. J. Gastroenterol.* **2013**, *24*, 30–35. [CrossRef] [PubMed]
68. Kim, C.J.; Kovacs-Nolan, J.A.; Yang, C.; Archbold, T.; Fan, M.Z.; Mine, Y. L-Tryptophan exhibits therapeutic function in a porcine model of dextran sodium sulfate (DSS)-induced colitis. *J. Nutr. Biochem.* **2010**, *21*, 468–475. [CrossRef] [PubMed]
69. Islam, J.; Sato, S.; Watanabe, K.; Watanabe, T.; Ardiansyah; Hirahara, K.; Aoyama, Y.; Tomita, S.; Aso, H.; Komai, M.; et al. Dietary tryptophan alleviates dextran sodium sulfate-induced colitis through aryl hydrocarbon receptor in mice. *J. Nutr. Biochem.* **2017**, *42*, 43–50. [CrossRef] [PubMed]
70. Tsune, I.; Ikejima, K.; Hirose, M.; Yoshikawa, M.; Enomoto, N.; Takei, Y.; Sato, N. Dietary glycine prevents chemical-induced experimental colitis in the rat. *Gastroenterology* **2003**, *125*, 775–785. [CrossRef]
71. Andou, A.; Hisamatsu, T.; Okamoto, S.; Chinen, H.; Kamada, N.; Kobayashi, T.; Hashimoto, M.; Okutsu, T.; Shimbo, K.; Takeda, T.; et al. Dietary histidine ameliorates murine colitis by inhibition of proinflammatory cytokine production from macrophages. *Gastroenterology* **2009**, *136*, 564–574. [CrossRef] [PubMed]
72. Sido, B.; Seel, C.; Hochlehnert, A.; Breitkreutz, R.; Dröge, W. Low intestinal glutamine level and low glutaminase activity in Crohn's disease: A rational for glutamine supplementation? *Dig. Dis. Sci.* **2006**, *51*, 2170–2179. [CrossRef] [PubMed]
73. Fasina, Y.O.; Bowers, J.B.; Hess, J.B.; McKee, S.R. Effect of dietary glutamine supplementation on Salmonella colonization in the ceca of young broiler chicks. *Poult. Sci.* **2010**, *89*, 1042–1048. [CrossRef] [PubMed]
74. Zhang, Y.; Lu, T.; Han, L.; Zhao, L.; Niu, Y.; Chen, H. L-glutamine supplementation alleviates constipation during late gestation of mini sows by modifying the microbiota composition in feces. *BioMed Res. Int.* **2017**, *2017*. [CrossRef] [PubMed]
75. Benjamin, J.; Makharia, G.; Ahuja, V.; Anand Rajan, K.D.; Kalaivani, M.; Gupta, S.D.; Joshi, Y.K. Glutamine and whey protein improve intestinal permeability and morphology in patients with Crohn's disease: A randomized controlled trial. *Dig. Dis. Sci.* **2012**, *57*, 1000–1012. [CrossRef] [PubMed]
76. Ockenga, J.; Borchert, K.; Stüber, E.; Lochs, H.; Manns, M.P.; Bischoff, S.C. Glutamine-enriched total parenteral nutrition in patients with inflammatory bowel disease. *Eur. J. Clin. Nutr.* **2005**, *59*, 1302–1309. [CrossRef] [PubMed]
77. Den Hond, E.; Hiele, M.; Peeters, M.; Ghoos, Y.; Rutgeerts, P. Effect of long-term oral glutamine supplements on small intestinal permeability in patients with Crohn's disease. *JPEN J. Parenter. Enter. Nutr.* **1999**, *23*, 7–11. [CrossRef] [PubMed]

78. Akobeng, A.K.; Elawad, M.; Gordon, M. Glutamine for induction of remission in Crohn's disease. *Cochrane Database Syst. Rev.* **2016**, *2*, CD007348. [PubMed]
79. Newsholme, P.; Lima, M.M.; Procopio, J.; Pithon-Curi, T.C.; Doi, S.Q.; Bazotte, R.B.; Curi, R. Glutamine and glutamate as vital metabolites. *Braz. J. Med. Biol. Res.* **2003**, *36*, 153–163. [CrossRef] [PubMed]
80. Tapiero, H.; Mathé, G.; Couvreur, P.; Tew, K.D., II. Glutamine and glutamate. *Biomed. Pharmacother.* **2002**, *56*, 446–457. [CrossRef]
81. Blachier, F.; Boutry, C.; Bos, C.; Tomé, D. Metabolism and functions of L-glutamate in the epithelial cells of the small and large intestines. *Am. J. Clin. Nutr.* **2009**, *90*, 814S–821S. [CrossRef] [PubMed]
82. Jiao, N.; Wu, Z.; Ji, Y.; Wang, B.; Dai, Z.; Wu, G. L-Glutamate enhances barrier and antioxidative functions in intestinal porcine epithelial cells. *J. Nutr.* **2015**, *145*, 2258–2264. [CrossRef] [PubMed]
83. Wu, M.; Xiao, H.; Ren, W.; Yin, J.; Tan, B.; Liu, G.; Li, L.; Nyachoti, C.M.; Xiong, X.; Wu, G. Therapeutic effects of glutamic acid in piglets challenged with deoxynivalenol. *PLoS ONE* **2014**, *9*, e100591. [CrossRef] [PubMed]
84. Wang, X.Y. Regulative Effect of Glutamate on Intestinal Injury and Muscle Protein Synthesis and Degradation of Piglets after Lipopolysaccharide Challenge. Master's Thesis, Wuhan Polytechnic University, Wuhan, China, 2015.
85. Ren, X.R. Regulatory Effect of Glutamic Acid or Glycine on Intestinal Mucosal Immune Barrier Injury in Piglets after Lipopolysaccharide Challenge. Master's Thesis, Wuhan Polytechnic University, Wuhan, China, 2015.
86. Ren, W.; Chen, S.; Yin, J.; Duan, J.; Li, T.; Liu, G.; Feng, Z.; Tan, B.; Yin, Y.; Wu, G. Dietary arginine supplementation of mice alters the microbial population and activates intestinal innate immunity. *J. Nutr.* **2014**, *144*, 988–995. [CrossRef] [PubMed]
87. Wu, G.; Meininger, C.J.; Knabe, D.A.; Bazer, F.W.; Rhoads, J.M. Arginine nutrition in development, health and disease. *Curr. Opin. Clin. Nutr. Metab. Care* **2000**, *3*, 59–66. [CrossRef] [PubMed]
88. Coburn, L.A.; Horst, S.N.; Allaman, M.M.; Brown, C.T.; Williams, C.S.; Hodges, M.E.; Druce, J.P.; Beaulieu, D.B.; Schwartz, D.A.; Wilson, K.T. L-Arginine availability and metabolism is altered in ulcerative colitis. *Inflamm. Bowel Dis.* **2016**, *22*, 1847–1858. [CrossRef] [PubMed]
89. Zhu, H.L.; Liu, Y.L.; Xie, X.L.; Huang, J.J.; Hou, Y.Q. Effect of L-arginine on intestinal mucosal immune barrier function in weaned pigs after *Escherichia coli* LPS challenge. *Innate Immun.* **2013**, *19*, 242–252. [CrossRef] [PubMed]
90. Liu, Y.L.; Han, J.; Huang, J.J.; Wang, X.Q.; Wang, F.L.; Wang, J.J. Dietary L-Arginine supplementation improves intestinal function in weaned pigs after an *Escherichia coli* lipopolysaccharide. *Asian-Aust. J. Anim. Sci.* **2009**, *22*, 1667–1675. [CrossRef]
91. Liu, Y.; Huang, J.; Hou, Y.; Zhu, H.; Zhao, S.; Ding, B.; Yin, Y.; Yi, G.; Shi, J.; Fan, W. Dietary arginine supplementation alleviates intestinal mucosal disruption induced by *Escherichia coli* lipopolysaccharide in weaned pigs. *Br. J. Nutr.* **2008**, *100*, 552–560. [CrossRef] [PubMed]
92. Lecleire, S.; Hassan, A.; Marion-Letellier, R.; Antonietti, M.; Savoye, G.; Bôle-Feysot, C.; Lerebours, E.; Ducrotté, P.; Déchelotte, P.; Coëffier, M. Combined glutamine and arginine decrease proinflammatory cytokine production by biopsies from Crohn's patients in association with changes in nuclear factor-kappaB and p38 mitogen-activated protein kinase pathways. *J. Nutr.* **2008**, *138*, 2481–2486. [CrossRef] [PubMed]
93. Chen, Y.; Li, D.; Dai, Z.; Piao, X.; Wu, Z.; Wang, B.; Zhu, Y.; Zeng, Z. L-methionine supplementation maintains the integrity and barrier function of the small-intestinal mucosa in post-weaning piglets. *Amino Acids* **2014**, *46*, 1131–1142. [CrossRef] [PubMed]
94. Shen, Y.B.; Weaver, A.C.; Kim, S.W. Effect of feed grade L-methionine on growth performance and gut health in nursery pigs compared with conventional DL-methionine. *J. Anim. Sci.* **2014**, *92*, 5530–5539. [CrossRef] [PubMed]
95. Ramalingam, A.; Wang, X.; Gabello, M.; Valenzano, M.C.; Soler, A.P.; Ko, A.; Morin, P.J.; Mullin, J.M. Dietary methionine restriction improves colon tight junction barrier function and alters claudin expression pattern. *Am. J. Physiol. Cell Physiol.* **2010**, *299*, C1028–C1035. [CrossRef] [PubMed]
96. Komninou, D.; Leutzinger, Y.; Reddy, B.S.; Richie, J.P., Jr. Methionine restriction inhibits colon carcinogenesis. *Nutr. Cancer* **2006**, *54*, 202–208. [CrossRef] [PubMed]
97. Rao, Y.X.; Chen, J.; Chen, L.L.; Gu, W.Z. The impact of dietary methionine-restriction on tight junction expression and function in a rat colonitis model. *Zhonghua Nei Ke Za Zhi* **2013**, *52*, 503–509. [PubMed]

98. Tang, Y.; Tan, B.; Xiong, X.; Li, F.; Ren, W.; Kong, X.; Qiu, W.; Hardwidge, P.R.; Yin, Y. Methionine deficiency reduces autophagy and accelerates death in intestinal epithelial cells infected with enterotoxigenic *Escherichia coli*. *Amino Acids* **2015**, *47*, 2199–2204. [CrossRef] [PubMed]
99. Li, T.W.; Yang, H.; Peng, H.; Xia, M.; Mato, J.M.; Lu, S.C. Effects of *S*-adenosylmethionine and methylthioadenosine on inflammation-induced colon cancer in mice. *Carcinogenesis* **2012**, *33*, 427–435. [CrossRef] [PubMed]
100. Ji, Y.; Wu, Z.; Dai, Z.; Sun, K.; Zhang, Q.; Wu, G. Excessive L-cysteine induces vacuole-like cell death by activating endoplasmic reticulum stress and mitogen-activated protein kinase signaling in intestinal porcine epithelial cells. *Amino Acids* **2016**, *48*, 149–156. [CrossRef] [PubMed]
101. Song, Z.H.; Tong, G.; Xiao, K.; Jiao, L.F.; Ke, Y.L.; Hu, C.H. L-cysteine protects intestinal integrity, attenuates intestinal inflammation and oxidant stress, and modulates NF-κB and Nrf2 pathways in weaned piglets after LPS challenge. *Innate Immun.* **2016**, *22*, 152–161. [CrossRef] [PubMed]
102. Hou, Y.; Wang, L.; Yi, D.; Wu, G. *N*-acetylcysteine and intestinal health: A focus on its mechanism of action. *Front. Biosci.* **2015**, *20*, 872–891. [CrossRef]
103. Xu, C.C.; Yang, S.F.; Zhu, L.H.; Cai, X.; Sheng, Y.S.; Zhu, S.W.; Xu, J.X. Regulation of *N*-acetyl cysteine on gut redox status and major microbiota in weaned piglets. *J. Anim. Sci.* **2014**, *92*, 1504–1511. [CrossRef] [PubMed]
104. Xie, X.; Zhao, Y.; Ma, C.Y.; Xu, X.M.; Zhang, Y.Q.; Wang, C.G.; Jin, J.; Shen, X.; Gao, J.L.; Li, N.; et al. Dimethyl fumarate induces necroptosis in colon cancer cells through GSH depletion/ROS increase/MAPKs activation pathway. *Br. J. Pharmacol.* **2015**, *172*, 3929–3943. [CrossRef] [PubMed]
105. Yi, D.; Hou, Y.Q.; Xiao, H.; Wang, L.; Zhang, Y.; Chen, H.B.; Wu, T.; Ding, B.Y.; Hu, C.A.; Wu, G.Y. *N*-Acetylcysteine improves intestinal function in lipopolysaccharides-challenged piglets through multiple signaling pathways. *Amino Acids* 2017. [CrossRef] [PubMed]
106. Mao, X.; Zeng, X.; Qiao, S.; Wu, G.; Li, D. Specific roles of threonine in intestinal mucosal integrity and barrier function. *Front. Biosci.* **2011**, *3*, 1192–1200. [CrossRef]
107. Chen, Y.P.; Cheng, Y.F.; Li, X.H.; Yang, W.L.; Wen, C.; Zhuang, S.; Zhou, Y.M. Effects of threonine supplementation on the growth performance, immunity, oxidative status, intestinal integrity, and barrier function of broilers at the early age. *Poult. Sci.* **2017**, *96*, 405–413. [CrossRef] [PubMed]
108. Baird, C.H.; Niederlechner, S.; Beck, R.; Kallweit, A.R.; Wischmeyer, P.E. L-Threonine induces heat shock protein expression and decreases apoptosis in heat-stressed intestinal epithelial cells. *Nutrition* **2013**, *29*, 1404–1411. [CrossRef] [PubMed]
109. Corfield, A.P.; Myerscough, N.; Longman, R.; Sylvester, P.; Arul, S.; Pignatelli, M. Mucins and mucosal protection in the gastrointestinal tract: New prospects for mucins in the pathology of gastrointestinal disease. *Gut* **2000**, *47*, 589–594. [CrossRef] [PubMed]
110. Faure, M.; Mettraux, C.; Moennoz, D.; Godin, J.P.; Vuichoud, J.; Rochat, F.; Breuillé, D.; Obled, C.; Corthésy-Theulaz, I. Specific amino acids increase mucin synthesis and microbiota in dextran sulfate sodium-treated rats. *J. Nutr.* **2006**, *136*, 1558–1564. [PubMed]
111. Wang, H.; Ji, Y.; Wu, G.; Sun, K.; Sun, Y.; Li, W.; Wang, B.; He, B.; Zhang, Q.; Dai, Z.; Wu, Z. L-Tryptophan activates mammalian target of rapamycin and enhances expression of tight junction proteins in intestinal porcine epithelial cells. *J. Nutr.* **2015**, *145*, 1156–1162. [CrossRef] [PubMed]
112. Messori, S.; Trevisi, P.; Simongiovanni, A.; Priori, D.; Bosi, P. Effect of susceptibility to enterotoxigenic *Escherichia coli* F4 and of dietary tryptophan on gut microbiota diversity observed in healthy young pigs. *Vet. Microbiol.* **2013**, *162*, 173–179. [CrossRef] [PubMed]
113. Etienne-Mesmin, L.; Chassaing, B.; Gewirtz, A.T. Tryptophan: A gut microbiota-derived metabolites regulating inflammation. *World J. Gastrointest. Pharmacol. Ther.* **2017**, *8*, 7–9. [CrossRef] [PubMed]
114. Ghia, J.E.; Li, N.; Wang, H.; Collins, M.; Deng, Y.; El-Sharkawy, R.T.; Côté, F.; Mallet, J.; Khan, W.I. Serotonin has a key role in pathogenesis of experimental colitis. *Gastroenterology* **2009**, *137*, 1649–1660. [CrossRef] [PubMed]
115. Nikolaus, S.; Al-Massad, N.; Bethge, J.; Waetzig, G.H.; Rosenstiel, P.C.; Junker, R.; Thieme, F.; Schreiber, S. Su1079 Tryptophan deficiency in Crohn disease. *Gastroenterology* **2014**, *146*, S366–S367. [CrossRef]
116. Schröcksnadel, K.; Wirleitner, B.; Winkler, C.; Fuchs, D. Monitoring tryptophan metabolism in chronic immune activation. *Clin. Chim. Acta* **2006**, *364*, 82–90. [CrossRef] [PubMed]
117. Petrat, F.; Boengler, K.; Schulz, R.; de Groot, H. Glycine, a simple physiological compound protecting by yet puzzling mechanism(s) against ischaemia-reperfusion injury: Current knowledge. *Br. J. Pharmacol.* **2012**, *165*, 2059–2072. [CrossRef] [PubMed]

118. Wang, W.; Wu, Z.; Lin, G.; Hu, S.; Wang, B.; Dai, Z.; Wu, G. Glycine stimulates protein synthesis and inhibits oxidative stress in pig small intestinal epithelial cells. *J. Nutr.* **2014**, *144*, 1540–1548. [CrossRef] [PubMed]
119. Effenberger-Neidnicht, K.; Jägers, J.; Verhaegh, R.; de Groot, H. Glycine selectively reduces intestinal injury during endotoxemia. *J. Surg. Res.* **2014**, *192*, 592–598. [CrossRef] [PubMed]
120. Meyer, K.F.; Martins, J.L.; de Freitas Filho, L.G.; Oliva, M.L.; Patrício, F.R.; Macedo, M.; Wang, L. Glycine reduces tissue lipid peroxidation in hypoxia-reoxygenation-induced necrotizing enterocolitis in rats. *Acta Cir. Bras.* **2006**, *21*, 161–167. [CrossRef] [PubMed]
121. Zhong, Z.; Wheeler, M.D.; Li, X.; Froh, M.; Schemmer, P.; Yin, M.; Bunzendaul, H.; Bradford, B.; Lemasters, J.J. L-Glycine: A novel antiinflammatory, immunomodulatory, and cytoprotective agent. *Curr. Opin. Clin. Nutr. Metab. Care* **2003**, *6*, 229–240. [CrossRef] [PubMed]
122. Wu, H.T. Regulative Effect of Glycine on Intestinal Injury and Muscle Protein Sythesis and Degradation of Piglets after Lipopolysaccharide Challenge. Master's Thesis, Wuhan Polytechnic University, Wuhan, China, 2015.
123. Liu, Y.; Wang, X.; Wu, H.; Chen, S.; Zhu, H.; Zhang, J.; Hou, Y.; Hu, C.A.; Zhang, G. Glycine enhances muscle protein mass associated with maintaining Akt-mTOR-FOXO1 signaling and suppressing TLR4 and NOD2 signaling in piglets challenged with LPS. *Am. J. Physiol. Regul. Integr. Comp. Physiol.* **2016**, *311*, R365–R373. [CrossRef] [PubMed]
124. Wade, A.M.; Tucker, H.N. Antioxidant characteristics of L-histidine. *J. Nutr. Biochem.* **1998**, *9*, 308–315. [CrossRef]
125. Jutel, M.; Akdis, M.; Akdis, C.A. Histamine, histamine receptors and their role in immune pathology. *Clin. Exp. Allergy* **2009**, *39*, 1786–1800. [CrossRef] [PubMed]
126. Son, D.O.; Satsu, H.; Shimizu, M. Histidine inhibits oxidative stress- and TNF-alpha-induced interleukin-8 secretion in intestinal epithelial cells. *FEBS Lett.* **2005**, *579*, 4671–4677. [CrossRef] [PubMed]
127. Hasegawa, S.; Ichiyama, T.; Sonaka, I.; Ohsaki, A.; Hirano, R.; Haneda, Y.; Fukano, R.; Hara, M.; Furukawa, S. Amino acids exhibit anti-inflammatory effects in human monocytic leukemia cell line, THP-1 cells. *Inflamm. Res.* **2011**, *60*, 1013–1019. [CrossRef] [PubMed]
128. Hisamatsu, T.; Ono, N.; Imaizumi, A.; Mori, M.; Suzuki, H.; Uo, M.; Hashimoto, M.; Naganuma, M.; Matsuoka, K.; Mizuno, S.; et al. Decreased plasma histidine level predicts risk of relapse in patients with ulcerative colitis in remission. *PLoS ONE* **2015**, *10*, e0140716. [CrossRef] [PubMed]
129. Li, P.; Yin, Y.L.; Li, D.; Kim, S.W.; Wu, G. Amino acids and immune function. *Br. J. Nutr.* **2007**, *98*, 237–252. [CrossRef] [PubMed]
130. Pi, D.; Liu, Y.; Shi, H.; Li, S.; Odle, J.; Lin, X.; Zhu, H.; Chen, F.; Hou, Y.; Leng, W. Dietary supplementation of aspartate enhances intestinal integrity and energy status in weanling piglets after lipopolysaccharide challenge. *J. Nutr. Biochem.* **2014**, *25*, 456–462. [CrossRef] [PubMed]
131. Wang, X.; Liu, Y.; Li, S.; Pi, D.; Zhu, H.; Hou, Y.; Shi, H.; Leng, W. Asparagine attenuates intestinal injury, improves energy status and inhibits AMP-activated protein kinase signalling pathways in weaned piglets challenged with *Escherichia coli* lipopolysaccharide. *Br. J. Nutr.* **2015**, *114*, 553–565. [CrossRef] [PubMed]
132. Wang, H.; Liu, Y.; Shi, H.; Wang, X.; Zhu, H.; Pi, D.; Leng, W.; Li, S. Aspartate attenuates intestinal injury and inhibits TLR4 and NODs/NF-κB and p38 signaling in weaned pigs after LPS challenge. *Eur. J. Nutr.* **2017**, *56*, 1433–1443. [CrossRef] [PubMed]
133. Chen, S.; Liu, Y.; Wang, X.; Wang, H.; Li, S.; Shi, H.; Zhu, H.; Zhang, J.; Pi, D.; Hu, C.A.; Lin, X.; Odle, J. Asparagine improves intestinal integrity, inhibits TLR4 and NOD signaling, and differently regulates p38 and ERK1/2 signaling in weanling piglets after LPS challenge. *Innate Immun.* **2016**, *22*, 577–587. [CrossRef] [PubMed]
134. Kang, P.; Zhang, L.; Hou, Y.; Ding, B.; Yi, D.; Wang, L.; Zhu, H.; Liu, Y.; Yin, Y.; Wu, G. Effects of L-proline on the growth performance, and blood parameters in weaned lipopolysaccharide (LPS)-challenged pigs. *Asian-Australas. J. Anim. Sci.* **2014**, *27*, 1150–1156. [CrossRef] [PubMed]
135. Coëffier, M.; Marion-Letellier, R.; Déchelotte, P. Potential for amino acids supplementation during inflammatory bowel diseases. *Inflamm. Bowel Dis.* **2010**, *16*, 518–524. [CrossRef] [PubMed]

3

Diet, Gut Microbiome and Epigenetics: Emerging Links with Inflammatory Bowel Diseases and Prospects for Management and Prevention

Krasimira Aleksandrova [1,*], Beatriz Romero-Mosquera [2] and Vicent Hernandez [2]

[1] Nutrition, Immunity and Metabolism Start-up Lab, Department of Epidemiology, German Institute of Human Nutrition Potsdam-Rehbrücke, Arthur-Scheunert Allee 114-116, 14558 Nuthetal, Germany

[2] Department of Gastroenterology, Instituto Investigación Sanitaria Galicia Sur, Estrutura Organizativa de Xestión Integrada de Vigo, 36312 Vigo, Spain; beatriz.romero.mosquera@sergas.es (B.R.-M.); vicenthernandez@yahoo.es (V.H.)

* Correspondence: krasimira.aleksandrova@dife.de

Abstract: Inflammatory bowel diseases (IBD) represent a growing public health concern due to increasing incidence worldwide. The current notion on the pathogenesis of IBD is that genetically susceptible individuals develop intolerance to dysregulated gut microflora (dysbiosis) and chronic inflammation develops as a result of environmental triggers. Among the environmental factors associated with IBD, diet plays an important role in modulating the gut microbiome, influencing epigenetic changes, and, therefore, could be applied as a therapeutic tool to improve the disease course. Nevertheless, the current dietary recommendations for disease prevention and management are scarce and have weak evidence. This review summarises the current knowledge on the complex interactions between diet, microbiome and epigenetics in IBD. Whereas an overabundance of calories and some macronutrients increase gut inflammation, several micronutrients have the potential to modulate it. Immunonutrition has emerged as a new concept putting forward the importance of vitamins such as vitamins A, C, E, and D, folic acid, beta carotene and trace elements such as zinc, selenium, manganese and iron. However, when assessed in clinical trials, specific micronutrients exerted a limited benefit. Beyond nutrients, an anti-inflammatory dietary pattern as a complex intervention approach has become popular in recent years. Hence, exclusive enteral nutrition in paediatric Crohn's disease is the only nutritional intervention currently recommended as a first-line therapy. Other nutritional interventions or specific diets including the Specific Carbohydrate Diet (SCD), the low fermentable oligosaccharides, disaccharides, monosaccharides, and polyol (FODMAP) diet and, most recently, the Mediterranean diet have shown strong anti-inflammatory properties and show promise for improving disease symptoms. More work is required to evaluate the role of individual food compounds and complex nutritional interventions with the potential to decrease inflammation as a means of prevention and management of IBD.

Keywords: diet; gut microbiota; epigenetics; inflammatory bowel diseases

---

1. Introduction

The inflammatory bowel diseases (IBD)—Crohn's disease (CD) and ulcerative colitis (UC)—are two diseases characterised by chronic relapsing inflammation of the gastrointestinal tract. They represent an increasing public health concern and an aetiological enigma due to unknown causal factors. Despite suggested differences in pathology, both diseases are believed to share a common aetiology. The strongest IBD risk factor identified to date is a family history of IBD [1]. The current notion on the pathogenesis of IBD is that genetically susceptible individuals develop intolerance to dysregulated gut microflora (dysbiosis) and chronic inflammation develops as a result of environmental triggers [2]. Current research in the field of IBD largely focusses on establishing the role of causal variants on gene expression and various pathological pathways have been already uncovered [3]. However, genetic risk loci identified to date only explain a small part of the genetic variance in disease risk and more factors need to be taken into account for understanding the multifactorial pathology of IBD [4]. Impaired immune response in genetically susceptible individuals as the result of a complex interaction between impaired intestinal barrier function and dysfunctional microbe–host interactions has therefore been suggested as a major unifying aetiological background [5]. While the identification of IBD environmental risk factors remains a subject of intensive research, diet remains one of the best candidates. Diet participates in the regulation of intestinal inflammation, either directly or indirectly by modifying the gut microbiota [6,7]. A greater understanding of the contribution of dietary factors to dysbiosis is therefore critical as a healthy microbiome is pivotal in preventing the development of IBD and its complications [8]. Most recently, the fast-evolving field of epigenetics has offered new explanations on the mechanisms by which environmental changes induce pathological gene expression and determine cell phenotype and function in IBD [9]. Collectively, the pathogenic mechanisms for IBD could be largely imposed by gene–environment interactions switching on a cascade of induced effects on the microbiota, the immune system, and the mucosal barrier (Figure 1).

Here, we review the recent developments in understanding the role of the gut microbiome, epigenetics, and dietary factors in IBD that outline directions for disease management and prevention.

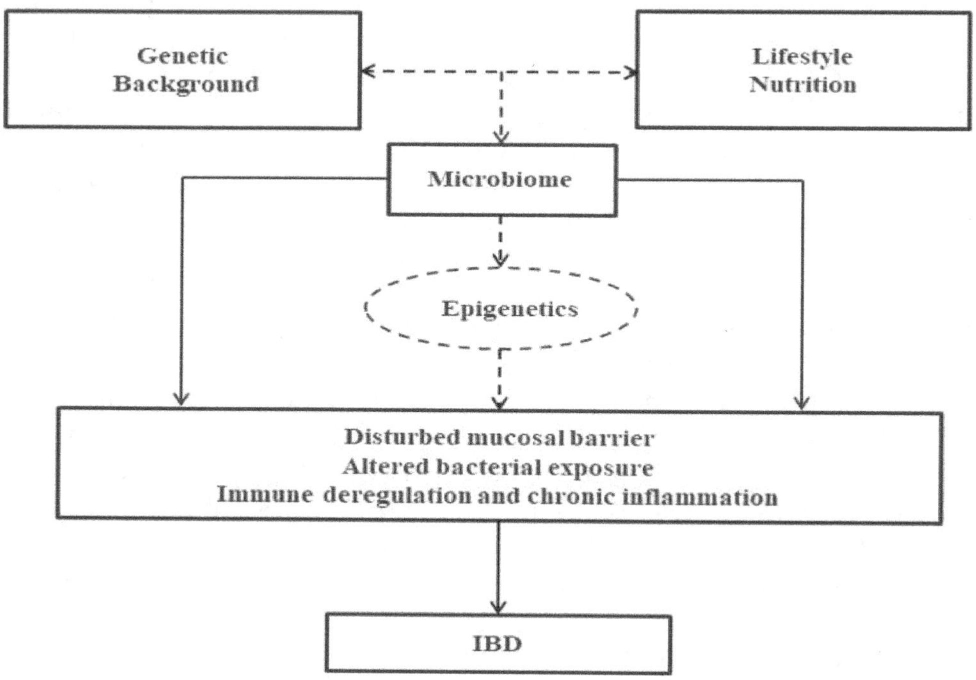

Figure 1. Proposed patho-physilogical mechanisms for inflammatory bowel disease (IBD). Complex interaction between genetic and lifestyle factors and the putative role of epigenetics on the interplay between microbiota, the immune system and the mucosal barrier.

2. Epidemiology of IBD and Environmental Exposures

IBDs occur worldwide with differences in epidemiology, exposures to risk factors and phenotypes between regions. The prevalence of IBD is higher in industrialised countries (e.g., Western Europe, United States of America, Canada, Australia and New Zealand) than in developing countries (in Asia, the Middle East, South America and Africa) [10]. The incidence of IBD steadily increased in industrialised countries during the 20th century and, although some studies indicated that a plateau was reached in some regions during the 21st century [10], recent reports suggest that it could be still increasing in these countries [11–13]. In developing countries, traditionally considered low-incidence areas, increasing incidence has been described since the beginning of the 21st century [8–10,14]. These observed increases in incidence rates could be partially accounted for by pragmatic reasons such as increased media coverage and health awareness in both developed and developing countries, improved access to medical technology and health care providers, and the development of sophisticated disease surveillance systems [15,16]. However, the parallel of higher incidence rates with the Westernisation of affected societies points to the potential important role of the environment [15,16]. In that regard, environmental factors (also known as "exposome") have been thoroughly studied and many of the factors related to Westernisation have been linked to the risk of IBD development. The list of putative factors so far includes environmental pollution, medication, psychological stress, infections and lifestyle. Certain differences in environmental risk for CD and UC have been reported. For example, cigarette smoking has been shown to increase the risk of developing CD, while smoking is less common in people at risk for UC [17]. Studies of migrant populations moving from regions of low to high IBD incidence point to early life as a key time for environmental triggers [18]. In these populations, the second generation, i.e., those born in high-incidence regions, have been shown to have higher incidence rates compared to their parents. Early life environmental exposures, such as breast feeding, have been also implicated in IBD risk [18]. However, an important obstacle to identifying the role of environmental factors in IBD is a lack of methodological standardisation among studies [19].

3. Intestinal Microbiome in the Pathogenesis of IBD

The gut microbiome interacts with the host in a symbiotic way and exerts a variety of beneficial effects including digestion of substrates and nutrient production; development, maturation and regulation of the immune system (both the local and the systemic response); and prevention of the growth of harmful microorganisms [20]. The human microbiota has been classified into clusters of well-balanced, defined microbial community compositions, known as "enterotypes" [21]. While the enterotypes are stable, environmental factors (i.e., diet) can influence microbiome composition without affecting the enterotype entity [22,23]. IBD is associated with alterations in the composition of the intestinal microbiota, characterised by decreased diversity, reduced proportions of Firmicutes, and increased proportions of Proteobacteria and Actinobacteria [6]. Some of the bacterial species with pro-inflammatory actions are enriched in patients with IBD (Escherichia, Fusobacterium), while anti-inflammatory species (Faecalibacterium, Roseburia) are largely reduced in IBD [6]. Patients with active IBD have different microbial composition as compared to patients in remission. For example, patients with active IBD have been shown to have lower abundance of *Clostridium coccoides*, *Clostridium leptum*, *Faecalibacterium prausnitzii* and Bifidobacterium [24]. Prospective studies investigating microbiome changes during disease course have been scarce. A Dutch study based on 10 CD and nine UC patients reported on patient-specific shifts in microbial composition, but could not demonstrate general changes in microbial composition or diversity [25]. A Spanish study followed up with 18 UC patients over the course of one year; in those who remained in remission *Faecalibacterium prausnitzii* increased steadily, while in those who relapsed it remained low [26].

Several factors could potentially influence the microbiome's composition. The intestinal colonisation begins immediately after birth, and beyond genetic predisposition is influenced very early in life by the route of delivering, the infant diet (breastfeeding or formula) and by hygiene. Apart from environmental factors such as drugs, stress and toxins (i.e., tobacco), diet was suggested to play a decisive role in modulating the microbiome composition [6,20,27]. Dietary composition was shown to affect the microbiota balance; therefore, it is conceivable that altering the diet can impact the inflammatory response [28]. For example, diets rich in saturated fats are shown to induce damage of the intestinal epithelial cell layer, leading to a loss of barrier function in animal studies [29,30]. In contrast, diets high in fibre predispose short-chain fatty acid production by the microbiota and lead to improved energy expenditure [31]. Thus, a balanced low-fat and high-fibre diet may be important in preventing dysbiosis and preserving the immune system [32]. Targeting microbiota through nutritional interventions could represent a promising therapeutic approach. So far, several nutritional interventions have been evaluated such as dietary supplementation with prebiotics and contrabiotics, phosphatidylcholine and the use of genetically modified bacteria [33]. Among these, therapies such as prebiotics and probiotics that selectively manipulate the intestinal microbiota have been evaluated as an attractive therapeutic option with few side effects [34]. Prebiotics represent non-digestible carbohydrates that promote the growth of beneficial bacteria in the gut. They may increase the production of short-chain fatty acids and the modulation of cytokine production within the gut mucosa [35]. Diets deficient or low in fibre were shown to exacerbate colitis development, while a very high intake of dietary fibre or short-chain fatty acids may protect against colitis [36]. Despite evidence from animal studies that suggested the beneficial actions of prebiotics in IBD [32,35], evidence from human studies is insufficient. A recent review summarised existing evidence from human randomised trials on the effect of prebiotics in UC [37]. Overall, 17 studies reported inconsistent findings for the effect of five prebiotic groups, including fructo-oligosaccharides, barley foodstuff, galacto-oligosaccharides, lactulose and resveratrol, in modulating ulcerative colitis.

Probiotics contain living bacteria that are suggested to exert positive health effects in the human intestine, modulating mucosal permeability and strengthening the immune system keeping away pathogens from intestinal mucosa surface. In particular, animal research has suggested that Lactobacillus and Bifidobacteria produce harmful substances for Gram-positive and Gram-negative bacteria and compete with pathogenic bacteria [32,38]. Further, human studies suggested that *Clostridium coccodies* and *C. leptum* exert protective effects against IBD [32]. The multispecies products VSL#3 and *E. coli* Nissle have been revealed as particularly effective in maintaining remission in UC [31]. Probiotic yogurt intake was associated with significant anti-inflammatory effects that paralleled the expansion of peripheral pool of putative T(reg) cells in IBD patients and had few effects in controls [39]. Recently, a meta-analysis based on 22 randomised control trials compared effects of administering probiotics with 5-aminosalicylates (5-ASAs) or placebo in relation to IBD [40]. Overall the meta-analysis suggested that probiotics, and VSL#3 in particular, may be as effective as 5-ASAs in preventing a relapse of quiescent UC. However, the overall efficacy of probiotics in IBD should be confirmed by further research. In addition, long-term benefits from probiotics may be limited without an overall modification of the person's diet. Thus, single pre-/probiotic administration may not prove useful outside of the context of switching to an overall healthy diet plan. Probiotics and other commercial interventions such as tea or berry extracts would be unlikely to counteract an unhealthy diet and, used alone, may, analogous to other medicinal products such as antioxidant supplements, fail to improve primary or secondary disease prevention [41]. More effort should be put into evaluating complex lifestyle and nutritional approaches for modulating the gut microbiome. Much work remains before the understanding of the effects of dysbiosis in humans reaches that of mice; however, while definitive statements may be lacking, the preponderance of current evidence strongly suggests that the gut microbiome is a major contributor to human health and disease [32].

4. Epigenetics and IBD

Research in recent years has contributed to an improved understanding of the role of epigenetic modifications—i.e., non-coding RNAs and DNA methylation—in defining the molecular basis of IBD [42,43]. Such research has been largely driven by observations that genetics alone cannot explain the onset of IBD. Thus, a meta-analysis of GWAS studies estimated that susceptibility loci for UC explained only 16% of UC heritability [44]. In this regard, gene–environment interactions have been suggested to play an important role in IBD pathogenesis and this is where epigenetics could offer new insights beyond genetic research [42,45]. Epigenetic factors were therefore suggested to mediate interactions between the environment and the genome, thereby providing new insights into the pathogenesis of IBD [46]. Earlier studies reported on the differential expression of specific microRNAs in the colonic mucosa samples of IBD patients compared to the mucosa of control patients [43]. miRNAs identified in peripheral blood were additionally suggested as new biomarkers of disease development [47]. Recent data have implicated miRNAs in immune response to bacteria invasion and the differential regulation of cytokines [48]. miRNA dysregulation, especially in Th17 cells, has been implicated in IBD. miRNAs have also been shown to regulate intestinal barrier integrity in UC. As previously reviewed, an increased expression of miR-21 is among the most consistently replicated novel therapeutic targets [47,48]. More recently, DNA methylation signatures for UC and CD have been also described. However, whether changes in DNA methylation systematically correlate with gene expression is not clear [49]. In addition, it remains challenging to identify aetiologically significant epigenetic alterations since epigenetic modification of DNA may differ between tissues, time of development within the same tissue, and environmental influences.

Initial evidence arising from epigenetic research is sometimes hard to prove in clinical practice. An example is the identified role of cytokines and subsequent development of biological drugs that fail to prove an important role in disease control. Thus, dysregulation of cytokine genes and increased mRNA levels of cytokines, including interleukin1-beta, interleukin-18 and tumour necrosis factor-alpha (TNFα), were reported in IBD patients compared with controls in the late 1990s [50–53]. This has led to introducing biologically based therapies (i.e., anti-TNFα) in IBD patients. However, achieving adequate response levels still remains elusive as stand-alone anti-TNFα therapies have not proven completely useful at predicting disease progression and drug response [54]. Recently, animal models suggested that the lack of response could be related to differences in the gut microbiome before and after disease initiation. Thus, alternative strategies are needed to account for the interplay between immunity, epigenetics and dietary factors.

Diet is known to influence epigenetic changes associated with disease and to modify gene expression patterns in a state of disturbed immunity [45]. Poor dietary choices are encoded into the human gut and genetic make-up, and could be transferred to the offspring [55]. A number of nutrients have been shown to modulate immune responses and may potentially counteract inflammatory processes [56]. Recent research suggested secondary plant metabolites, such as polyphenols, may modulate gene expression, chromatin remodelling and DNA methylation [57]. Polyphenols in green tea or soybean such as epigallocatechin-3-gallate or genistein have been demonstrated to inhibit DNA methyltransferases activity. Epigenetic effects have also been shown for other dietary components such as curcumin [58]. Nutrition provides substrates necessary for DNA methylation and can regulate the activity of the enzymes involved in the one-carbon cycle. Thus, precursors of S-adenosylmethionine, such as methionine, folate, choline, betaine and vitamins B2, B6 and B12, have been suggested to influence DNA methylation patterns [59].

Immune cells are rapidly dividing and have increased sensitivity to impaired DNA replication. Dietary factors act differently to modulate immune response, but all appear to have the potential to modulate inflammation [60]. Furthermore, active immunisation against the outer membrane protein of bacteria present in the gut was recently shown to enhance local and systemic immune control via apoE-mediated immune-modulation [61]. Immunonutrition was therefore suggested as a less invasive alternative to immunotherapy in protection against chronic inflammation predisposing IBD [60].

Gut microbiota may alter host histone acetylation and methylation in human colon tissues [62]. Fermentation end products, especially short-chain fatty acids such as acetate, butyrate and propionate, which are mostly produced by microbial fermentation of fibre, may be particularly important for the epigenetic regulation of inflammatory reactions [62]. A diet poor in fibre leads to a suppression in microbiota-driven short-chain fatty acid production and disturbed chromatin effects [62]. Of note is the finding previously mentioned, that butyrate-producing bacteria (Faecalibacterium) and SCFA-producing bacteria (Roseburia) are decreased in IBD [6]. However, the therapeutic value of butyrate-producing bacteria as pharmabiotics in humans has been questioned because of the difficulty of growing them in vitro [63]. The current state of research does not allow for definitive statements on which exact changes in the diet affect epigenetics via the microbiota. Nevertheless, accumulating lines of research reveal certain microbes that communicate with their hosts by sending out metabolites influencing gene transcription in the colon and potentially driving disease development.

5. Diet, Immunity and IBD

Western diet is characterised by overconsumption of refined sugars, salt, and saturated fat and low consumption of dietary fibre, as well as overall low food variability. New features of human nutrition in modern society include artificial sweeteners, gluten, and genetically modified foods. Western societies seem to have dealt with micro- and macronutrient deficiencies; however, overabundance of calories and macronutrients poses new challenges of increased inflammation, infection susceptibility, and increased risk for auto-inflammatory diseases such as IBD [64,65]. Several micronutrients are especially important for immunonutrition, among which vitamins such as vitamins A, C, D and E, folic acid, beta carotene and trace elements such as zinc, selenium, manganese and iron have garnered much research interest. Deficiencies in zinc and vitamins A and D may reduce the natural killer cell function, whereas supplemental zinc or vitamin C may enhance their activity [66,67]. Vitamin D has been shown to play a role in intestinal defence by suppressing the microbial invasion into the epithelium. Vitamin D deficiency has been identified in 82% of IBD patients, compared to the 31% national average, and has been linked to defective epithelial processes. Therapy targeting vitamin D3 signalling was suggested for treatment of inflammatory diseases, affecting both innate and adaptive immune functions. The overall impact of vitamins on IBD is still not well understood. So far, only two randomised clinical trials were conducted to evaluate the effect of vitamin D supplementation on IBD outcomes. In a Danish study, 94 patients were randomised to receive oral vitamin D3 or a placebo; patients receiving vitamin D3 had a non-significant reduced risk of relapse [68]. A more recent Iranian study conducted among 108 IBD patients reported that oral supplementation with vitamin D3 reduced serum TNF-alpha levels, though not substantially [69]. More studies with larger samples would be beneficial to assess effects of vitamin supplementation in IBD. Trace elements represent another important avenue for research in the prevention and control of inflammatory diseases. Zinc is involved in the control of DNA replication and transcription and controls signal transduction during T-cell activation [70]. Selenium deficiency decreases antibody production, while selenium supplementation enhances T-cell responses and increases antibody synthesis. It is also known to exert antioxidative effects and protect against the deteriorating effects of reactive oxygen species [71]. Iron deficiency leads to defective T-cell proliferative response and impaired cytokine production by lymphocytes. It should be noted that iron supports pathogen development and iron supplementation can also result in increased susceptibility to infections [72]. Of note, dietary iron has also been shown to enhance IBD and carcinogenesis by augmenting oxidative and nitrosative stress. In an experimental animal study, an iron-enriched diet significantly increased colorectal tumour incidence as compared with the control diet [73]. Despite the fact that micronutrient deficiency may theoretically influence the immune system and predispose one to the onset and development of IBD, more research is needed to understand optimal micronutrient levels and specific therapeutic implications [28]. Beyond micronutrients, specific food compounds such as green tea [74–76] or Echinacea [77–79] have also been suggested to reduce or enhance immune stimulation and play a role in IBD prevention.

6. Dietary Patterns in IBD Management and Prevention

Despite years of research, the role of diet in the prevention and control of IBD is not well understood [80–82]. Overall, no concerted effort has been made to provide nutritional guidelines for IBD patients and the existing guidelines largely follow the principle "If it hurts, don't do it". Dietary recommendations include patient advice to self-monitor and avoid foods that may worsen symptoms, eating smaller meals at more frequent intervals, drinking adequate fluids, avoiding caffeine and alcohol, taking vitamin/mineral supplementation, eliminating dairy if lactose intolerant, limiting excess fat, reducing carbohydrates and reducing high-fibre foods during flares. Mixed advice exists regarding pre-/probiotics. Recommendations are different across regions/countries. For example, enteral nutrition is recommended for Crohn's disease patients in Japan, which differs from practices in the USA [82]. A potential reason for the lack of solid dietary recommendations is the scarcity of studies evaluating the role of diet in IBD [83]. So far, only one study has assessed nutritional factors and their influence on disease outcome in newly diagnosed IBD patients [84]. In this inception cohort study, high intake of caffeine was associated with an increased risk of surgery, severe disease course and higher treatment step in CD patients; in UC patients, daily fast food intake was associated with an increased risk of surgery and high intake of caffeine was associated with a higher risk of extra-intestinal manifestations and lower treatment step.

In an attempt to fill this gap, in recent years more effort has gone into evaluating specific diets for the management of IBD, such as the Specific Carbohydrate Diet (SCD) and the low fermentable oligosaccharides, disaccharides, monosaccharides, and polyol (FODMAP) diet. Exclusive enteral nutrition is recommended as a first-line therapy to induce remission in children with active luminal CD [85]. In adults, long-term diet interventions such as total parenteral nutrition or the elemental diet [86] have also shown promise; however, their administration is more complicated and does not allow patients to lead a normal life. The SCD is a dietary regime that aims to induce and maintain drug-free remission in patients with IBD, initially developed by gastroenterologist Sidney Haas in 1951 and later popularised by biochemist Elaine Gottschall in the book *Breaking the Vicious Cycle: Intestinal Health Through Diet* [87]. The SCD diet is based on the hypothesis that patients with IBD and other intestinal diseases present a dysfunction of the disaccharidases, which are necessary to digest and absorb disaccharides and amylopectin; therefore, higher amounts of disaccharides would enter into the colon, which may lead to bacterial overgrowth and bowel injury with increased intestinal permeability. The diet allows carbohydrate foods consisting of monosaccharides only (fruit and honey) and excludes disaccharides and most polysaccharides; therefore it includes vegetables with a high amylose-to-amylopectin ratio, fruits, nuts, solid proteins and fats [87]. So far, several case-series studies have suggested an important potential of the SCD diet in the control and remission maintenance in IBD [65,88–90]. The low FODMAP diet gained much attention in research as means for IBD treatment. A recent meta-analysis including two randomised control trials and four before–after studies with a total of 319 patients (96% in remission) reported overall improvement in gastrointestinal symptoms such as diarrhoea response abdominal bloating fatigue and nausea [91]. Recently, plant-based dietary patterns were suggested as valid means of long-term inflammation control [92]. In particular, the Mediterranean diet was suggested to exert strong immunomodulatory effects and even showing a potential to modulate epigenetic mechanisms. Recent data from the Predimed study, a randomised, controlled, parallel trial in high cardiovascular risk volunteers, revealed that over five years of intervention the Mediterranean diet was associated with the methylation of genes related to inflammation and exerted high regulatory effects [93]. Further intervention trials utilising transcriptomics analyses revealed the potential of Mediterranean to modulate gene expression and to normalise microbiota in IBD patients [94]. Similarly, semi-vegetarian diet (SVD) was shown to exert preventive effects against IBD relapse in patients who have achieved remission in a prospective, single-centre, two-year clinical trial [95]. In summary, the current evidence on specific diets in the IBD course remains to be confirmed and updated by further well-designed and long-term follow-up studies, in which the complex interactions between nutrients and microbiota should be taken into account.

7. Ongoing Research

Several research projects have been recently launched or are being launched that aim to assess diet and the microbiome as related to IBD. These include the Food and Resulting Microbial Metabolites (FARMM) study by the Crohn's and Colitis Foundation of America (CCFA) [96], the Study on the Genetic, Environmental and Microbial Interactions that Cause IBD (GEM Project) by the Crohn's and Colitis Canada [97], the Prognostic effect of Environmental factors in Crohn's and Colitis (PREdiCCt) study [98] and the Diet, microbiome and inflammatory bowel disease course (microIBDiet) study. The FARMM study, part of the CCFA's Microbiome Initiative, is a controlled feeding experiment among healthy volunteers, with the objective of examining how different diets (the "Western" diet, exclusive enteral nutrition and a vegan diet for two weeks) influence the gut microbiota and faecal metabolomics. The GEM Project is recruiting healthy first-degree relatives of CD patients, and will assess genetic and environmental factors and the gut microbiome; participants will be followed up to assess the risk of developing CD and the factors associated with the disease. The PREdiCCT study will recruit IBD patients in remission, and will assess diet, lifestyle, genetics and microbiome; participants will be followed up for two years to study the factors associated with relapse. The microIBDiet study will recruit newly diagnosed IBD patients, and will assess diet and the microbiome; patients will be followed up for five years to study the factors associated with an impaired outcome (personal communication from the principal investigator). These projects promise to shed more light on the role of dietary and nutritional factors in IBD as a basis for further dietary intervention trials.

8. Conclusions

In summary, rapid technological bioscience development has opened up new horizons for an improved understanding of the role of gene–environment interactions in the onset and development of IBD. Targeted nutrition taking into account individual genetic make-up, epigenetics and microbiota composition may represent a novel platform for successful prevention and disease control. More work is required to evaluate the role of individual food compounds and complex nutritional interventions with potential to decrease inflammation, modulate immune-modulatory epigenetic traits and maintain intestinal microbial balance as a means of prevention and management of IBD.

Acknowledgments: Krasimira Aleksandrova was supported by the German Research Foundation (DFG) Grant AL 1784/3-1. Vicent Hernandez received the GETECCU's "V Antonio Obrador" Grant, devoted to epidemiological studies in IBD.

Author Contributions: All the authors participated in the literature research. K.A. and V.H. wrote the manuscript. All the authors approved the final version of the manuscript.

References

1. Russell, R.K.; Satsangi, J. IBD: A family affair. *Best Pract. Res. Clin. Gastroenterol.* **2004**, *18*, 525–539. [CrossRef] [PubMed]
2. Zanello, G.; Kevans, D.; Goethel, A.; Silverberg, M.; Tyler, A.; Croitoru, K. Genetics and innate and adaptive immunity in IBD. *Nestle Nutr. Inst. Workshop Ser.* **2014**, *79*, 41–55. [PubMed]
3. Van Limbergen, J.; Radford-Smith, G.; Satsangi, J. Advances in IBD genetics. *Nat. Rev. Gastroenterol. Hepatol.* **2014**, *11*, 372–385. [CrossRef] [PubMed]
4. Tamboli, C.P. How do genetics help an understanding of IBD epidemiology? *Inflamm. Bowel Dis.* **2008**, *14*, S29–S30. [CrossRef] [PubMed]
5. Danese, S.; Fiocchi, C. Etiopathogenesis of inflammatory bowel diseases. *World J. Gastroenterol.* **2006**, *12*, 4807–4812. [PubMed]
6. Kostic, A.D.; Xavier, R.J.; Gevers, D. The microbiome in inflammatory bowel disease: Current status and the future ahead. *Gastroenterology* **2014**, *146*, 1489–1499. [CrossRef] [PubMed]
7. Lee, D.; Albenberg, L.; Compher, C.; Baldassano, R.; Piccoli, D.; Lewis, J.D.; Wu, G.D. Diet in the pathogenesis and treatment of inflammatory bowel diseases. *Gastroenterology* **2015**, *148*, 1087–1106. [CrossRef] [PubMed]
8. Lovasz, B.D.; Golovics, P.A.; Vegh, Z.; Lakatos, P.L. New trends in inflammatory bowel disease epidemiology and disease course in eastern europe. *Dig. Liver Dis.* **2013**, *45*, 269–276. [CrossRef] [PubMed]
9. Malekzadeh, M.M.; Vahedi, H.; Gohari, K.; Mehdipour, P.; Sepanlou, S.G.; Daryani, N.E.; Zali, M.R.; Mansour-Ghanaei, F.; Safarpour, A.R.; Aghazadeh, R.; et al. Emerging epidemic of inflammatory bowel disease in a middle income country: A nation-wide study from Iran. *Arch. Iran. Med.* **2016**, *19*, 2–15. [PubMed]
10. Molodecky, N.A.; Soon, I.S.; Rabi, D.M.; Ghali, W.A.; Ferris, M.; Chernoff, G.; Benchimol, E.I.; Panaccione, R.; Ghosh, S.; Barkema, H.W.; et al. Increasing incidence and prevalence of the inflammatory bowel diseases with time, based on systematic review. *Gastroenterology* **2012**, *142*, 46–54. [CrossRef] [PubMed]
11. Fernández, A.; Hernández, V.; Martínez-Ares, D.; Sanromán, L.; de Castro, M.L.; Pineda, J.R.; Carmona, A.; González-Portela, C.; Salgado, C.; Martínez-Cadilla, J.; et al. Incidence and phenotype at diagnosis of inflammatory bowel disease. Results in Spain of the EpiCom study. *Gastroenterol. Hepatol.* **2015**, *38*, 534–540. [CrossRef] [PubMed]

12. Lophaven, S.N.; Lynge, E.; Burisch, J. The incidence of inflammatory bowel disease in Denmark 1980–2013: A nationwide cohort study. *Aliment. Pharmacol. Ther.* **2017**, *45*, 961–972. [CrossRef] [PubMed]
13. Shivashankar, R.; Tremaine, W.J.; Harmsen, W.S.; Loftus, E.V. Incidence and prevalence of Crohn's disease and ulcerative colitis in Olmsted county, Minnesota from 1970 through 2010. *Clin. Gastroenterol. Hepatol.* **2017**, *15*, 857–863. [CrossRef] [PubMed]
14. Ng, S.C.; Tang, W.; Ching, J.Y.; Wong, M.; Chow, C.M.; Hui, A.J.; Wong, T.C.; Leung, V.K.; Tsang, S.W.; Yu, H.H.; et al. Incidence and phenotype of inflammatory bowel disease based on results from the Asia-Pacific Crohn's and Colitis Epidemiology Study. *Gastroenterology* **2013**, *145*, 158–165. [CrossRef] [PubMed]
15. Kaplan, G.G. The global burden of IBD: From 2015 to 2025. *Nat. Rev. Gastroenterol. Hepatol.* **2015**, *12*, 720–727. [CrossRef] [PubMed]
16. Saro Gismera, C. ¿Por qué está aumentando la incidencia de la EIIC? *Enferm. Inflam. Intest. Al Día* **2010**, *9*, 139–149.
17. Rogler, G.; Vavricka, S. Exposome in IBD: Recent insights in environmental factors that influence the onset and course of IBD. *Inflamm. Bowel Dis.* **2015**, *21*, 400–408. [CrossRef] [PubMed]
18. Gearry, R.B. IBD and environment: Are there differences between east and west. *Digest. Dis.* **2016**, *34*, 84–89. [CrossRef] [PubMed]
19. Molodecky, N.A.; Panaccione, R.; Ghosh, S.; Barkema, H.W.; Kaplan, G.G.; Alberta Inflammatory Bowel Disease Consortium. Challenges associated with identifying the environmental determinants of the inflammatory bowel diseases. *Inflamm. Bowel Dis.* **2011**, *17*, 1792–1799. [CrossRef] [PubMed]
20. O'hara, A.M.; Shanahan, F. The gut flora as a forgotten organ. *EMBO Rep.* **2006**, *7*, 688–693. [CrossRef] [PubMed]
21. Arumugam, M.; Raes, J.; Pelletier, E.; Le Paslier, D.; Yamada, T.; Mende, D.R.; Fernandes, G.R.; Tap, J.; Bruls, T.; Batto, J.-M.; et al. Enterotypes of the human gut microbiome. *Nature* **2011**, *473*, 174–180. [CrossRef] [PubMed]
22. Roager, H.M.; Licht, T.R.; Poulsen, S.K.; Larsen, T.M.; Bahl, M.I. Microbial enterotypes, inferred by the prevotella-to-bacteroides ratio, remained stable during a 6-month randomized controlled diet intervention with the new nordic diet. *Appl. Environ. Microbiol.* **2014**, *80*, 1142–1149. [CrossRef] [PubMed]
23. Wu, G.D.; Chen, J.; Hoffmann, C.; Bittinger, K.; Chen, Y.-Y.; Keilbaugh, S.A.; Bewtra, M.; Knights, D.; Walters, W.A.; Knight, R.; et al. Linking long-term dietary patterns with gut microbial enterotypes. *Science* **2011**, *334*, 105–108. [CrossRef] [PubMed]
24. Prosberg, M.; Bendtsen, F.; Vind, I.; Petersen, A.M.; Gluud, L.L. The association between the gut microbiota and the inflammatory bowel disease activity: A systematic review and meta-analysis. *Scand. J. Gastroenterol.* **2016**, *51*, 1407–1415. [CrossRef] [PubMed]
25. Wills, E.S.; Jonkers, D.M.A.E.; Savelkoul, P.H.; Masclee, A.A.; Pierik, M.J.; Penders, J. Fecal microbial composition of ulcerative colitis and Crohn's disease patients in remission and subsequent exacerbation. *PLoS ONE* **2014**, *9*, e90981. [CrossRef] [PubMed]
26. Varela, E.; Manichanh, C.; Gallart, M.; Torrejón, A.; Borruel, N.; Casellas, F.; Guarner, F.; Antolin, M. Colonisation by *Faecalibacterium prausnitzii* and maintenance of clinical remission in patients with ulcerative colitis. *Aliment. Pharmacol. Ther.* **2013**, *38*, 151–161. [CrossRef] [PubMed]
27. Dominguez-Bello, M.G.; Costello, E.K.; Contreras, M.; Magris, M.; Hidalgo, G.; Fierer, N.; Knight, R. Delivery mode shapes the acquisition and structure of the initial microbiota across multiple body habitats in newborns. *Proc. Natl. Acad. Sci. USA* **2010**, *107*, 11971–11975. [CrossRef] [PubMed]
28. Malavia, D.; Crawford, A.; Wilson, D. Nutritional immunity and fungal pathogenesis: The struggle for micronutrients at the host-pathogen interface. *Adv. Microb. Phys.* **2017**, *70*, 85–103.
29. Benoit, B.; Bruno, J.; Kayal, F.; Estienne, M.; Debard, C.; Ducroc, R.; Plaisancie, P. Saturated and unsaturated fatty acids differently modulate colonic goblet cells in vitro and in rat pups. *J. Nutr.* **2015**, *145*, 1754–1762. [CrossRef] [PubMed]
30. Devkota, S.; Wang, Y.; Musch, M.W.; Leone, V.; Fehlner-Peach, H.; Nadimpalli, A.; Antonopoulos, D.A.; Jabri, B.; Chang, E.B. Dietary-fat-induced taurocholic acid promotes pathobiont expansion and colitis in IL10$^{-/-}$ mice. *Nature* **2012**, *487*, 104–108. [CrossRef] [PubMed]
31. Brandsma, E.; Houben, T.; Fu, J.; Shiri-Sverdlov, R.; Hofker, M.H. The immunity-diet-microbiota axis in the development of metabolic syndrome. *Curr. Opin. Lipidol.* **2015**, *26*, 73–81. [CrossRef] [PubMed]

32. Brown, K.; DeCoffe, D.; Molcan, E.; Gibson, D.L. Diet-induced dysbiosis of the intestinal microbiota and the effects on immunity and disease. *Nutrients* **2012**, *4*, 1095–1119. [CrossRef] [PubMed]
33. Simpson, H.L.; Campbell, B.J.; Rhodes, J.M. IBD: Microbiota manipulation through diet and modified bacteria. *Digest. Dis.* **2014**, *32*, 18–25. [CrossRef] [PubMed]
34. Sinagra, E.; Tomasello, G.; Cappello, F.; Leone, A.; Cottone, M.; Bellavia, M.; Rossi, F.; Facella, T.; Damiani, P.; Zeenny, M.N.; et al. Probiotics, prebiotics and symbiotics in inflammatory bowel diseases: State-of-the-art and new insights. *J. Biol. Regul. Homeost. Agents* **2013**, *27*, 919–933. [PubMed]
35. Scaldaferri, F.; Gerardi, V.; Lopetuso, L.R.; Del Zompo, F.; Mangiola, F.; Boskoski, I.; Bruno, G.; Petito, V.; Laterza, L.; Cammarota, G.; et al. Gut microbial flora, prebiotics, and probiotics in IBD: Their current usage and utility. *BioMed Res. Int.* **2013**, *2013*, 435268. [CrossRef] [PubMed]
36. Macia, L.; Tan, J.; Vieira, A.T.; Leach, K.; Stanley, D.; Luong, S.; Maruya, M.; Ian McKenzie, C.; Hijikata, A.; Wong, C.; et al. Metabolite-sensing receptors GPR43 and GPR109A facilitate dietary fibre-induced gut homeostasis through regulation of the inflammasome. *Nat. Commun.* **2015**, *6*, 6734. [CrossRef] [PubMed]
37. Laurell, A.; Sjoberg, K. Prebiotics and synbiotics in ulcerative colitis. *Scand. J. Gastroenterol.* **2017**, *52*, 477–485. [CrossRef] [PubMed]
38. Hidalgo-Cantabrana, C.; Delgado, S.; Ruiz, L.; Ruas-Madiedo, P.; Sanchez, B.; Margolles, A. Bifidobacteria and their health-promoting effects. *Microbiol. Spectr.* **2017**, *5*. [CrossRef] [PubMed]
39. Lorea Baroja, M.; Kirjavainen, P.V.; Hekmat, S.; Reid, G. Anti-inflammatory effects of probiotic yogurt in inflammatory bowel disease patients. *Clin. Exp. Immunol.* **2007**, *149*, 470–479. [CrossRef] [PubMed]
40. Derwa, Y.; Gracie, D.J.; Hamlin, P.J.; Ford, A.C. Systematic review with meta-analysis: The efficacy of probiotics in inflammatory bowel disease. *Aliment. Pharmacol. Ther.* **2017**, *46*, 389–400. [CrossRef] [PubMed]
41. Bjelakovic, G.; Nikolova, D.; Gluud, L.L.; Simonetti, R.G.; Gluud, C. Mortality in randomized trials of antioxidant supplements for primary and secondary prevention: Systematic review and meta-analysis. *JAMA* **2007**, *297*, 842–857. [CrossRef] [PubMed]
42. Scarpa, M.; Stylianou, E. Epigenetics: Concepts and relevance to IBD pathogenesis. *Inflamm. Bowel Dis.* **2012**, *18*, 1982–1996. [CrossRef] [PubMed]
43. Ventham, N.T.; Kennedy, N.A.; Nimmo, E.R.; Satsangi, J. Beyond gene discovery in inflammatory bowel disease: The emerging role of epigenetics. *Gastroenterology* **2013**, *145*, 293–308. [CrossRef] [PubMed]
44. Anderson, C.A.; Boucher, G.; Lees, C.W.; Franke, A.; D'Amato, M.; Taylor, K.D.; Lee, J.C.; Goyette, P.; Imielinski, M.; Latiano, A.; et al. Meta-analysis identifies 29 additional ulcerative colitis risk loci, increasing the number of confirmed associations to 47. *Nat. Genet.* **2011**, *43*, 246–252. [CrossRef] [PubMed]
45. Beaudet, A.L. Epigenetics and complex human disease: Is there a role in IBD? *J. Pediatr. Gastroenterol. Nutr.* **2008**, *46*, E2. [PubMed]
46. Dabritz, J.; Menheniott, T.R. Linking immunity, epigenetics, and cancer in inflammatory bowel disease. *Inflamm. Bowel Dis.* **2014**, *20*, 1638–1654. [CrossRef] [PubMed]
47. Chapman, C.G.; Pekow, J. The emerging role of mirnas in inflammatory bowel disease: A review. *Ther. Adv. Gastroenterol.* **2015**, *8*, 4–22. [CrossRef] [PubMed]
48. Kalla, R.; Ventham, N.T.; Kennedy, N.A.; Quintana, J.F.; Nimmo, E.R.; Buck, A.H.; Satsangi, J. MicroRNAs: New players in IBD. *Gut* **2015**, *64*, 504–517. [CrossRef] [PubMed]
49. Harris, R.A.; Nagy-Szakal, D.; Pedersen, N.; Opekun, A.; Bronsky, J.; Munkholm, P.; Jespersgaard, C.; Andersen, P.; Melegh, B.; Ferry, G.; et al. Genome-wide peripheral blood leukocyte DNA methylation microarrays identified a single association with inflammatory bowel diseases. *Inflamm. Bowel Dis.* **2012**, *18*, 2334–2341. [CrossRef] [PubMed]
50. Bouma, G.; Xia, B.; Crusius, J.B.; Bioque, G.; Koutroubakis, I.; Von Blomberg, B.M.; Meuwissen, S.G.; Pena, A.S. Distribution of four polymorphisms in the tumour necrosis factor (TNF) genes in patients with inflammatory bowel disease (IBD). *Clin. Exp. Immunol.* **1996**, *103*, 391–396. [CrossRef] [PubMed]
51. Dionne, S.; Hiscott, J.; D'Agata, I.; Duhaime, A.; Seidman, E.G. Quantitative PCR analysis of TNF-alpha and IL-1 beta mRNA levels in pediatric IBD mucosal biopsies. *Digest. Dis. Sci.* **1997**, *42*, 1557–1566. [CrossRef] [PubMed]
52. Greenberg, G.R. Bugs, TNF-alpha and IBD: More fuel for the fire. *Can. J. Gastroenterol.* **2002**, *16*, 127–128. [CrossRef] [PubMed]
53. Ludwiczek, O.; Kaser, A.; Novick, D.; Dinarello, C.A.; Rubinstein, M.; Tilg, H. Elevated systemic levels of free interleukin-18 (IL-18) in patients with Crohn's disease. *Eur. Cytokine Netw.* **2005** *16*, 27–33. [PubMed]

54. Tighe, D.; Hall, B.; Jeyarajah, S.K.; Smith, S.; Breslin, N.; Ryan, B.; McNamara, D. One-year clinical outcomes in an IBD cohort who have previously had anti-TNFα trough and antibody levels assessed. *Inflamm. Bowel Dis.* **2017**, *23*, 1154–1159. [CrossRef] [PubMed]
55. Mochizuki, K.; Hariya, N.; Honma, K.; Goda, T. Relationship between epigenetic regulation, dietary habits, and the developmental origins of health and disease theory. *Congenit. Anom.* **2017**. [CrossRef] [PubMed]
56. Burdge, G.C.; Hoile, S.P.; Lillycrop, K.A. Epigenetics: Are there implications for personalised nutrition? *Curr. Opin. Clin. Nutr. Metab. Care* **2012**, *15*, 442–447. [CrossRef] [PubMed]
57. Remely, M.; Lovrecic, L.; de la Garza, A.L.; Migliore, L.; Peterlin, B.; Milagro, F.I.; Martinez, A.J.; Haslberger, A.G. Therapeutic perspectives of epigenetically active nutrients. *Br. J. Pharm.* **2015**, *172*, 2756–2768. [CrossRef] [PubMed]
58. Reuter, S.; Gupta, S.C.; Park, B.; Goel, A.; Aggarwal, B.B. Epigenetic changes induced by curcumin and other natural compounds. *Genes Nutr.* **2011**, *6*, 93–108. [CrossRef] [PubMed]
59. Anderson, O.S.; Sant, K.E.; Dolinoy, D.C. Nutrition and epigenetics: An interplay of dietary methyl donors, one-carbon metabolism and DNA methylation. *J. Nutr. Biochem.* **2012**, *23*, 853–859. [CrossRef] [PubMed]
60. Philpott, M.; Ferguson, L.R. Immunonutrition and cancer. *Mutat. Res.* **2004**, *551*, 29–42. [CrossRef] [PubMed]
61. Saita, D.; Ferrarese, R.; Foglieni, C.; Esposito, A.; Canu, T.; Perani, L.; Ceresola, E.R.; Visconti, L.; Burioni, R.; Clementi, M.; et al. Adaptive immunity against gut microbiota enhances apoE-mediated immune regulation and reduces atherosclerosis and western-diet-related inflammation. *Sci. Rep.* **2016**, *6*, 29353. [CrossRef] [PubMed]
62. Krautkramer, K.A.; Kreznar, J.H.; Romano, K.A.; Vivas, E.I.; Barrett-Wilt, G.A.; Rabaglia, M.E.; Keller, M.P.; Attie, A.D.; Rey, F.E.; Denu, J.M. Diet-microbiota interactions mediate global epigenetic programming in multiple host tissues. *Mol. Cell* **2016**, *64*, 982–992. [CrossRef] [PubMed]
63. Eeckhaut, V.; Ducatelle, R.; Sas, B.; Vermeire, S.; Van Immerseel, F. Progress towards butyrate-producing pharmabiotics: Butyricicoccus pullicaecorum capsule and efficacy in TNBS models in comparison with therapeutics. *Gut* **2014**, *63*, 367. [CrossRef] [PubMed]
64. Myles, I.A. Fast food fever: Reviewing the impacts of the western diet on immunity. *Nutr. J.* **2014**, *13*, 61. [CrossRef] [PubMed]
65. Andersen, V.; Hansen, A.K.; Heitmann, B.L. Potential impact of diet on treatment effect from anti-TNF drugs in inflammatory bowel disease. *Nutrients* **2017**, *9*, 286. [CrossRef] [PubMed]
66. Erickson, K.L.; Medina, E.A.; Hubbard, N.E. Micronutrients and innate immunity. *J. Infect. Dis.* **2000**, *182*, S5–S10. [CrossRef] [PubMed]
67. Shaik-Dasthagirisaheb, Y.B.; Varvara, G.; Murmura, G.; Saggini, A.; Caraffa, A.; Antinolfi, P.; Tete, S.; Tripodi, D.; Conti, F.; Cianchetti, E.; et al. Role of vitamins D, E and C in immunity and inflammation. *J. Biol. Regul. Homeost. Agents* **2013**, *27*, 291–295. [PubMed]
68. Jorgensen, S.P.; Agnholt, J.; Glerup, H.; Lyhne, S.; Villadsen, G.E.; Hvas, C.L.; Bartels, L.E.; Kelsen, J.; Christensen, L.A.; Dahlerup, J.F. Clinical trial: Vitamin D3 treatment in Crohn's disease—A randomized double-blind placebo-controlled study. *Aliment. Pharmacol. Ther.* **2010**, *32*, 377–383. [CrossRef] [PubMed]
69. Dadaei, T.; Safapoor, M.H.; Asadzadeh Aghdaei, H.; Balaii, H.; Pourhoseingholi, M.A.; Naderi, N.; Zojaji, H.; Azimzadeh, P.; Mohammadi, P.; Zali, M.R. Effect of vitamin D3 supplementation on TNF-alpha serum level and disease activity index in iranian IBD patients. *Gastroenterol. Hepatol. Bed Bench* **2015**, *8*, 49–55. [PubMed]
70. Crawford, A.; Wilson, D. Essential metals at the host-pathogen interface: Nutritional immunity and micronutrient assimilation by human fungal pathogens. *FEMS Yeast Res.* **2015**, *15*, fov071. [CrossRef] [PubMed]
71. Huang, Z.; Rose, A.H.; Hoffmann, P.R. The role of selenium in inflammation and immunity: From molecular mechanisms to therapeutic opportunities. *Antioxid. Redox Signal.* **2012**, *16*, 705–743. [CrossRef] [PubMed]
72. Seril, D.N.; Liao, J.; West, A.B.; Yang, G.Y. High-iron diet: Foe or feat in ulcerative colitis and ulcerative colitis-associated carcinogenesis. *J. Clin. Gastroenterol.* **2006**, *40*, 391–397. [CrossRef] [PubMed]
73. Seril, D.N.; Liao, J.; Ho, K.L.; Warsi, A.; Yang, C.S.; Yang, G.Y. Dietary iron supplementation enhances dss-induced colitis and associated colorectal carcinoma development in mice. *Digest. Dis. Sci.* **2002**, *47*, 1266–1278. [CrossRef] [PubMed]
74. Bayer, J.; Gomer, A.; Demir, Y.; Amano, H.; Kish, D.D.; Fairchild, R.; Heeger, P.S. Effects of green tea polyphenols on murine transplant-reactive t cell immunity. *Clin. Immunol.* **2004**, *110*, 100–108. [CrossRef] [PubMed]

75. Kuo, C.L.; Chen, T.S.; Liou, S.Y.; Hsieh, C.C. Immunomodulatory effects of EGCG fraction of green tea extract in innate and adaptive immunity via T regulatory cells in murine model. *Immunopharmacol. Immunotoxicol.* **2014**, *36*, 364–370. [CrossRef] [PubMed]
76. Santilli, G.; Anderson, J.; Thrasher, A.J.; Sala, A. Catechins and antitumor immunity: Not MDSC's cup of tea. *Oncoimmunology* **2013**, *2*, e24443. [CrossRef] [PubMed]
77. Balan, B.J.; Sokolnicka, I.; Skopinska-Rozewska, E.; Skopinski, P. The modulatory influence of some Echinacea-based remedies on antibody production and cellular immunity in mice. *Cent.-Eur. J. Immunol.* **2016**, *41*, 12–18. [CrossRef] [PubMed]
78. Barbour, E.K.; Assi, C.A.; Shaib, H.; Hamadeh, S.; Murtada, M.; Mahmoud, G.; Yaghmoor, S.; Iyer, A.; Harakeh, S.; Kumosani, T. Evaluation of a Salmonella enteritidis vaccine and related ELISA for respective induction and assessment of acquired immunity to the vaccine and/or Echinacea purpurea in Awassi Ewes. *Vaccine* **2015**, *33*, 2228–2231. [CrossRef] [PubMed]
79. Hall, H.; Fahlman, M.M.; Engels, H.J. Echinacea purpurea and mucosal immunity. *Int. J. Sports Med.* **2007**, *28*, 792–797. [CrossRef] [PubMed]
80. Yamamoto, T.; Nakahigashi, M.; Saniabadi, A.R. Review article: Diet and inflammatory bowel disease—Epidemiology and treatment. *Aliment. Pharmacol. Ther.* **2009**, *30*, 99–112. [CrossRef] [PubMed]
81. Richman, E.; Rhodes, J.M. Review article: Evidence-based dietary advice for patients with inflammatory bowel disease. *Aliment. Pharmacol. Ther.* **2013**, *38*, 1156–1171. [CrossRef] [PubMed]
82. Brown, A.C.; Rampertab, S.D.; Mullin, G.E. Existing dietary guidelines for Crohn's disease and ulcerative colitis. *Expert Rev. Gastroenterol. Hepatol.* **2011**, *5*, 411–425. [CrossRef] [PubMed]
83. Spooren, C.E.; Pierik, M.J.; Zeegers, M.P.; Feskens, E.J.; Masclee, A.A.; Jonkers, D.M. Review article: The association of diet with onset and relapse in patients with inflammatory bowel disease. *Aliment. Pharmacol. Ther.* **2013**, *38*, 1172–1187. [CrossRef] [PubMed]
84. Burisch, J.; Pedersen, N.; Cukovic-Cavka, S.; Turk, N.; Kaimakliotis, I.; Duricova, D.; Bortlik, M.; Shonova, O.; Vind, I.; Avnstrom, S.; et al. Environmental factors in a population-based inception cohort of inflammatory bowel disease patients in Europe—An ECCO-EpiCom study. *J. Crohn's Colitis* **2014**, *8*, 607–616. [CrossRef] [PubMed]
85. Ruemmele, F.M.; Veres, G.; Kolho, K.L.; Griffiths, A.; Levine, A.; Escher, J.C.; Amil Dias, J.; Barabino, A.; Braegger, C.P.; Bronsky, J.; et al. Consensus guidelines of ECCO/ESPGHANn on the medical management of pediatric Crohn's disease. *J. Crohn's Colitis* **2014**, *8*, 1179–1207. [CrossRef] [PubMed]
86. Jones, V.A. Comparison of total parenteral nutrition and elemental diet in induction of remission of Crohn's disease. Long-term maintenance of remission by personalized food exclusion diets. *Digest. Dis. Sci.* **1987**, *32*, 100S–107S. [CrossRef] [PubMed]
87. Nieves, R.; Jackson, R.T. Specific carbohydrate diet in treatment of inflammatory bowel disease. *Tenn. Med.* **2004**, *97*, 407. [PubMed]
88. Olendzki, B.C.; Silverstein, T.D.; Persuitte, G.M.; Ma, Y.; Baldwin, K.R.; Cave, D. An anti-inflammatory diet as treatment for inflammatory bowel disease: A case series report. *Nutr. J.* **2014**, *13*, 5. [CrossRef] [PubMed]
89. Suskind, D.L.; Wahbeh, G.; Gregory, N.; Vendettuoli, H.; Christie, D. Nutritional therapy in pediatric Crohn disease: The specific carbohydrate diet. *J. Pediatr. Gastroenterol. Nutr.* **2014**, *58*, 87–91. [CrossRef] [PubMed]
90. Kakodkar, S.; Farooqui, A.J.; Mikolaitis, S.L.; Mutlu, E.A. The specific carbohydrate diet for inflammatory bowel disease: A case series. *J. Acad. Nutr. Diet.* **2015**, *115*, 1226–1232. [CrossRef] [PubMed]
91. Zhan, Y.L.; Zhan, Y.A.; Dai, S.X. Is a low FODMAP diet beneficial for patients with inflammatory bowel disease? A meta-analysis and systematic review. *Clin. Nutr.* **2017**. [CrossRef] [PubMed]
92. Eichelmann, F.; Schwingshackl, L.; Fedirko, V.; Aleksandrova, K. Effect of plant-based diets on obesity-related inflammatory profiles: A systematic review and meta-analysis of intervention trials. *Obes. Rev.* **2016**, *17*, 1067–1079. [CrossRef] [PubMed]
93. Arpon, A.; Riezu-Boj, J.I.; Milagro, F.I.; Razquin, C.; Martinez-Gonzalez, M.A.; Corella, D.; Estruch, R.; Casas, R.; Fito, M.; Ros, E.; et al. Adherence to Mediterranean diet is associated with methylation changes in inflammation-related genes in peripheral blood cells. *J. Phys. Biochem.* **2017**, *73*, 455. [CrossRef] [PubMed]
94. Marlow, G.; Ellett, S.; Ferguson, I.R.; Zhu, S.; Karunasinghe, N.; Jesuthasan, A.C.; Han, D.Y.; Fraser, A.G.; Ferguson, L.R. Transcriptomics to study the effect of a Mediterranean-inspired diet on inflammation in Crohn's disease patients. *Hum. Genom.* **2013**, *7*, 24. [CrossRef] [PubMed]

95. Chiba, M.; Abe, T.; Tsuda, H.; Sugawara, T.; Tsuda, S.; Tozawa, H.; Fujiwara, K.; Imai, H. Lifestyle-related disease in Crohn's disease: Relapse prevention by a semi-vegetarian diet. *World J. Gastroenterol.* **2010**, *16*, 2484–2495. [CrossRef] [PubMed]
96. Crohn's and Colitis Foundation. Available online: http://www.crohnscolitisfoundation.org/science-and-professionals/research/current-research-studies/microbiome-initiative.html (accessed on 14 August 2017).
97. The Gem Project. Available online: http://www.gemproject.ca/ (accessed on 13 August 2017).
98. Predicct Study. Available online: http://www.predicct.co.uk/ (accessed on 13 August 2017).

Antioxidative Efficacy of a *Pistacia Lentiscus* Supplement and its Effect on the Plasma Amino Acid Profile in Inflammatory Bowel Disease

Efstathia Papada [1], Alastair Forbes [2], Charalampia Amerikanou [1], Ljilja Torović [3], Nick Kalogeropoulos [1], Chara Tzavara [1], John K. Triantafillidis [4] and Andriana C. Kaliora [1,*]

1 Department of Dietetics and Nutritional Science, School of Health Science and Education, Harokopio University, 17671 Athens, Greece; efpapada@gmail.com (E.P.); amerikanou@windowslive.com (C.A.); nickal@hua.gr (N.K.); htzavara@med.uoa.gr (C.T.)
2 Norwich Medical School, University of East Anglia, Bob Champion Building, James Watson Road, Norwich NR4 7UQ, UK; Alastair.Forbes@uea.ac.uk
3 Department of Pharmacy, Faculty of Medicine, University of Novi Sad, 21000 Novi Sad, Serbia; ljilja.torovic@izjzv.org.rs
4 Inflammatory Bowel Disease Unit, IASO General Hospital, 15562 Athens, Greece; jktrian@gmail.com
* Correspondence: akaliora@hua.gr or andrianakaliora@gmail.com

Abstract: Oxidative stress is present in patients with Inflammatory Bowel Disease (IBD), and natural supplements with antioxidant properties have been investigated as a non-pharmacological approach. The objective of the present study was to assess the effects of a natural *Pistacia lentiscus* (PL) supplement on oxidative stress biomarkers and to characterise the plasma-free amino acid (AA) profiles of patients with active IBD (Crohn's disease (CD) $N = 40$, ulcerative colitis (UC) $N = 20$). The activity was determined according to $5 \leq$ Harvey Bradshaw Index ≤ 16 or $2 \leq$ Partial Mayo Score ≤ 6. This is a randomised, double-blind, placebo-controlled clinical trial. IBD patients ($N = 60$) were randomly allocated to PL (2.8 g/day) or to placebo for 3 months being under no treatment ($N = 21$) or under stable medical treatment (mesalamine $N = 24$, azathioprine $N = 14$, and corticosteroids $N = 23$) that was either single medication ($N = 22$) or combined medication ($N = 17$). Plasma oxidised, low-density lipoprotein (oxLDL), total serum oxidisability, and serum uric acid were evaluated at baseline and follow-up. OxLDL/LDL and oxLDL/High-Density Lipoprotein (HDL) ratios were calculated. The plasma-free AA profile was determined by applying a gas chromatography/mass spectrometry analysis. oxLDL ($p = 0.031$), oxLDL/HDL ($p = 0.020$), and oxLDL/LDL ($p = 0.005$) decreased significantly in the intervention group. The mean change differed significantly in CD between groups for oxLDL/LDL ($p = 0.01$), and, in the total sample, both oxLDL/LDL ($p = 0.015$) and oxLDL/HDL ($p = 0.044$) differed significantly. Several changes were reported in AA levels. PL ameliorated a decrease in plasma-free AAs seen in patients with UC taking placebo. In conclusion, this intervention resulted in favourable changes in oxidative stress biomarkers in active IBD.

Keywords: oxidative stress; amino acids; inflammatory bowel disease; Crohn's disease; ulcerative colitis; *pistacia lentiscus* (mastiha)

---

1. Introduction

Inflammatory bowel disease (IBD) is a chronic gastrointestinal disease that includes Crohn's disease (CD) and ulcerative colitis (UC). Patients face several intestinal and extraintestinal complications (e.g., hepatobiliary and ocular complications). In addition, IBD patients in relapse are at increased risk of acute arterial events even at a young age [1] and at increased risk of acute myocardial infarction and heart failure even if they do not meet the traditional risk factors for cardiovascular disease [2].

Oxidative stress has been proposed as both a putative causal and perpetuating factor for IBD [3]. Oxidative stress plays a critical role in the pathogenesis, progression, and severity of IBD, serving as an immunoregulatory factor. Chronic inflammation of the intestinal mucosa stimulates excessive reactive oxygen species (ROS)/reactive nitrogen species (RNS) production leading to oxidative stress [4,5]. Alterations in RNS levels recruit phagocytes and Nitric Oxide Synthases (NOS), which affect the nitric oxide levels of the intestinal mucosa [6], lead to overproduction of cytotoxic reactive oxygen metabolites, and inhibit the antioxidative system. The above results in oxidative injury of the intestinal mucous membrane [7]. Additionally, the link between IBD severity and duration with the pathogenesis of atherosclerosis [8] has been explained by the release of inflammatory cytokines that lead to endothelial dysfunction [9].

Amino acids (AAs) control and protect intestinal health, and not only act as substrates for proteinosynthesis in intestinal mucosal cells [10], but also as regulators of major metabolic pathways [11,12]. Their protective function may be linked to intestinal epithelial cells apoptosis and proliferation, as well as inhibition of inflammation and oxidative stress through blocking of the NF-κB signaling pathway [13]. Recently, it has been shown that variations in the levels of some AAs may be involved in the pathogenesis of IBD [14]. Data on circulating AAs in active IBD patients are limited and sometimes conflicting; however, it seems that the AA profile differentiates IBD patients from healthy controls, pointing towards a link between the AAs and the disease process [15–17]. Aminograms and multivariate indexes using AA molar ratios have been proven to be useful in reflecting the nutritional status, assessing disease activity, and monitoring disease progression [15,18].

Pistacia lentiscus L. var latifolius Coss or *Pistacia lentiscus* var. Chia is an evergreen shrub of the *pistacia* genus that is cultivated for its aromatic resin mainly on the Greek island of Chios. Previous studies of *Pistacia lentiscus* resin have documented the presence of phenolics [19], terpenes [20,21], their bioavailability in humans [22], as well as antioxidant [23], anti-inflammatory [24], lipid-lowering [25], and immunomodulating properties [26,27] of this natural product.

The European Medicines Agency has recognised *Pistacia lentiscus* resin as a herbal medicinal product with the following indications: (a) mild dyspeptic disorders, (b) symptomatic treatment of minor inflammations of the skin, and (c) as an aid in the healing of minor wounds [28].

In previous research, it has been reported that a 3-month intervention with a supplement containing the natural resinous product of *Pistacia lentiscus* (the supplement herein given as PL), adjunctive to stable medical treatment, regulated faecal biomarkers and improved quality of life in active IBD patients compared with a placebo [29]. Herein, the aim was to explore the effects of this intervention on biomarkers of oxidative stress in active IBD. Additionally, another study in healthy adults has shown that AA profiles are modified in response to acute supplementation with PL resin [30]. AAs are key regulators in metabolic pathways that affect intestinal health, and are also implicated in oxidative stress and inflammatory cytokines production [31,32]. Therefore, a second aim was to assess whether PL administration could have an impact on the health of patients reflected in the plasma-free AA profile after an assessment of AAs in the diet.

2. Materials and Methods

2.1. Study Design

The Harokopio University Ethics Committee (49/29-10-2015) reviewed and approved the protocol, and the trial was conducted according to the rules of the Declaration of Helsinki of 1975 as revised in 2008. All subjects gave their informed consent before they participated in the study. The trial was registered with ClinicalTrials.gov, where the full trial protocol can be accessed (Identifier:

NCT02796339). Patients were recruited between May 2016 and June 2017. Follow-up visits were completed on September 2017. The study took place in Athens, Greece.

IBD patients in relapse were enrolled in this randomised, double-blind, placebo-controlled, parallel-group clinical trial (Appendix A Figure A1). The primary endpoint was attenuation of oxidative stress biomarkers. The secondary endpoints were plasma-free AAs profile and quality of life assessment. In brief, IBD patients in relapse, with endoscopically confirmed UC or CD, were enrolled based on certain inclusion and exclusion criteria. In detail, both males and females, of age ranging between 18 and 67 years old, with a diagnosis of IBD established by endoscopy, and with consistent histology and clinical course were included. To avoid hospitalisation, surgeries, and major changes in drug treatments, the study was designed to include moderately active patients. Active disease was assessed by applying the Harvey Bradshaw Index ($5 \leq \text{HBI} \leq 16$) [33] for CD patients or the Partial Mayo Score ($2 \leq \text{PMS} \leq 6$) for UC patients [34]. Medication included treatment with steroids for at least 2 weeks before the initiation of the trial, mesalamine and mesalamine analogues for 4 weeks, and immunosuppressants for 8 weeks before the start of the trial. Patients were excluded from trial enrollment in the case of positive stool culture for enteric pathogens or Clostridium difficile toxin or when treated with antibiotics during and 2 months prior to screening. Also, patients who had undergone bowel surgery ≤3 months prior to screening or a planned elective surgery or hospitalisation during the study were excluded. Additionally, clinically significant short bowel syndrome, the presence of an intra-abdominal abscess or a fistula with clinical or radiological evidence of an associated abscess, ileostomy, and colostomy were exclusion criteria. Enteral or parenteral nutrition, alcohol or drug abuse, vitamin or inorganic supplement use <6 months prior to screening, a vegan or macrobiotic diet <5 years prior to screening, any malignancy in the year prior to screening or cancer survivors >10 years, the presence of a cardiovascular disease or peptic ulcer, pregnancy, and lactation were set as exclusion criteria. Patients who changed their medication or diet or who initiated nutritional supplement intake during the trial were considered to be protocol violators. The recruitment of patients was conducted according to the above criteria in the IASO IBD Unit. A qualified and independent (unrelated to the project) gastroenterologist was responsible for all trial-related medical decisions, for ensuring that the selection of patients at baseline was unbiased, and for the unbiased follow-up assessment according to the protocol. Demographical data, medical history, including such data as the date of disease onset, duration, and medical treatment, and anthropometrics (body weight, height, body mass index) were documented.

After the baseline assessment, patients were randomly allocated to an intervention, either verum or a placebo. Randomisation was achieved by a computer-generated random number list that was prepared by an investigator with no clinical involvement in the trial. Blinding of intervention staff and participants was strictly maintained. The PL group received a natural PL supplement at a dose of 2.8 g daily (four tabs × 700 mg PL), while the placebo group received identical placebo tablets. This dose was chosen based on a previous pilot study in CD patients experiencing no side effects and a bioavailability study in healthy humans [22,26,27]. The intervention lasted 3 months. Both groups continued their usual medical treatment, which had to remain unaltered throughout the trial.

The verum tablets weighed 0.98 g and consisted of 70% PL, 14% microcrystalline cellulose, 14% dibasic calcium phosphate anhydrous, and 2% magnesium stearate. The supplement was standardised to 14 mg mastihadienonic acid and 13 mg isomastihadienonic acid. The placebo tablets weighed 0.99 g and consisted of 49% microcrystalline cellulose with a characteristic off-white to yellowish colour for similarity to verum, 49% dibasic calcium phosphate anhydrous, and 2% magnesium stearate. The verum and placebo tablets had an identical appearance and shared organoleptic characteristics.

2.2. Laboratory Analyses

2.2.1. Evaluation of Oxidative Stress

The Total Serum Oxidisability Assay

Serum samples were oxidised with copper sulfate as described by Aurrekoetxea and colleagues [35]. After dilution with phosphate-buffered saline (PBS, Arlington, TX, USA), samples were placed in the wells of a flat-bottomed plate. Copper sulfate was added at time zero and the plate was placed in an ELISA reader (Biotek PowerWave XS2, Winuski, VT, USA). The conjugated dienic hydroperoxides that were produced were measured at 245 nm. The increase in absorbance was plotted against time. The kinetics of oxidation were analysed in terms of the lag-time preceding oxidation and expressed in seconds (tLAG). All samples were measured in duplicate.

The oxLDL Assay

The levels of oxLDL in plasma were measured photometrically in an ELISA reader (Biotek PowerWave XS2) applying an ELISA Sandwich Kit according to the instructions of the manufacturer (Mercodia, AB, Uppsala, Sweden). Additionally, the oxLDL/HDL and oxLDL/LDL ratios were calculated. All samples were measured in duplicate.

The Uric Acid Assay

Uric acid (UA) was quantified in serum (Biosis, GR). The assay is based on the oxidation of UA in the presence of the enzyme uricase that results in the production of H_2O_2. The red-coloured product of the reaction of H_2O_2 with a phenolic derivative and 4-aminophenazone is proportional to the concentration of UA and was measured at 510 nm in a microplate spectrophotometer (Biotek PowerWave XS2). All samples were measured in duplicate.

2.2.2. AA Analysis

Free (physiological) plasma AAs in an overnight fasting state were determined by gas chromatography-mass spectrometry (GC-MS), employing the Phenomenex® EZ:faast kit (California, CA, USA). The procedure involves a solid phase extraction followed by derivatisation and subsequent liquid/liquid extraction. The derivatised AAs are then analysed by GC-MS.

An Agilent (Wallborn, Germany) series GC 6890 N gas chromatograph, coupled with an HP5973 Mass Spectrometer detector (EI, 70 eV), a split-splitess injector, and an HP7683 autosampler were used for analysis. An aliquot (2 μL) of derivatised samples was injected into the GC at a split ratio of 1:15. AA separation was achieved using a Phenomenex Zebron ZB-A AA analysis-dedicated column (length = 10 m, internal diameter = 0.25 mm, film thickness = 25 μm). The carrier gas was helium at a constant flow of 1.1 mL/min. The injector and transfer line temperatures were 250 °C and 340 °C, respectively. The initial oven temperature was 110 °C, which was then increased (30 °C/min), and held at 320 °C for 3 min. A selective ion monitoring (SIM) GC-MS method was applied for the detection of 26 AAs based on the ± 0.05 retention time presence of target and qualifier ions at the predetermined ratios. The retention times and the target and qualifier ions of AAs are shown in Supplementary Table S1. Quantification was carried out employing norvaline as an internal standard and constructing reference curves for each AA by standard solutions.

2.3. Statistical Analysis

Continuous variables are presented with the mean and the standard deviation (SD) or with the median and the interquartile range (IQR). Quantitative variables are presented with the absolute and relative frequencies. All analyses were conducted on an intention-to-treat basis. For the comparison of proportions, chi-squared and Fisher's exact tests were used. For the comparison of means between the control group and the intervention group, the Student's *t*-test was computed. To reduce the bias implicit in utilising only complete cases, multiple imputation procedures for all of the data were implemented. Differences in changes of study variables during the follow-up period between the two study groups were evaluated using repeated measurements analysis of variance (ANOVA). The Kolmogorov–Smirnov test was applied to examine the normal distribution. For variables with a skewed distribution, the ranks were used for the analysis of variance. Statistical significance was set at 0.05, and all analyses were conducted using the SPSS statistical software (version 22.0).

The study had a power of 0.90 for the between-subjects main effect at an effect size of 0.37; a power of 0.95 for the within-subjects main effect at an effect size of 0.25; and a power of 0.95 for the interaction effect at an effect size of 0.25.

3. Results

Sixty IBD patients met the criteria for recruitment. Out of the 60 patients, 27 (45.0%) were randomised to the placebo group and 33 (55.0%) to the verum group, while 40 (66.7%) of them were diagnosed with CD and 20 (33.3%) with UC. Clinical, anthropometric, and demographic characteristics for all groups are presented in Tables 1 and 2. No adverse events were reported in either treatment arm. Additionally, 24-h recalls were analysed applying the Nutritionist Pro software and no significant differences were observed in macronutrient or micronutrient intake between the mean changes in groups (Supplementary Material, Table S2). No significant changes were observed in the AAs of diet between the mean changes in groups either (Supplementary Material, Table S3).

Table 3 presents the oxidative stress markers before and after the intervention. The levels of oxLDL/LDL decreased significantly in CD patients, and the difference in mean changes between the placebo and intervention groups was significant. The mean changes were unaltered for lag time and uric acid; however, the lag time of serum oxidation significantly increased and this was paralleled by attenuation in the decrease of uric acid in serum. In the total sample, apart from oxLDL/LDL, the mean changes were significantly different between the control and intervention groups also for oxLDL/HDL. In UC, no significant differences were reported. The effect of therapy, as well as the effect of the type of disease (UC, CD) on changes in oxidative stress markers, was explored via repeated measurements models and no significant associations were found ($p > 0.05$).

Significant differences in levels of AAs are presented in Table 4. In CD patients, the levels of thioproline and lysine decreased in the PL arm; however, the difference in mean changes in PL and placebo remained insignificant. Nevertheless, in patients with UC, some interesting results were extracted. The levels of the following AAs were significantly decreased in UC patients receiving a placebo compared with their baseline, but remained largely unchanged in the UC patients receiving PL: allo-isoleucine, isoleucine, lysine, tyrosine, and tryptophane. Tyrosine rose significantly in the UC verum group compared with the baseline. In the cases of allo-leucine, glutamine, isoleucine, leucine, lysine, ornithine, serine, tryptophan, and tyrosine, the end-of-study levels in placebo patients were statistically distinct from the results in the verum group ($p < 0.05$ in each case). In the total sample, aspartic acid fell significantly in the PL group and glutamic acid rose significantly, but there was no significant difference between the two groups, and cysteine rose only in the verum group. No other significant changes were reported.

Table 1. Demographics in Inflammatory Bowel Disease (IBD) patients or in the Crohn's disease (CD) and ulcerative colitis (UC) subgroups. The results are given as *N* (%) of the total number.

	IBD (N = 60)			CD (N = 40)			UC (N = 20)		
	Placebo (27)	**PL (33)**	***P***	**Placebo (18)**	**PL (22)**	***P***	**Placebo (9)**	**PL (11)**	***P***
Sex									
Females	9 (33.3)	18 (54.5)	0.100 $^{+}$	7 (38.9)	11 (50)	0.482 $^{+}$	2 (22.2)	7 (63.6)	0.092 $^{++}$
Males	18 (66.7)	15 (45.5)		11 (61.1)	11 (50)		7 (77.8)	4 (36.4)	
Age (years), mean (SD)	45 (17.4)	38.2 (11.9)	0.076 ‡	48.1 (17.6)	36 (10.7)	0.011 ‡	38.9 (16.1)	42.5 (13.6)	0.597 ‡
Marital status									
Unmarried/Divorced	14 (51.9)	14 (42.4)	0.466 $^{+}$	9 (50)	11 (50)	1.000 $^{+}$	5 (55.6)	3 (27.3)	0.362 $^{++}$
Married	13 (48.1)	19 (57.6)		9 (50)	11 (50)		4 (44.4)	8 (72.7)	
Education (years)									
1–9	3 (11.1)	7 (21.2)	0.510 $^{+}$	2 (11.1)	2 (9.1)	0.884 $^{++}$	1 (11.1)	5 (45.5)	0.326 $^{++}$
10–12	5 (18.5)	7 (21.2)		3 (16.7)	6 (27.3)		2 (22.2)	1 (9.1)	
>12	19 (70.4)	19 (57.6)		13 (72.2)	14 (63.6)		6 (66.7)	5 (45.5)	
Smoking $^{\#}$									
No	20 (74.1)	23 (69.7)	0.653 $^{+}$	11 (61.1)	15 (68.2)	0.641 $^{+}$	9 (100)	8 (72.7)	0.211 $^{++}$
Yes	7 (25.9)	10 (30.3)		7 (38.9)	7 (31.8)		0 (0)	3 (27.3)	

$^{\#}$ Smoking habits are presented herein at baseline; $^{+}$ Pearson's chi-square test; $^{++}$ Fisher's exact test; ‡ Student's *t*-test. PL, *Pistacia lentiscus*.

Table 2. Anthropometrics and clinical characteristics in IBD patients. The results are given as *N* (%) of the total number.

	IBD (*N* = 60)		*P*	CD (*N* = 40)		*P*	UC (*N* = 20)		*P*
	Placebo (27)	Mastiha (33)		Placebo (18)	Mastiha (22)		Placebo (9)	Mastiha (11)	
BMI (kg/m^2) mean (SD)	24.5 (6.6)	23.4 (5.3)	0.481 ‡	24.4 (6.1)	22 (4.2)	0.149 ‡	24.7 (7.8)	26.2 (6.2)	0.628 ‡
Normal	17 (63.0)	23 (69.7)	0.863 ++	11 (61.1)	17 (77.3)	0.292 ++	6 (66.7)	6 (54.5)	0.830 ++
Overweight	5 (18.5)	6 (18.2)		3 (16.7)	4 (18.2)		2 (22.2)	2 (18.2)	
Obese	5 (18.5)	4 (12.1)		4 (22.2)	1 (4.5)		1 (11.1)	3 (27.3)	
Disease duration (years), mean (SD)	13.9 (10.7)	9.4 (7.0)	0.061 ‡	14.8 (12.0)	10.2 (6.9)	0.131 ‡	12.0 (7.7)	7.9 (7.4)	0.240 ‡
Age of first symptoms, mean (SD)	29.6 (16.1)	27.0 (11.9)	0.480 ‡	31.2 (16.6)	25.0 (10.3)	0.152 ‡	26.4 (15.7)	31.6 (14.2)	0.463 ‡
Age of diagnosis, mean (SD)	32.0 (17.4)	27.9 (11.9)	0.290 ‡	34.5 (18.0)	25.8 (10.6)	0.065 ‡	26.9 (15.9)	32.4 (13.9)	0.431 ‡
Disease extent									
Ileal				9 (50.0)	8 (36.4)				
Ileocolonic				7 (39.0)	9 (40.9)				
Colonic				1 (5.5)	3 (13.6)				
Colonic and duodenum				1 (5.5)	0 (0.0)				
Colonic and upper GI-				0 (0.0)	2 (9.1)				
Pancolitis							6 (66.7)	8 (72.7)	
Left-sided							3 (33.3)	2 (18.2)	
Rectitis							0 (0)	1 (9.1)	
Surgical therapy in the past	12 (44.4)	12 (36.4)	0.525 +	10 (55.5)	10 (45.5)	0.525 +	2 (22.2)	2 (18.2)	1.000 ++
Concomitant treatment									
None	9 (33.3)	12 (36.4)	0.966 +	7 (38.9)	10 (45.5)	0.783 +	2 (22.2)	2 (18.2)	0.850 ++
One	10 (37.0)	12 (36.4)		5 (27.8)	7 (31.8)		5 (55.6)	5 (45.5)	
Combined	8 (29.6)	9 (27.3)		6 (33.3)	5 (22.7)		2 (22.2)	4 (36.4)	
Medication									
Mesalamine	11 (40.7)	13 (39.4)	0.916 +	5 (27.8)	4 (18.2)	0.705 ++	6 (66.7)	9 (81.8)	0.617 ++
Azathioprine	7 (25.9)	7 (21.2)	0.668 +	5 (27.8)	4 (18.2)	0.705 ++	2 (22.2)	3 (27.3)	1.000 ++
Corticosteroids	9 (33.3)	14 (42.4)	0.807 +	7 (38.9)	10 (45.5)	0.676 +	2 (22.2)	4 (36.4)	1.000 ++

+ Pearson's chi-square test; ++ Fisher's exact test; ‡ Student's *t*-test. BMI, body mass index.

Table 3. The oxidative stress markers at baseline and at follow-up. Values are expressed as the mean ± SD.

	IBD (N = 60)					CD (N = 40)					UC (N = 20)				
	Pre-	Post-	Change	p^1	p^2	Pre-	Post-	Change	p^1	p^2	Pre-	Post-	Change	p^1	p^2
oxLDL (U/L)															
Placebo	135.3 (48.38)	135.45 (38.92)	0.15 (52.76)	ns	ns	122.7 (47.1)	128.3 (43)	5.6 (50.4)	ns	ns	160.4 (42.8)	149.7 (25.4)	−10.7 (58.8)	ns	ns
PL	160.42 (34.26)	140.12 (41.91)	−20.3 (51.7)	0.031		159.4 (34.5)	138.2 (44.1)	−21.2 (55.3)	ns		162.4 (35.3)	144 (39)	−18.4 (46)	ns	
p^3	0.022	ns				0.007	ns				ns	ns			
oxLDL/HDL															
Placebo	2.44 (1.22)	2.63 (1.38)	0.19 (1.67)	ns	0.044	2.44 (1.2)	2.51 (1.51)	0.07 (1.63)	ns	ns	2.45 (1.33)	2.88 (1.11)	0.43 (1.83)	ns	ns
PL	3.06 (0.91)	2.37 (1.42)	−0.69 (1.63)	0.020		2.98 (0.85)	2.45 (1.42)	−0.53 (1.46)	ns		3.23 (1.03)	2.2 (1.45)	−1.03 (1.96)	ns	
p^3	0.028	ns				ns	ns				ns	ns			
oxLDL/LDL															
Placebo	1.62 (0.88)	1.7 (0.88)	0.07 (0.82)	ns	0.015	1.55 (0.99)	1.79 (0.96)	0.24 (0.73)	ns	0.010	1.78 (0.63)	1.51 (0.73)	−0.27 (0.92)	ns	ns
PL	1.84 (0.73)	1.3 (0.85)	−0.54 (1.03)	0.005		1.95 (0.84)	1.34 (0.94)	−0.61 (1.15)	0.006		1.62 (0.38)	1.23 (0.65)	−0.39 (0.76)	ns	
p^3	ns	ns				ns	ns				ns	ns			
Lagtime (s)															
Placebo	4279.8 (2573.79)	4889.15 (2094.22)	609.31 (2159.4)	ns	ns	4014.1 (2335.6)	4619.9 (1869.8)	605.8 (2210)	ns	ns	4811.3 (3075.8)	5427.6 (2516.9)	616.3 (2185.5)	ns	ns
PL	4271.12 (2236.36)	4959.46 (1760.57)	688.34 (2327.7)	ns		3823.2 (1763.5)	4852.6 (1793.3)	1029.4 (2119)	0.031		5166.9 (2854.6)	5173.2 (1757.7)	6.3 (2672.4)	ns	
p^3	ns	ns				ns	ns				ns	ns			
UA (mg/dL)															
Placebo	4.99 (1.92)	4.45 (1.22)	−0.54 (1.79)	ns	ns	5.25 (2.22)	4.39 (1.29)	−0.9 (2)	0.037	ns	4.46 (1.04)	4.58 (1.12)	0.1 (0.9)	ns	ns
PL	5.76 (4.9)	4.64 (1.11)	−1.12 (4.82)	ns		5.14 (1.45)	4.58 (1.15)	−0.6 (1.4)	ns		7.01 (8.36)	4.76 (1.08)	−2.3 (8.3)	ns	
p^3	ns	ns				ns	ns				ns	ns			

[1] p-value for the time effect; [2] The effects reported include differences between the groups in the degree of change (repeated measurements ANOVA); [3] p-value for the group effect; ns, non-significant.

Table 4. Significant differences in amino acids (AAs) levels (nmoL/mL). Values are expressed as the mean (SD) or median (interquartile range, IQR).

	Pre-	Post-	Change	p^1	p^2
		IBD (N = 60)			
Aspartic acid					
Placebo	7 (4.1)	6.7 (4.2)	−0.3 (6.2)	ns	ns
PL	8.2 (4.5)	5.3 (3.3)	−2.9 (6)	0.009	
p^3	ns	ns			
Cysteine ‡					
Placebo	27.9 (26.5; 28.8)	27.5 (26.3; 29.6)	0 (−2; 2.1)	ns	ns
PL	27.1 (25.4; 28.5)	28.7 (26.2; 29.5)	1.3 (−0.7; 3.5)	0.042	
p^3	ns	ns			
Glutamic acid ‡					
Placebo	12.3 (5.1; 26.5)	20.2 (9.5; 30)	3.6 (−7.4; 15.1)	0.039	ns
PL	18.6 (10.4; 26.6)	25.7 (21.7; 28.2)	4 (−3.6; 16.3)	0.045	
p^3	ns	0.042			
Glutamine ‡					
Placebo	433.9 (392.9; 461.8)	385 (375.1; 446.4)	−34.4 (−60.4; −13.8)	ns	ns
PL	368.4 (303.1; 428.4)	385.4 (311; 413.1)	−7.4 (−53.7; −67.6)	ns	
p^3	0.011	ns			
Lysine ‡					
Placebo	185.3 (160.1; 222.3)	171.3 (153.4; 177.1)	−25.8 (−58.5; −0.9)	ns	ns
PL	188.1 (163.3; 220.8)	164.3 (150.3; 172.2)	−27 (−55.8; 1.9)	ns	
p^3	ns	ns			
Thioproline					
Placebo	16.7 (4.1)	14.1 (2.3)	−2.7 (5.2)	0.006	ns
PL	18.1 (4.2)	13.7 (2.8)	−4.4 (4.6)	<0.001	
p^3	ns	ns			
		CD (N = 40)			
Cysteine ‡					
Placebo	28.3 (26.9; 29.3)	27.2 (26.3; 29.3)	−0.8 (−2.2; 1.7)	ns	ns
PL	27.2 (25.6; 28.5)	27.7 (25; 29.2)	0.2 (−1.9; 3.7)	ns	
p^3	0.050	ns			
Lysine ‡					
Placebo	165.3 (142.8; 218.4)	173.4 (155; 178.2)	−9.9 (−50.1; 1.5)	ns	ns
PL	192.6 (175.3; 221.6)	160.8 (142.7; 171.4)	−30.6 (−62.2; −4)	0.036	
p^3	ns	ns			

Table 4. *Cont.*

	Pre-	Post-	Change	P^1	P^2
Thioproline					
Placebo	15.6 (3.6)	14.4 (2.4)	−1.2 (4.9)	ns	ns
PL	17.8 (4.8)	13.4 (3.1)	−4.4 (5)	<0.001	
p^3	ns	ns			
		UC (N = 20)			
Alo-isoleucine ‡					
Placebo	58.4 (53; 68.9)	48.7 (41.4; 55.5)	−14.4 (−15.4; −11.6)	0.038	0.016
PL	45.5 (32; 52.4)	51.8 (47.3; 55.6)	7.9 (−4.2; 17.2)	ns	
p^3	0.007	ns			
β-Aminobutyric acid ‡					
Placebo	98.1 (96.8; 99.9)	98 (97; 98.8)	−1.1 (−2.5; −0.4)	ns	ns
PL	98.7 (97.3; 99.4)	98.8 (98.1; 101.7)	1 (−0.9; 3.8)	ns	
p^3	ns	0.022			
Aspartic acid					
Placebo	6.4 (2.4)	5.6 (2.5)	−0.8 (4.4)	0.672	ns
PL	9.7 (4.6)	5.6 (3.5)	−4.1 (5.6)	0.016	
p^3	ns	ns			
Cysteine ‡					
Placebo	27.7 (26.5; 27.9)	28.8 (26.5; 29.6)	1.2 (0.2; 2.3)	ns	ns
PL	26.4 (25.1; 28.6)	29.2 (28.1; 31.5)	2.1 (0.8; 3.5)	<0.001	
p^3	ns	ns			
Glutamic acid ‡					
Placebo	4.1 (2.9; 17.1)	14.9 (9.1; 19.6)	2.2 (−2.8; 6.6)	ns	ns
PL	21.1 (10.4; 34.1)	24.4 (21.7; 30.3)	2.2 (−3; 19.9)	ns	
p^3	ns	0.005			
Glutamine ‡					
Placebo	427.2 (401.8; 456.3)	385 (375.1; 394.7)	−37.5 (−47.9; −22.7)	ns	0.038
PL	330.6 (255.4; 428.4)	387.1 (311; 413.1)	50.3 (−50.2; 129.8)	ns	
p^3	0.048	ns			
Isoleucine ‡					
Placebo	68.3 (61.8; 80.2)	51.5 (49.1; 63.6)	−16.9 (−17.6; −10.4)	0.019	0.009
PL	55.4 (38.1; 61.5)	60.4 (55.2; 67.8)	0.8 (−3.3; −24.4)	ns	
p^3	0.008	ns			

Table 4. *Cont.*

	Pre-	Post-	Change	p^1	p^2
Leucine ‡					
Placebo	132.3 (115.2; 146.6)	117.7 (92.3; 139.3)	−23.8 (−29.9; −7.9)	ns	0.043
PL	102.1 (85; 123.7)	127.8 (120.1; 137.3)	16.1 (0.7; 42.8)	ns	
p^3	ns	ns			
Lysine ‡					
Placebo	207.2 (190.5; 222.3)	164.1 (153.4; 174.3)	−47.5 (−69.1; −41.6)	0.002	0.009
PL	163.3 (129.9; 209.9)	166.7 (159.5; 182.8)	−0.6 (−33.4; 26.5)	ns	
p^3	ns	ns			
Ornithine ‡					
Placebo	103.5 (77.8; 125.5)	75.2 (69.1; 82.9)	−20.8 (−50.3; −3.8)	ns	0.036
PL	77.1 (47.1; 96.1)	85 (68.5; 92.9)	15.2 (−27.6; 22.4)	ns	
p^3	ns	ns			
Proline					
Placebo	257.9 (55.7)	223.6 (56.1)	−34.3 (92.2)	ns	ns
PL	240.6 (90.9)	275.7 (49.6)	35.1 (114.8)	ns	
p^3	ns	0.041			
Serine					
Placebo	130.4 (36.2)	114.1 (19.8)	−16.3 (32.8)	ns	0.028
PL	94.8 (28.1)	108.3 (15.3)	13.5 (23)	ns	
p^3	0.023	ns			
Thioproline					
Placebo	19.1 (4.4)	13.3 (1.8)	−5.8 (4.8)	0.001	0.047
PL	18.7 (2.7)	14.1 (2.1)	−4.6 (4)	0.003	
p^3	ns	ns			
Tryptophane					
Placebo	65.3 (12.3)	57 (12.8)	−8.3 (12)	0.050	0.037
PL	55.1 (13.9)	58.8 (9)	3.7 (11.7)	ns	
p^3	ns	ns			
Tyrosine					
Placebo	71 (18.4)	58.1 (17.2)	−12.9 (17.3)	0.045	0.005
PL	50.4 (18.6)	63.3 (11.9)	12.9 (18.6)	0.029	
p^3	0.023	ns			

[1] *p*-value for the time effect; [2] The effects reported include differences between the groups in mean changes (repeated measurements ANOVA); [3] *p*-value for the group effect; ‡ The analyses were based on ranks, and variables are presented with the median (IQR); ns, non-significant.

4. Discussion

Herein, the effect of a natural supplement prepared with PL on biomarkers of oxidative stress in IBD patients in relapse has been investigated. Furthermore, the AA profiles in patients as potential biomarkers of metabolic changes have been characterised. There are pre-clinical and pilot clinical data supporting PL administration in IBD [26,27,36]. The results described herein are part of a larger survey, which is to our knowledge the first one that evaluates the effectiveness of PL on the basis of a Phase-II randomised placebo-controlled clinical trial of IBD patients in relapse.

OxLDL is considered to be the most specific biomarker for oxidative stress evaluation in humans; most recently, its measurement by immunological methods (i.e., antibodies) has been recognised by the European Food Safety Authority (EFSA) as a reliable method to assess oxidative damage with appropriate specificity [37]. In this study, oxLDL fell significantly only in patients receiving PL, even if the mean change between the two groups remained insignificant. However, data on oxLDL levels in IBD patients are limited. A previous study in eight patients with active CD and eight controls showed that CD patients had elevated levels of oxLDL compared with the controls, reflecting the increased oxidative stress and the higher risk for atherosclerosis [38]. The decreased levels of oxLDL after PL intervention could point towards an antioxidant effect of this natural supplement in active IBD patients. Future research on its mechanism of action is justified, since its main bioactive compounds, which are mostly triterpenes (i.e., mastihadienonic and isomastihadeinonic acids), are bioavailable and exhibit antioxidant effects in vivo [22]. Azathioprine is an immunosuppressant drug that, despite its severe short- and long-term adverse effects, is most frequently used to induce and maintain remission in IBD. Although the number of patients treated with azathioprine was low and equal to seven for each trial arm, a subgroup analysis for patients treated with azathioprine showed no significant changes in oxidative stress markers.

Another interesting result of the present study was the significant reduction in the ratios of oxLDL/LDL and oxLDL/HDL in the PL arm compared with the placebo arm. A decrease in feacal lysozyme in the PL arm has been reported in the study of Papada and coworkers [29], and this parallels the decrease in the oxLDL/LDL and oxLDL/HDL ratios. Herein, when changes in oxidative stress were assessed separately for CD and UC patients, significant changes were reported for patients with CD, showing possibly a most promising response to this antioxidant supplement in CD compared with UC. In CD, the increased oxidative stress has been documented as a key factor of the disease's pathogenesis [39], and evidence supports the implication of ROS in oxidative damage in peripheral blood of naïve and treated patients with CD as well as the role of antioxidant mechanisms in the regulation of cellular processes [40–42]. As such, elevated hydrogen peroxide levels have been correlated with inflammation in CD and oxidative damage is insistent in the immune cells of active and inactive CD patients, whereas catalase activity is permanently inhibited [40]. However, despite the indisputable presence of oxidative stress in CD and although these patients are at increased risk for cardiovascular disease [1,43], data on the above ratios are scarce. Overall, the level of oxLDL and the oxLDL/LDL and oxLDL/HDL ratios seem to be better biomarkers than total cholesterol, triglycerides, HDL-C, and LDL-C for discrimination between patients with increased cardiovascular risk and healthy subjects [43]. In addition, they seem to be the most useful clinical parameters of lipoprotein oxidation in other pathologies as well, such as type II diabetes, reflecting the association between lipids in the state of oxidative stress [44]. A study in elderly patients with type II diabetes showed that oxLDL/HDL was directly associated with advanced glycation end products and advanced oxidation protein products, which enhance oxidative stress [45]. A more recent study in a population with a high prevalence of cardiovascular disease and type II diabetes showed that these ratios were significantly associated with HbA1c, glucose, and CRP [46]. To our knowledge, this is the first study evaluating these ratios in patients with active CD and UC in the context of a randomised clinical trial that is designed to assess the effectiveness of a natural supplement. These results in CD could point towards a favourable effect of an antioxidant supplement on the mechanisms of systemic inflammation that increase the risk of cardiovascular disease.

AAs are both substrates and regulators in several metabolic pathways. Circulating AA levels may reflect not only nutritional status, but also the inflammatory state and disease activity. In this study of patients with active IBD, no significant changes in dietary AAs were reported and this was paralleled by no significantly different changes in plasma-free AAs between the groups at baseline and at follow-up. However, some stimulating results regarding AAs changes in UC have been revealed. As such, levels of allo-isoleucine, isoleucine, cysteine, and tryptophane significantly decreased in the placebo group, whereas in the PL group they remained unchanged, with the mean changes between the groups being significant. The mean changes between the two UC groups differed significantly for leucine, serine, and glutamine. Plasma-free AA normalisation paralleled the improvement in oxidative stress biomarkers; however, no significant correlation was reported ($p > 0.05$). The general tendency for plasma AAs to increase in UC patients on the placebo may indicate increased de novo AA synthesis in the presence of inflammation. The fact that AA alterations were present predominantly in the group of UC patients may indicate a more favourable effect of PL in patients with active UC.

Several AAs are implicated in oxidative stress. Cysteine is a precursor of glutathione. Cysteine was significantly lower in the placebo group and correlated negatively with levels of oxLDL ($r = -0.26$, $p = 0.044$). This is in accordance with previous findings that oxidative stress in vivo could be translated as a deficiency of glutathione and/or cysteine [47]. Tryptophane, which was significantly decreased in the placebo group, is metabolised along the oxidative kynurenine pathway leading to the generation of quinolinic acid, 3-hydroxykynurenine, and 3-hydroxyanthranilic acid, all of which are known to generate free radicals [48]. In addition, proline is upregulated as an oxidative stress response in mammalian cells [49]. Previous studies in intestinal cell culture models have shown that the presence of sulfhydryl-containing AAs, branched-chain AAs (BCAAs), heterocyclic-group-containing AAs, or other AAs is associated with attenuation of oxidative-stress-induced inflammation [50,51].

While this study has interesting results and the quality of being double-blinded, it has limitations, including the absence of endoscopy at follow-up, precluding the ability to comment on histological alterations, and the absence of an identification of the full metabolic profile. Arginine, the immediate precursor of nitric oxide, which regulates vasodilation, was not within the group of AAs targeted, limiting the knowledge on PL's effect on vasodilation. It is also compromised by the fact that no specific diet was recommended the day before the assessment. Additionally, treatments included steroids, ASA, and immunosupressants, and patients were in relapse for different time periods. However, these limitations are compensated by the very tight control of the verum and placebo groups to ensure compliance of patients with the protocol, as well as the adequate power of the study overall, which ensued from the total number of participants that were recruited.

5. Conclusions

Given the increasing interest in the use of natural supplements with antioxidant and anti-inflammatory properties in IBD, herein the effects of a PL supplement on oxidative stress biomarkers in active IBD patients were explored. These results showed, for the first time, that PL could exhibit favourable effects in oxidative stress biomarkers in patients with active CD that could be of clinical importance.

Supplementary Materials: Supplementary Table S1: Retention times and target and qualifier ions of the AAs and the internal standard. Supplementary Table S2: Nutritional intake in IBD patients in relapse before and after intervention. Values are median (IQR). Table S3: Dietary AAs (mg) in IBD patients in relapse before and after intervention. Values are median (IQR).

Author Contributions: Conceptualization, A.C.K.; Methodology, A.C.K.; Investigation, E.P. (Data collection, analysis, and interpretation), C.A. (Contribution to laboratory work, data analysis, and interpretation), L.T. and N.K. (Set up of the chromatographic analysis protocol and in charge of analysis), J.K.T. (Participation in patient recruitment); Resources, A.C.K.; Formal Analysis, C.T. Writing—Original Draft Preparation, E.P.; Writing—Review & Editing, A.C.K. and A.F.; Visualization, E.P.; Supervision, A.C.K.; Project Administration, A.C.K.; Funding Acquisition, A.C.K.

Acknowledgments: All authors have approved the final article. We are grateful to the patients for participating in this study and for the funder for financial support.

Appendix A

CONSORT

TRANSPARENT REPORTING of TRIALS

CONSORT 2010 Flow Diagram

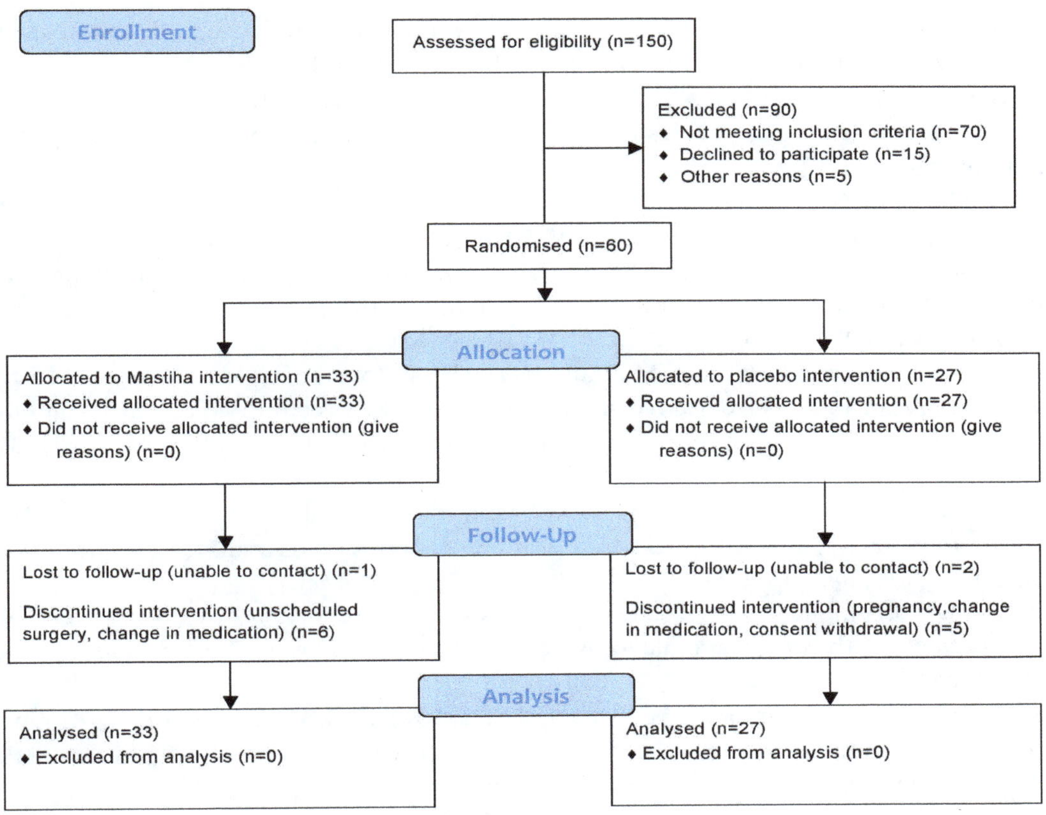

Figure A1. CONSORT 2010 flow diagram.

References

1. Kirchgesner, J.; Beaugerie, L.; Carrat, F.; Andersen, N.N.; Jess, T.; Schwarzinger, M. BERENICE study group, Increased risk of acute arterial events in young patients and severely active IBD: A nationwide French cohort study. *Gut* **2018**, *67*, 1261–1268. [CrossRef] [PubMed]
2. Aniwan, S.; Pardi, D.S.; Tremaine, W.J.; Loftus, E.V., Jr. Increased risk of acute myocardial infarction and heart failure in patients with inflammatory bowel diseases. *Clin. Gastroenterol. Hepatol.* **2018**. [CrossRef] [PubMed
3. Pereira, C.; Grácio, D.; Teixeira, J.P.; Magro, F. Oxidative stress and DNA damage: Implications in inflammatory bowel disease. *Inflamm. Bowel. Dis.* **2015**, *21*, 2403–2417. [CrossRef] [PubMed]
4. Ng, S.C.; Tang, W.; Ching, J.Y.; Wong, M.; Chow, C.M.; Hui, A.J.; Wong, T.C.; Leung, V.K.; Tsang, S.W.; Yu, H.H.; et al. Asia–Pacific Crohn's and Colitis Epidemiologic Study (ACCESS) Study Group. Incidence and phenotype of inflammatory bowel disease based on results from the Asia-pacific Crohn's and colitis epidemiology study. *Gastroenterology* **2013**, *145*, 158–165. [CrossRef] [PubMed]

5. Zeng, Z.; Zhu, Z.; Yang, Y.; Ruan, W.; Peng, X.; Su, Y.; Peng, L.; Chen, J.; Yin, Q.; Zhao, C.; et al. Incidence and clinical characteristics of inflammatory bowel disease in a developed region of Guangdong Province, China: A prospective population-based study. *J. Gastroenterol. Hepatol.* **2013**, *28*, 1148–1153. [CrossRef] [PubMed]
6. Matheson, P.J.; Wilson, M.A.; Garrison, R.N. Regulation of intestinal blood flow. *J. Surg. Res.* **2000**, *93*, 182–196. [CrossRef] [PubMed]
7. Almenier, H.A.; Al Menshawy, H.H.; Maher, M.M.; Al Gamal, S. Oxidative stress and inflammatory bowel disease. *Front. Biosci. (Elite Ed.)* **2012**, *4*, 1335–1344. [CrossRef] [PubMed]
8. Singh, S.; Kullo, I.J.; Pardi, D.S.; Loftus, E.V., Jr. Epidemiology, risk factors and management of cardiovascular diseases in IBD. *Nat. Rev. Gastroenterol. Hepatol.* **2015**, *12*, 26–35. [CrossRef] [PubMed]
9. Wu, P.; Jia, F.; Zhang, B.; Zhang, P. Risk of cardiovascular disease in inflammatory bowel disease. *Exp. Ther. Med.* **2017**, *13*, 395–400. [CrossRef] [PubMed]
10. Liu, Y.; Wang, X.; Hu, C.A. Therapeutic Potential of Amino Acids in Inflammatory Bowel Disease. *Nutrients* **2017**, *9*, 920. [CrossRef] [PubMed]
11. Bao, X.; Feng, Z.; Yao, J.; Li, T.; Yin, Y. Roles of Dietary Amino Acids and Their Metabolites in Pathogenesis of Inflammatory Bowel Disease. *Mediat. Inflamm.* **2017**. [CrossRef] [PubMed]
12. Wang, T.J.; Larson, M.G.; Vasan, R.S.; Cheng, S.; Rhee, E.P.; McCabe, E.; Lewis, G.D.; Fox, C.S.; Jacques, P.F.; Fernandez, C.; et al. Metabolite profiles and the risk of developing diabetes. *Nat. Med.* **2011**, *17*, 448–453. [CrossRef] [PubMed]
13. He, F.; Wu, C.; Li, P.; Li, N.; Zhang, D.; Zhu, Q.; Ren, W.; Peng, Y. Functions and signaling pathways of amino acids in intestinal inflammation. *Biomed. Res. Int.* **2018**. [CrossRef] [PubMed]
14. Shiomi, Y.; Nishiumi, S.; Ooi, M.; Hatano, N.; Shinohara, M.; Yoshie, T.; Kondo, Y.; Furumatsu, K.; Shiomi, H.; Kutsumi, H.; et al. GCMS-based metabolomic study in mice with colitis induced by dextran sulfate sodium. *Inflamm. Bowel Dis.* **2011**, *17*, 2261–2274. [CrossRef] [PubMed]
15. Hisamatsu, T.; Okamoto, S.; Hashimoto, M.; Muramatsu, T.; Andou, A.; Uo, M.; Kitazume, M.T.; Matsuoka, K.; Yajima, T.; Inoue, N.; et al. Novel, objective, multivariate biomarkers composed of plasma amino acid profiles for the diagnosis and assessment of inflammatory bowel disease. *PLoS ONE* **2012**, *7*, e31131. [CrossRef] [PubMed]
16. Ooi, M.; Nishiumi, S.; Yoshie, T.; Shiomi, Y.; Kohashi, M.; Fukunaga, K.; Nakamura, S.; Matsumoto, T.; Hatano, N.; Shinohara, M.; et al. GC/MS-based profiling of amino acids and TCA cycle-related molecules in ulcerative colitis. *Inflamm. Res.* **2011**, *60*, 831–840. [CrossRef] [PubMed]
17. Zhang, Y.; Lin, L.; Xu, Y.; Lin, Y.; Jin, Y.; Zheng, C. 1H NMR-based spectroscopy detects metabolic alterations in serum of patients with early-stage ulcerative colitis. *Biochem. Biophys. Res. Commun.* **2013**, *433*, 547–551. [CrossRef] [PubMed]
18. Noguchi, Y.; Zhang, Q.W.; Sugimoto, T.; Furuhata, Y.; Sakai, R.; Mori, M.; Takahashi, M.; Kimura, T. Network analysis of plasma and tissue amino acids and the generation of an amino index for potential diagnostic use. *Am. J. Clin. Nutr.* **2016**, *83*, 513S–519S. [CrossRef] [PubMed]
19. Kaliora, A.C.; Mylona, A.; Chiou, A.; Petsios, D.G.; Andrikopoulos, N.K. Detection and identification of simple phenolics in pistacia lentiscus resin. *J. Liq. Chromatogr. Relat. Technol.* **2004**, *27*. [CrossRef]
20. Assimopoulou, A.N.; Papageorgiou, V.P. GC-MS analysis of penta- and tetra-cyclic triterpenes from resins of Pistacia species. Part I. Pistacia lentiscus var. Chia. *Biomed. Chromatogr.* **2005**, *19*, 285–311. [CrossRef] [PubMed]
21. Paraschos, S.; Magiatis, P.; Mitakou, S.; Petraki, K.; Kalliaropoulos, A.; Maragkoudakis, P.; Mentis, A.; Sgouras, D.; Skaltsounis, A.L. In vitro and in vivo activities of Chios mastic gum extracts and constituents against Helicobacter pylori. *Antimicrob. Agents Chemother.* **2007**, *51*, 551–559. [CrossRef] [PubMed]
22. Papada, E.; Gioxari, A.; Brieudes, V.; Amerikanou, C.; Halabalaki, M.; Skaltsounis, A.L.; Smyrnioudis, I.; Kaliora, A.C. Bioavailability of terpenes and postprandial effect on human antioxidant potential. An open–label study in healthy subjects. *Mol. Nutr. Food Res.* **2018**, *62*. [CrossRef]
23. Dedoussis, G.V.; Kaliora, A.C.; Psarras, S.; Chiou, A.; Mylona, A.; Papadopoulos, N.G.; Andrikopoulos, N.K. Antiatherogenic effect of Pistacia lentiscus via GSH restoration and downregulation of CD36 mRNA expression. *Atherosclerosis* **2004**, *174*, 293–303. [CrossRef] [PubMed]
24. Heo, C.; Kim, S.W.; Kim, K.J.; Kim, D.W.; Kim, H.J.; Do, J.H.; Chang, S.K. Protective effects of mastic in non- steroidal anti-inflammatory drug induced gut damage and bacterial translocation in a rat model. *Korean J. Med.* **2006**, *71*, 354–361.

25. Kartalis, A.; Didagelos, M.; Georgiadis, I.; Benetos, G.; Smyrnioudis, N.; Marmaras, H.; Voutas, P.; Zotika, C.; Garoufalis, S.; Andrikopoulos, G. Effects of Chios mastic gum on cholesterol and glucose levels of healthy volunteers: A prospective, randomised, placebo-controlled, pilot study (CHIOS-MASTIHA). *Eur. J. Prev. Cardiol.* **2016**, *23*, 722–729. [CrossRef] [PubMed]
26. Kaliora, A.C.; Stathopoulou, M.G.; Triantafillidis, J.K.; Dedoussis, G.V.; Andrikopoulos, N.K. Alterations in the function of circulating mononuclear cells derived from patients with Crohn's disease treated with mastic. *World J. Gastroenterol.* **2007**, *13*, 6031–6036. [PubMed]
27. Kaliora, A.C.; Stathopoulou, M.G.; Triantafillidis, J.K.; Dedoussis, G.V.; Andrikopoulos, N.K. Chios mastic treatment of patients with active Crohn's disease. *World J. Gastroenterol.* **2007**, *13*, 748–753. [CrossRef] [PubMed]
28. EMA. Committee on Herbal Medicinal Products European Union Herbal Monograph on *Pistacia lentiscus* L., Resin (Mastix). London, UK, 2015. Available online: http://www.ema.europa.eu/docs/en_GB/document_library/Herbal_-_Herbal_monograph/2015/07/WC500190099.pdf (accessed on 8 January 2018).
29. Papada, E.; Gioxari, A.; Amerikanou, C.; Forbes, A.; Tzavara, C.; Smyrnioudis, I.; Kaliora, A.C. Regulation of faecal biomarkers in inflammatory bowel disease patients treated with oral mastiha (*Pistacia lentiscus*) supplement: A double-blind and placebo-controlled randomised trial. *Phytother. Res.* **2018**. [CrossRef]
30. Papada, E.; Torović, L.; Amerikanou, C.; Kalogeropoulos, N.; Smyrnioudis, I.; Kaliora, A.C. Modulation of free amino acid profile in healthy humans administered with mastiha terpenes. An open-label trial. *Nutrients* **2018**, *10*, 715. [CrossRef] [PubMed]
31. Li, P.; Yin, Y.L.; Li, D.; Kim, S.W.; Wu, G. Amino acids and immune function. *Br. J. Nutr.* **2007**, *98*, 237–252. [CrossRef] [PubMed]
32. Nakaya, M.; Xiao, Y.; Zhou, X.; Chang, J.H.; Chang, M.; Cheng, X.; Blonska, M.; Lin, X.; Sun, S.C. Inflammatory T cell responses rely on amino acid transporter ASCT2 facilitation of glutamine uptake and mTORC1 kinase activation. *Immunity* **2014**, *40*, 692–705. [CrossRef] [PubMed]
33. Harvey, R.F.; Bradshaw, J.M. A simple index of Crohn's-disease activity. *Lancet* **1980**, *8167*, 514. [CrossRef]
34. Lewis, J.D.; Chuai, S.; Nessel, L.; Lichtenstein, G.R.; Aberra, F.N.; Ellenberg, J.H. Use of the noninvasive components of the Mayo score to assess clinical response in ulcerative colitis. *Inflamm. Bowel Dis.* **2008**, *14*, 1660–1666. [CrossRef] [PubMed]
35. Aurrekoetxea, I.; Ruiz-Sanz, J.I.; del Agua, A.R.; Navarro, R.; Hernández, M.L.; Matorras, R.; Prieto, B.; Ruiz-Larrea, M.B. Serum oxidizability and antioxidant status in patients undergoing in vitro fertilization. *Fertil. Steril.* **2010**, *94*, 1279–1286. [CrossRef] [PubMed]
36. Gioxari, A.; Kaliora, A.C.; Papalois, A.; Agrogiannis, G.; Triantafillidis, J.K.; Andrikopoulos, N.K. Pistacia lentiscus resin regulates intestinal damage and inflammation in trinitrobenzene sulfonic acid-induced colitis. *J. Med. Food.* **2011**, *14*, 1403–1411. [CrossRef] [PubMed]
37. EFSA Panel on Dietetic Products, Nutrition and Allergies (NDA). Guidance on the scientific requirements for health claims related to antioxidants, oxidative damage and cardiovascular health. *EFSA J.* **2011**, *9*, 474. [CrossRef]
38. Grip, O.; Janciauskiene, S.; Lindgren, S. Circulating monocytes and plasma inflammatory biomarkers in active Crohn's disease: Elevated oxidised low-density lipoprotein and the anti-inflammatory effect of atorvastatin. *Inflamm. Bowel Dis.* **2004**, *10*, 193–200. [CrossRef] [PubMed]
39. Rezaie, A.; Parker, R.D.; Abdollahi, M. Oxidative stress and pathogenesis of inflammatory bowel disease: An epiphenomenon or the cause? *Dig. Dis. Sci.* **2007**, *52*, 2015–2021. [CrossRef] [PubMed]
40. Beltran, B.; Nos, P.; Dasi, F.; Iborra, M.; Bastida, G.; Martinez, M.; O'Connor, J.E.; Saez, G.; Moret, I.; Ponce, J. Mitochondrial dysfunction, persistent oxidative damage, and catalase inhibition in immune cells of naive and treated Crohn's disease. *Inflamm. Bowel Dis.* **2010**, *16*, 76–86. [CrossRef] [PubMed]
41. Iborra, M.; Moret, I.; Rausell, F.; Bastida, G.; Aguas, M.; Cerrillo, E.; Nos, P.; Beltran, B. Role of oxidative stress and antioxidant enzymes in Crohn's disease. *Biochem. Soc. Trans.* **2011**, *39*, 1102–1106. [CrossRef] [PubMed]
42. Moret-Tatay, I.; Iborra, M.; Cerrillo, E.; Tortosa, L.; Nos, P.; Beltran, B. Possible biomarkers in blood for Crohn's disease: Oxidative stress and microRNAs-current evidences and further aspects to unravel. *Oxid. Med. Cell Longev.* **2016**, *2016*. [CrossRef] [PubMed]
43. Huang, H.; Mai, W.; Liu, D.; Hao, Y.; Tao, J.; Dong, Y. The oxidation ratio of LDL: A predictor for coronary artery disease. *Dis. Mark.* **2008**, *24*, 341–349. [CrossRef]

44. Motamed, M.; Nargesi, A.A.; Heidari, B.; Mirmiranpour, H.; Esteghamati, A.; Nakhjavani, M. Oxidized low-lensity Lipoprotein (ox-LDL) to LDL Ratio (ox-LDL/LDL) and ox-LDL to high-density lipoprotein ratio (ox-LDL/HDL). *Clin. Lab.* **2016**, *62*, 1609–1617. [CrossRef] [PubMed]
45. Gradinaru, D.; Borsa, C.; Ionescu, C.; Margina, D. Advanced oxidative and glycoxidative protein damage markers in the elderly with type 2 diabetes. *J. Proteom.* **2013**, *92*, 313–322. [CrossRef] [PubMed]
46. Harmon, M.E.; Campen, M.J.; Miller, C.; Shuey, C.; Cajero, M.; Lucas, S.; Pacheco, B.; Erdei, E.; Ramone, S.; Nez, T.; et al. Associations of circulating oxidized LDL and conventional biomarkers of cardiovascular disease in a cross-sectional study of the Navajo population. *PLoS ONE* **2016**, *11*, e0143102. [CrossRef] [PubMed]
47. Atkuri, K.R.; Mantovani, J.J.; Herzenberg, L.A.; Herzenberg, L.A. N-Acetylcysteine—A safe antidote for cysteine/glutathione deficiency. *Curr. Opin. Pharmacol.* **2007**, *7*, 355–359. [CrossRef] [PubMed]
48. Forrest, C.M.; Mackay, G.M.; Stoy, N.; Egerton, M.; Christofides, J.; Stone, T.W.; Darlington, L.G. Tryptophan loading induces oxidative stress. *Free Radic. Res.* **2004**, *38*, 1167–1171. [CrossRef] [PubMed]
49. Krishnan, N.; Dickman, M.B.; Becker, D.F. Proline modulates the intracellular redox environment and protects mammalian cells against oxidative stress. *Free Radic. Biol. Med.* **2008**, *44*, 671–681. [CrossRef] [PubMed]
50. Katayama, S.; Mine, Y. Antioxidative activity of amino acids on tissue oxidative stress in human intestinal epithelial cell model. *J. Agric. Food Chem.* **2007**, *55*, 8458–8464. [CrossRef] [PubMed]
51. Son, D.O.; Satsu, H.; Shimizu, M. Histidine inhibits oxidative stress- and TNF-alpha-induced interleukin-8 secretion in intestinal epithelial cells. *FEBS Lett.* **2005**, *579*, 4671–4677. [CrossRef] [PubMed]

5

Synbiotic Supplementation Containing Whole Plant Sugar Cane Fibre and Probiotic Spores Potentiates Protective Synergistic Effects in Mouse Model of IBD

Tanvi Shinde [1,2,*], Agampodi Promoda Perera [2], Ravichandra Vemuri [2], Shakuntla V. Gondalia [3], Avinash V. Karpe [4], David J. Beale [4], Sonia Shastri [2], Benjamin Southam [2], Rajaraman Eri [2] and Roger Stanley [1,*]

1 Centre for Food Safety and Innovation, Tasmanian Institute of Agriculture, University of Tasmania, Launceston, TAS 7250, Australia

2 School of Health Sciences, College of Health and Medicine, University of Tasmania, Launceston, TAS 7250, Australia; agampodi.perera@utas.edu.au (A.P.P.); ravichandra.vemuri@utas.edu.au (R.V.); sonia.shastri@utas.edu.au (S.S.); benjamin.southam@utas.edu.au (B.S.); rajaraman.eri@utas.edu.au (R.E.)

3 Centre for Human Psychopharmacology, Swinburne University of Technology, Hawthorn, VIC 3122, Australia; sgondalia@swin.edu.au

4 Land and Water, Commonwealth Scientific and Industrial Research Organization (CSIRO), Ecosciences Precinct, Dutton Park, QLD 4102, Australia; Avinash.Karpe@csiro.au (A.V.K.); David.Beale@csiro.au (D.J.B.)

* Correspondence: tanvi.shinde@utas.edu.au (T.S.); roger.stanley@utas.edu.au (R.S.)

Abstract: Inflammatory bowel diseases (IBD) are a chronic inflammatory disorders with increasing global incidence. Synbiotic, which is a two-point approach carrying probiotic and prebiotic components in mitigating inflammation in IBD, is thought to be a pragmatic approach owing to the synergistic outcomes. In this study, the impacts of dietary supplementation with probiotic *Bacillus coagulans* MTCC5856 spores (*B. coagulans*) and prebiotic whole plant sugar cane fibre (PSCF) was assessed using a murine model of IBD. Eight-week-old C57BL/6 mice were fed a normal chow diet supplemented with either *B. coagulans*, PSCF or its synbiotic combination. After seven days of supplementation, colitis was induced with dextran sulfate sodium (DSS) in drinking water for seven days during the continuation of the supplemented diets. Synbiotic supplementation ameliorated disease activity index and histological score (−72%, 7.38, respectively), more effectively than either *B. coagulans* (−47%, 10.1) and PSCF (−53%, 13.0) alone. Synbiotic supplementation also significantly ($p < 0.0001$) prevented the expression of tight junction proteins and modulated the altered serum IL-1β (−40%), IL-10 (+26%), and C-reactive protein (CRP) (−39%) levels. Synbiotic supplementations also raised the short-chain fatty acids (SCFA) profile more extensively compared to the unsupplemented DSS-control. The synbiotic health outcome effect of the probiotic and prebiotic combinations may be associated with a synergistic direct immune-regulating efficacy of the components, their ability to protect epithelial integrity, stimulation of probiotic spores by the prebiotic fibre, and/or with stimulation of greater levels of fermentation of fibres releasing SCFAs that mediate the reduction in colonic inflammation. Our model findings suggest synbiotic supplementation should be tested in clinical trials.

Keywords: synbiotic; prebiotic; probiotic; IBD; *Bacillus* spores; dietary fibre; sugar cane fibre; ulcerative colitis

1. Introduction

Inflammatory bowel disease (IBD) is a chronic relapsing inflammatory condition of the gastrointestinal tract that comprises two partially overlapping but distinct clinical entities: Crohn's disease (CD) that involves the entire gastrointestinal tract and ulcerative colitis (UC) that is limited to colon and rectum [1]. The incidence of CD and UC has become a global disease with accelerating incidence in countries adopting a Westernised diet, highlighting the urgent need for research into prevention and management of this complex and costly pathology [2]. Although the aetiology and pathogenesis of IBD still remains unclear, emerging evidence supports the involvement of a recurrent tripartite pathophysiological circuit encompassing gut dysbiosis, altered epithelial integrity and defective immune responses [1]. Therefore, preventive and therapeutic approaches that impede or break this inflammatory circuit by resolving one or more of the pathophysiological circuit components are highly sought.

Dietary interventions are increasingly perceived as both preventive and corrective strategies to normalise the dysfunctional microbiome, altered immune and barrier integrity functions to normality in IBD [3–5]. In this regard, probiotic and prebiotic dietary fibres (DF) are thought to be useful in mitigating the inflammatory circuit thereby resolving or preventing the severity of IBD. Both bioactive ingredients can improve inflammatory parameters in the gut by modifying microbiota composition and metabolites, regulating secretion of immunomodulatory molecules and protecting the colonic epithelial barrier [1,6–8]. Synbiotics, being a combination of probiotic and prebiotic ingredients that positively interact, potentially offer prophylactic and therapeutic effects that could function synergistically to confer health benefits to the host.

DFs have shown particular promise in attenuating colonic inflammation in humans [9]. Meanwhile, the underlying mechanisms are likely to be multifactorial: they include dilution of toxins via stool bulking and the production of metabolites, particularly short-chain fatty acids (SCFA), as a result of microbial fermentation is frequently cited as a major potential contributor to the protective effect [10]. DFs consist of edible plant parts that resist digestion and absorption in the small intestine and undergo complete or partial fermentation in the colon. It is an extremely complex group of substances, including non-starch polysaccharides, resistant starch, cellulose and hemicellulose, oligosaccharides, pectins, gums, lignin, and waxes [11]. Much work on DFs, however, has examined various purified ingredients that represent limited chemical complexity, contrasting to those that naturally occur in fruits and vegetables [12]. Nevertheless, the biochemical complexity of DFs is recently being more appreciated to be a vital factor influencing the gut microbial complexity [12–14]. This highlights the prudence of application of prebiotic fibres that are representative of whole plant vegetables and fruits, prepared to retain fibre biochemical complexity. In this context, a process to produce sugar cane fibre by wet diffusion to remove most of the sucrose from cut cane, which is then dried and ground into a flour, has been reported to preserve the cell wall components and retain other intrinsic nutritional biologically active components [15,16]. Such fibre, in addition to retaining other micronutrients and polyphenols, also contains both soluble and insoluble benefits as well as rapid- and poor-fermentable fibres and at ratios that more accurately represent natural whole plant foods. In a recent study, such sugar cane fibre has been shown to impart positive effects on human gut microbiota in vitro [17]. The high content of total dietary fibre (87%) was accounted for with respect to its positive effect in this study. The relative similarity of this sugar cane fibre product to that in other whole plant foods indicates its potential as a convenient supplementary source of dietary fibre that could alter microbial ecology and have a positive influence for IBD attenuation.

Bacillus coagulans is a GRAS (generally recognised as safe) affirmed probiotic that can ferment a variety of plant substrates rich in insoluble cell wall components [18,19] more efficiently than most members of gut microbiota [20,21]. It is also known to be capable of modulating the innate immune system by binding and interacting with the gastrointestinal tract epithelium [22,23]. This makes it a suitable probiotic for its synbiotic combination with prebiotic whole plant sugar cane fibre (PSCF) rich in insoluble cell wall fractions. Probiotic *Bacillus coagulans* MTCC (Microbial Type Culture

Collection) 5856 spores in addition to exhibiting excellent immunomodulatory effects in vitro, have shown significant survival during simulated gastric transit with substantial adhesion capacity to human colonic epithelial cells [22]. Based on the aforementioned findings, we hypothesised that preconditioning with probiotic *B. coagulans* MTCC 5856 spores, prebiotic PSCF and its synbiotic combination might repress the onset and/or severity of DSS-induced colitis in mice. This study aimed to evaluate the efficacy of probiotic *B. coagulans* spores and PSCF, both alone and in combination as synbiotic to ameliorate the onset of experimental colitis in mice and further examine its underlying mechanisms.

2. Materials and Methods

2.1. Probiotic Bacteria and Prebiotic Dietary Fibre

LactoSpore® (Sabinsa Corporation, East Windsor, NJ, USA) containing the probiotic strain *Bacillus coagulans* MTCC 5856 (6×10^9 spores/gm) was produced by Sami Labs Limited (Bangalore, India) and supplied by Sabinsa Corporation (Australia). Kfibre™, prebiotic whole plant sugar cane fibre (PSCF) was supplied by KFSU Pty Ltd., Queensland, Australia.

2.2. Animals

Fifty C57BL/6J (seven week old) mice of both sexes of average weight 19g were obtained from the University of Tasmania animal breeding facility and housed in a temperature-controlled environment with a 12-h day/night light cycle. Individual body weights were assessed daily including over an initial acclimation period of seven days. All mice had ad libitum access to radiation-sterilised rodent feed pellets (Barastoc Rat and Mouse, Ridley AgProducts, Melbourne, Victoria, Australia) and autoclaved tap water for drinking during experiments. All animal experiments were approved by the Animal Ethics Committee of the University of Tasmania (ethics approval number: A0015840) and conducted in accordance with the Australian Code of Practice for Care and Use of Animals for Scientific Purposes (8th Edition, 2013). All efforts were made to minimize animals' suffering and to reduce the number of animals used.

2.3. Study Design and Treatments

Following one week of acclimation, mice at eight weeks of age were randomly allocated into the following five groups ($n = 10$ per group): (1) Healthy control (HC), (2) DSS-control, (3) probiotic *B. coagulans* MTCC 5856 spores (*B. coagulans*), (4) whole plant prebiotic sugar cane fibre (PSCF) supplement, and (5) synbiotic combined supplement. Mice in HC and DSS-control groups received 4 g chow mash (standard chow pellet blended with water). The *B. coagulans* group received 4 g chow mash supplemented with probiotic *B. coagulans* MTCC 5856 spores (2×10^9 CFU/day/mouse). The PSCF group received 4g chow mash supplemented with Kfibre™ (200 mg/day/mouse). Synbiotic treatment group mice received 4 g chow, each supplemented with *B. coagulans* MTCC 5856 spores (2×10^9 CFU/ day/mouse) and Kfibre (200 mg/day/mouse). The chow mash was prepared fresh each day. The mice were single-caged throughout the experiment to measure the defined daily intake of respective treatments from prepared chow mash. The mice were fed these treatments for 14 days. Colitis was induced during the last seven days of the experimental period as previously described [24], by administering 2% dextran sulfate sodium (DSS; MP Biomedicals, colitis grade average molecular weight: 36,000–50,000) in the drinking water of all groups except for the non-colitic DSS-control mice which received normal drinking water. Mice were sacrificed on day 15 by CO_2 asphyxiation.

2.4. Clinical Scoring and Histological Analysis

A Disease Activity Index (DAI) was determined daily in all mice by scoring for body weight, hemocult reactivity or presence of gross blood and stool consistency during the week of DSS induction, as detailed in [25]. Stool was collected from individual mice and tested for the presence of blood using

Hemoccult II slides (Beckman Coulter Inc., Brea, CA, USA). Briefly, the following parameters were used for calculation: (a) body weight loss (score 0 = 0%, score 1 = 1–5%, score 2 = 6–10%, score 3 = 11–15%); (b) stool consistency (score 0 = normal, score 1 = soft but still formed, score 2 = very soft/loose stool, score 3 = diarrhoea/watery stool); and (c) blood in stool (score 0 = negative hemoccult, score 1 = positive hemoccult, score 2 = Blood traces in stool visible, score 3 = rectal bleeding). DAI was determined by combining the scores from these three categories. Body weights were measured for each animal throughout the experiments and expressed as percent weight loss to the weight immediately before DSS treatment. Fecal samples were collected and stored at −80 °C on day 14 for metabolite analysis.

After sacrificing the mice, the colons were removed from the caecum to the anus following the method of Perera et al. [26]. The length of the colons from the ileocaecal junction to the rectum were recorded. The colon was subsequently opened along its longitudinal axis and the luminal (mucosal) contents were removed using sterilised 200 μL pipette tips prior to weighing the organ. The length and weight of colon and spleen were documented. Spleen weight, colon length, and colon weight/body weight ratio were calculated as macroscopic markers of inflammation. The mucosal and cecal contents were collected for metabolite profiling and stored at −80 °C. The colon was bisected longitudinally, and one half was prepared using the Swiss roll technique [27] whereas the remaining colonic tissue was dissected out, segregated into proximal colon (PC) and distal colon (DC) and snap-frozen for molecular analyses. Swiss rolls underwent 24 h fixation in 10% (*v/v*) neutral-buffered formalin. Swiss rolls were subsequently transferred to 70% ethanol prior to progressive dehydration, clearing and infiltration with HistoPrep paraffin wax (Fisher Scientific, Philadelphia, PA, USA). Swiss rolls were then embedded in wax and 5 μm sections were cut using a rotary microtome. Sections were stained with haematoxylin and eosin (H and E; HD Scientific, Sydney, Australia). Slides stained with H and E (n = 8 per group) graded blindly for the severity of tissue damage at distal and proximal regions as described previously [28,29]. Briefly, frequency of distribution of inflammation graded 0-3, crypt architectural distortion and ulceration graded 0–5, tissue damage graded 0-3, inflammatory infiltrate graded 0–3, goblet cell loss graded 0–3, mucosal thickening (oedema) were graded 0–3. All images were captured on a Leica DM500 microscope using a Leica ICC50 W camera (Leica Microsys-tems, Wetzlar, Germany).

2.5. Alcian Blue Staining

DSS-induced alterations in goblet cells and subsequent depletion in synthesis and secretion of mucin glycoprotein (MUC2) was analysed by Alcian blue staining (ab150662 Alcian Blue, pH 2.5 (Mucin Stain), Abcam, Australia) following the manufacturer's instructions. Briefly, paraffin-embedded colon sections (n = 4/group) were stained with Alcian blue, staining the acidic sulphated mucin blue and the counterstained with Safranin O, staining the nuclei red following the method previously described [30]. Computer-assisted image analysis was performed with a Leica DM500 microscope (Leica Microsystems, Wet-zlar, Germany) and Leica ICC50 W camera (Leica Microsys-tems, Wetzlar, Germany). The staining intensity (IOD) was assessed using Image Pro Plus 7.0 (Media Cybernetics, Inc., Rockville, MD, USA) and used for comparison among groups [31].

2.6. Immunohistochemical Detection of Tight Junction Proteins

Immunohistochemical detection of epithelial tight junction (TJ) proteins was performed using a Rabbit specific HRP/DAB (ABC) Detection IHC kit (ab64261, Abcam, Australia) following the manufacturer's instruction and as previously described [32]. Following removal of paraffin and rehydration, the tissue sections were exposed to heat-induced epitope retrieval (4 min at 121 °C) in a sodium citrate buffer, pH 6 in a Decloaking chamber (Biocare Medical, Pachico, CA, USA). After washing the slides in 1× phosphate buffered saline (PBS) 2 mins/wash, endogenous peroxidase activity was blocked by incubating the slides with hydrogen peroxide block for 10 min. Next, the slides were washed with PBS (2 × 2 min) washes and protein block was then applied for 30 min at room temperature to block non-specific background staining. Following PBS (1 × 2 min) wash, colon sections were then incubated with primary antibodies: anti-ZO-1 (NBP1-85046, Novus Biologicals, Australia,

1:400); anti-occludin (NBP1-87402, Novus, 1:600); anti-claudin-1 (NBP1-77036, Novus, 1 μg/mL) overnight at 4 °C. Sections were then washed with PBS (4 × 2 min) and biotinylated goat anti-rabbit IgG was applied and incubated for 10 min at room temperature. At the end of incubation, the slides were washed in PBS (4 × 2 min) and streptavidin peroxidase was applied to the sections and further incubated for 10 at room temperature. The slides were then thoroughly rinsed with PBS (4 × 2 min) before sections were covered with 3,3′-diaminobenzidine (DAB) chromogen and substrate solution for 10 min. Tissue sections were subsequently counterstained with hematoxylin, dehydrated, and mounted with DPX media (Sigma-Aldrich, Sydney, Australia).

Computer-assisted image analysis was performed with a Leica DM500 microscope (Leica Microsystems, Wet-zlar, Germany), Leica ICC50 W camera (Leica Microsys-tems, Wetzlar, Germany), and Image Pro Plus 7.0 (Media Cybernetics, Inc., Rockville, MD, USA) software. The expression of tight junction proteins (TJPs): ZO-1, occludin and claudin-1 was blindly assessed by choosing random five fields on each slide (n = 4/group). Barrier TJ protein expressions and staining intensity in colonic epithelium was expressed as the percentage expression of a respective TJ protein.

2.7. *Myeloperoxidase Activity*

The extent of the inflammatory cell invasion in the colon was examined by the assessment of myeloperoxidase (MPO) activity [24]. Weighed and snap frozen PC and DC specimens (n = 3) were analysed for MPO activity using a Myeloperoxidase Activity Assay kit (ab105136, colorimetric, Abcam®, Cambridge, UK). Briefly, frozen tissue after washing in cold PBS, was resuspended in MPO assay buffer, before homogenisation with 10–15 passes using an Omni TH tissue homogeniser (Omni International, US) with 10–15 passes. The homogenate was then centrifuged at 13,000× g (10 min) and the supernatant assayed for MPO activity as per the manufacturer's instructions. The values are expressed as MPO activity units/g tissue.

2.8. *Tissue Explant Culture and Cytokine Measurements*

PC and DC colon tissues of mice from each group were cut, weighed and washed with cold PBS before transferring to a 12 well plate containing 0.5 mL/well of RPMI1640 culture medium (In Vitro Technologies Pty Ltd, Melbourne, Australia) supplemented with 10% *v/v* fetal calf serum (Gibco, Life Technologies Pty Ltd, Melbourne, Australia), penicillin (100 mU/L), and streptomycin (100 mg/L) (Sigma-Aldrich Pty Ltd, Sydney, Australia) as described previously [26]. After 24 h of incubation, supernatant was collected from each well, centrifuged and stored at −80 °C until further analysis. Serum was collected from blood drawn by cardiac puncture at the end of the study for cytokine analysis.

The cytokine levels in colon tissue (n = 3) and serum (n = 3) were determined by immunoassay using a Bio-Plex Pro Mouse cytokine 23-plex kit (Bio-Rad #M60009RDPD, Bio-Rad Laboratories, Gladesville, NSW, Australia) following the manufacturer's instructions and concentrations analysed using a Bio-Plex 200 instrument (Bio-Rad) and Bioplex Manager software, version 6 (Bio-Rad Laboratories) respectively. For tissues, the cytokine levels were normalized by dividing the cytokine results (pg/mL) by the measured biopsy weight (g). The most significantly altered cytokines are presented as pg/g of tissue.

2.9. *iNOS Activity*

The expression of inducible isoform of nitric oxide synthase (iNOS) in colonic epithelial cells in response to pro-inflammatory stimuli [33] was determined in PC and DC specimens using a Nitic Oxide Synthase Activity Assay kit (ab211084, Fluorometric, Abcam®, Cambridge, UK). Snap frozen proximal and distal colonic tissues (n = 3) were washed in in cold PBS and resuspended in 200 μL NOS assay buffer then homogenised by 10–15 passes of an Omni TH tissue homogeniser (Omni International, Tulsa, OK, USA). The homogenate was then centrifuged at 10,000× g (10 min, 4 °C) and the supernatant then underwent iNOS activity assay activity assay as per the manufacturer's instructions. The amount of protein in the lysate was determined using DC™ Protein Assay (Bio-Rad Laboratories, Australia). The results are expressed as iNOS activity mU/mg.

2.10. Serum C-Reactive Protein Analysis

The levels of C-reactive protein (CRP) in serum from respective groups (n = 3 samples/group) were analysed using Mouse C-Reactive Protein/CRP Quantikine Elisa kit (MCRP00, R and D Systems, Australia) following the manufacturer's instructions. The results are expressed as μg/mL.

2.11. Volatile SCFA Analysis

Cecal, mucosal and fecal samples (n = 5 per group) were prepared and derivatized following the protocol developed by Furuhashi et al. [34] with some modifications. Briefly, cecal, mucosal and fecal samples of 100–150 mg fresh weight (stored at −80 °C) were weighed to ± 0.1 mg accuracy. These samples were added to a sterile 1.5 mL bead-beating tube (NAVY Rino Lysis tubes, Next Advance, Troy, NY, USA). A 1.0 mL aliquot isobutanol (10% MilliQ water), (LC-MS grade, Merck, Castle Hill, NSW, Australia) was added to each sample, followed by two 30 s, 4000 rpm homogenization pulses sandwiched between a 20-s pause interval (Precellys Evolution Homogenizer, Bertin Instruments, Montigny-le-Bretonneux, France). The samples were subsequently centrifuged at 16,000× g for 6 min.

The supernatant (675 μL) was transferred to a clean round bottomed 2 mL centrifuge tube (Eppendorf South Pacific Pty. Ltd., Macquarie Park, NSW, Australia) and NaOH (20 mM, 125 μL, Merck Pty Ltd., Castle Hill, NSW, Australia) and chloroform (400 μL, LC-MS grade, Merck Pty Ltd.,) were added. The samples were briefly vortexed and centrifuged at 16,000·g for 3 min. The aqueous phase (upper layer, 400 μL) was transferred to a new clean round bottomed 2 mL centrifuge tube (Eppendorf South Pacific Pty. Ltd., Macquarie Park, NSW, Australia) containing a boiling chip (Sigma Aldrich, Castle Hill, NSW, Australia). Pyridine (100μL), isobutanol (80 μL) (both LC-MS grade, Sigma Aldrich, Castle Hill, NSW, Australia), and MilliQ (Millipore Corporation) water (70 μL) were added and the samples were subjected to gentle hand vortexing (swirling action) followed by the addition of 50 μL isobutyl chloroformate (98% purity, Sigma Aldrich, Castle Hill, NSW, Australia). The tube was kept opened to release any generated gases and was allowed to stand for about one minute. Hexane (150 μL, LC-MS grade, Sigma Aldrich, Castle Hill, NSW, Australia) was then added to each tube, which was then capped and vortexed prior to centrifugation at 15,700× g for 4 min. The upper phase (100 μL) was subsequently transferred to clean gas chromatography (GC) autosampler vial fitted with silanized low volume glass inserts; Malathion (1 μL, equivalent to 2.5 μg dry weight) was added as an internal standard.

The GC-MS analysis was performed on an Agilent 6890B GC oven coupled to a 5977B mass spectrometer (MS) detector (Agilent Technologies, Mulgrave, VIC, Australia) fitted with an MPS autosampler (Gerstel GmbH & Co.KG, Mülheim an der Ruhr, Germany). The GC oven was fitted with two 15 m HP-5MS columns (0.25 mm ID and 0.25 μm film thickness; 19091S-431 UI (Ultra Inert), Agilent Technologies, VIC, Australia) coupled to each other through a purged ultimate union (PUU) for the use of post-run backflushing. The sample (1.0 μL) was introduced via a multimode inlet (MMI) operated in split mode (1:20). The column was maintained at 40 °C for 5 min, followed by an increase to 250 °C at a rate of 10 °C/min. This was followed by a second increment to 310 °C at a rate of 60 °C/min. The column was held at 310 °C for 1 min. The mass spectrometer was kept in extractor ion mode (EI mode) at 70 eV. The GC-MS ion source temperature and transfer line were kept at 250 °C and 280 °C, respectively. Detector voltage was kept at 1054 V. The MS detector was turned off for the first 3 min and, at 4.0–4.8 min and 12.5–13.2-min time windows until the excess derivatization reagent (chloroformate/hexane solvents) were eluted from the column. This ensured that the source filament was not saturated and damaged. The scan range was kept in the range of m/z 35–350 (35–350 Daltons). Data acquisition and spectral analysis were performed as described in a previous study [35] and qualitative identification of metabolites was performed according to the Metabolomics Standard Initiative (MSI) chemical analysis workgroup [36] using standard GC-MS reference metabolite libraries (NIST 17, and an in-house CF-based metabolomics library developed after Smart et al. [37] with the use of Kovats retention indices based on a reference n-alkane standard (C8-C40 Alkanes Calibration Standard, Sigma-Aldrich, Castle Hill, NSW, Australia).

2.12. Metabolic Phenotyping Analysis

Untargeted metabolomic profiling of cecal, mucosal and fecal samples (n = 5 per group) were performed using GC-MS analysis as described previously [35].

2.13. Statistical Analysis

The samples in the study were randomly chosen for all the analysis to avoid bias. All data are presented as means ± standard error of the mean (SEM). The statistical analysis was performed with the use of GraphPad Prism Software (Version 7.0, San Diego, CA, USA) The data were evaluated using One-way analysis of variance (ANOVA) followed by Tukey's post-hoc test to determine statistical differences between the groups against the DSS-control samples. For the analysis of DAI and body weight changes during the experimental period, two-way ANOVA followed by Tukey's post-hoc test was used, setting treatment and the time as the variables. A p-value of < 0.05 was considered significant.

3. Results

3.1. Effects of B. Coagulans, PSCF and Synbiotic Supplementation on DAI and Macroscopic Inflammatory Markers in DSS-Induced Mice

In comparison with the HC group, the administration of probiotic, prebiotic and synbiotic treatments in the respective groups did not show any sign of toxicity, which was evaluated by body weight increase, food intake and general appearance of the animals. DAI (cumulative score for body weight change, stool consistency and blood in feces) was evaluated to determine the efficacy of the treatments in reducing the severity of disease symptoms in DSS-induced colitis (Figure 1A). Compared with the DSS-control group that showed severe colitis symptoms, pre-conditioning with *B. coagulans*, PSCF and synbiotic combination significantly reduced the DAI levels as early as day2 until the end of experiment. At the end of the experiment, DAI of DSS-control group was significantly high (5.8 ± 0.5) ($p \leq 0.0001$) compared with that of *B. coagulans* (3.1 ± 0.6, 47% reduction), PSCF (2.7 ± 0.5, 53% reduction), and synbiotic (1.6 ± 0.2, 72% reduction) groups. DSS induction in DSS-control mice resulted in significant body weight loss until the end of experiment (−4.13 ± 1.4%). In contrast, mice maintained healthy body weight gain with *Bacillus* (2.84 ± 1.7%), PSCF (4.25 ± 1.0%), and synbiotic (4.7 ± 0.7%) treatments. Interestingly, PSCF was the more effective in reducing DAI starting from day 2 of DSS and in remediating the body weight loss as early as day 5 owing mainly to the impact of improvement in stool consistency on the DAI rating.

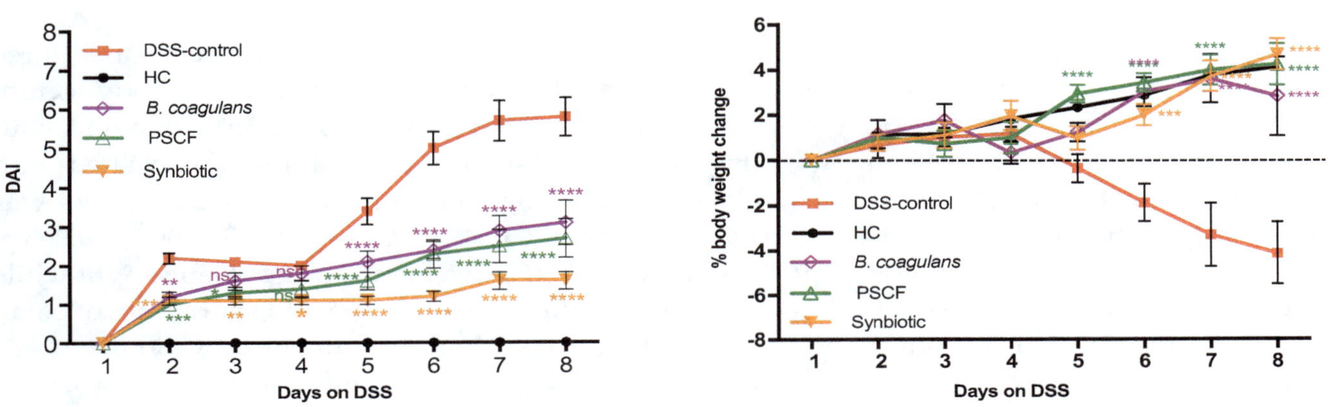

A B

Figure 1. *Cont.*

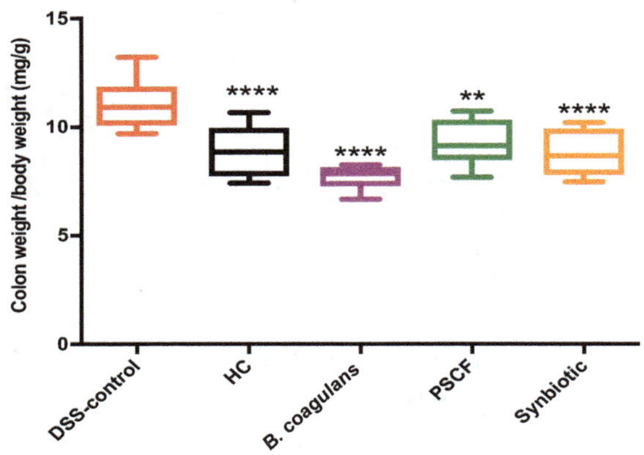

C

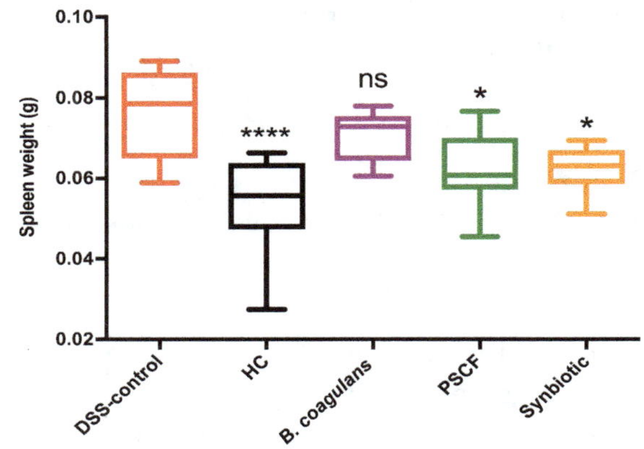

D

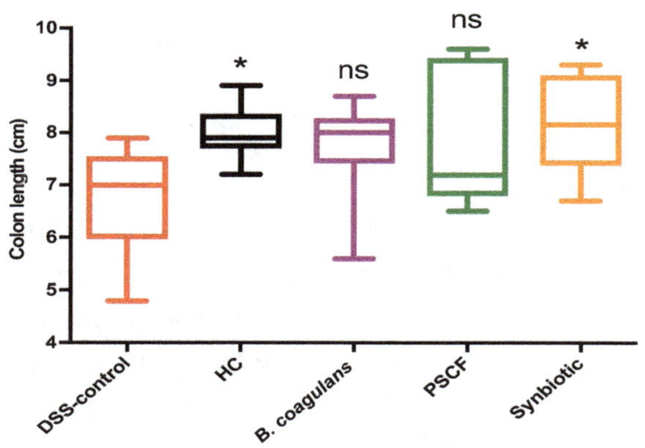

E

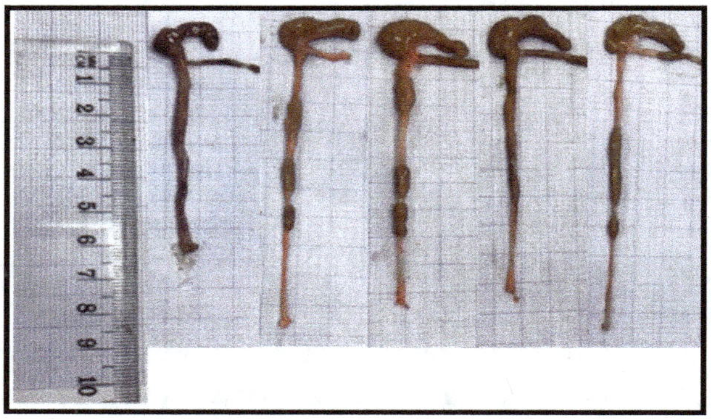

F

Figure 1. Effect of *B. coagulans* spores, PSCF and synbiotic in DSS-induced colitis model. (**A**) Disease Activity Index (DAI), (**B**) % body weight change. Statistical significance among groups evaluated by two-way repeated-measures analysis of variance (ANOVA) followed by Tukey's test. $^{*}p < 0.05$, $^{**}p < 0.01$, $^{***}p < 0.001$, $^{****}p < 0.0001$ vs. DSS-control group and data expressed as mean ± SEM (n =10 per group). Colon weight/body weight ratio (**C**), Spleen weight (**D**), Colon length (**E**) and Macroscopic appearance of colon (**F**). Data expressed as mean ± SEM (n =10 per group), evaluated by one-way ANOVA followed by Tukey's Test. ns-non-significant, HC-Healthy control, PSCF-Prebiotic sugar cane fibre.

The macroscopic evaluation of colonic segments determined the beneficial effects of all three treatments used in our study as evidenced by substantial reduction in colon weight/body weight ratio (*B. coagulans*, 7.68 ± 0.2; PSCF, 9.24 ± 0.3 and synbiotic, 8.74 ± 0.3 mg/g) compared with DSS-control group (11.12 ± 0.3 mg/gm) (Figure 1C). Intestinal inflammation is associated with spleen enlargement [24] and, as expected, relative spleen weight of untreated DSS-control mice was significantly higher (0.076 ± 0.004 g) than that of HC mice (0.054 ± 0.003 g). PSCF (0.062 ± 0.003 g) and synbiotic (0.063 ± 0.002 g) were equally significantly effective in reducing spleen weight while *B. coagulans* did not affect the relative spleen weight (Figure 1D). In contrast to shortening of colon length (Figure 1E,F) in DSS-control group (6.75 ± 0.3 cm), synbiotic treatment proved effective in reducing this outcome by maintaining the colon length (8.12 ± 0.2 cm), significantly equal (p = 0.99) to that of HC group (8.01 ± 0.2 cm). These markers are considered to be directly correlated to the severity of colonic damage in this experimental model of colitis [24].

3.2. *Effects of B. Coagulans, PSCF and Synbiotic Supplementation on Histological Alterations in DSS-Induced Mice*

Histological (H and E staining) examination of proximal colon (PC) and distal colon (DC) sections of DSS-induced mice showed altered erosion or destruction of epithelium, crypt distortion, depletion of goblet cells, submucosal oedema, and inflammatory cellular infiltration in the colon, mostly affecting the DC (Figure 2A). HC mice showed no signs of histological colon damage with score 0, while DSS induction in DSS-control mice resulted in a cumulative damage score of 10.5 ± 0.8 for the PC and 17.4 ± 0.5 for the DC (Figure 2B). Supplementation of DSS-induced mice with *B. coagulans*, PSCF and synbiotic induced protection and repair of the colonic mucosa. *B. coagulans* and synbiotic in particular were more effective in retention of colonic structure, protection of crypts and goblet cells and rescued infiltration of inflammatory cells, which resulted in a significant overall reduction of cumulative histological score of DC (10.1 ± 1.2 and 7.38 ± 0.7 respectively). Relatively, PSCF also provided partial significant protection with histological score of 13.0 ± 1.0. In contrast, PCSF had no effect in PC (10.1 ± 0.5) with only *B. coagulans* and synbiotic treatments being significantly successful in reducing damage to the PC with histological scores of 9.5 ± 0.7 and 7.8 ± 0.3 respectively. Unlike DSS-control group, there was reduced polymorphic inflammatory infiltrate in the lamina propria and submucosa in probiotic, prebiotic and synbiotic supplemented group. This observation corroborates with the significantly reduced MPO activity in the colon (Figure 2C) of all three treatments compared with the DSS-control group. The attenuation of colonic inflammation in pre-conditioned mice (*B. coagulans*, PSCF and synbiotic) is probably due to the anti-inflammatory properties of the functional dietary ingredients tested in this study.

3.3. *Effects of B. Coagulans, PSCF and Synbiotic Supplementation on Goblet Cells and Colonic Tight Junction Barrier*

Histological examination of distal colon from DSS mice showed a depletion of goblet cells when compared to HC and pre-conditioned mice. This suggested beneficial effects of probiotic and prebiotic ingredients on the intestinal epithelium potentially through stimulating mucus secretion by goblet cells. Specific staining with Alcian blue was therefore carried out to assess the mucus production following the administration of probiotic, prebiotic and synbiotic treatments. As depicted in Figure 3, in comparison with DSS-control group, there was a higher level of mucus staining with Alcian blue in supplemented mice samples. This implied that there has been an induction of higher levels of mucus secretion in the DSS-challenged mice that received *B. coagulans* spores, symbiotic, and PSCF supplementaions. Unlike the DSS-controlled samples where, goblet cells were almost entirely destroyed, the mice supplemented with synbiotic and *B. coagulans* showed protection of the goblet cells. PSCF also partially protected the goblet cells with mucus staining compared with DSS-control.

Immunohistochemical analysis was then performed to evaluate the assembly of the TJs and the integrity of the intestinal barrier. The presence of the TJ proteins-ZO-1, occludin, and claudin-1 on the tissue sections were analysed (Figure 4). In HC, ZO-1 (Figure 4A) staining was more intense in the apical tight junction complex both at the surface and in the crypts. In addition to showing their presence at the crypt surface, occludin (Figure 4B), and claudin-1 (Figure 4C) proteins stained more strongly at the basolateral membrane of crypts. As previously reported [38,39] such signals were weak or totally absent on the epithelium of DSS-control sections resulting in very low percentage TJ protein expressions. Basolateral and partial apical staining of ZO-1, occludin and claudin-1 was maintained with *B. coagulans* and synbiotic supplementation in DSS-treated animals. While PSCF was able to partially maintain ZO-1 and claudin-1 staining, such an effect was less evident for occludin. Synbiotic treatment was most effective in preserving the TJ protein expressions in DSS-induced mice further confirming its beneficial effects on the intestinal integrity.

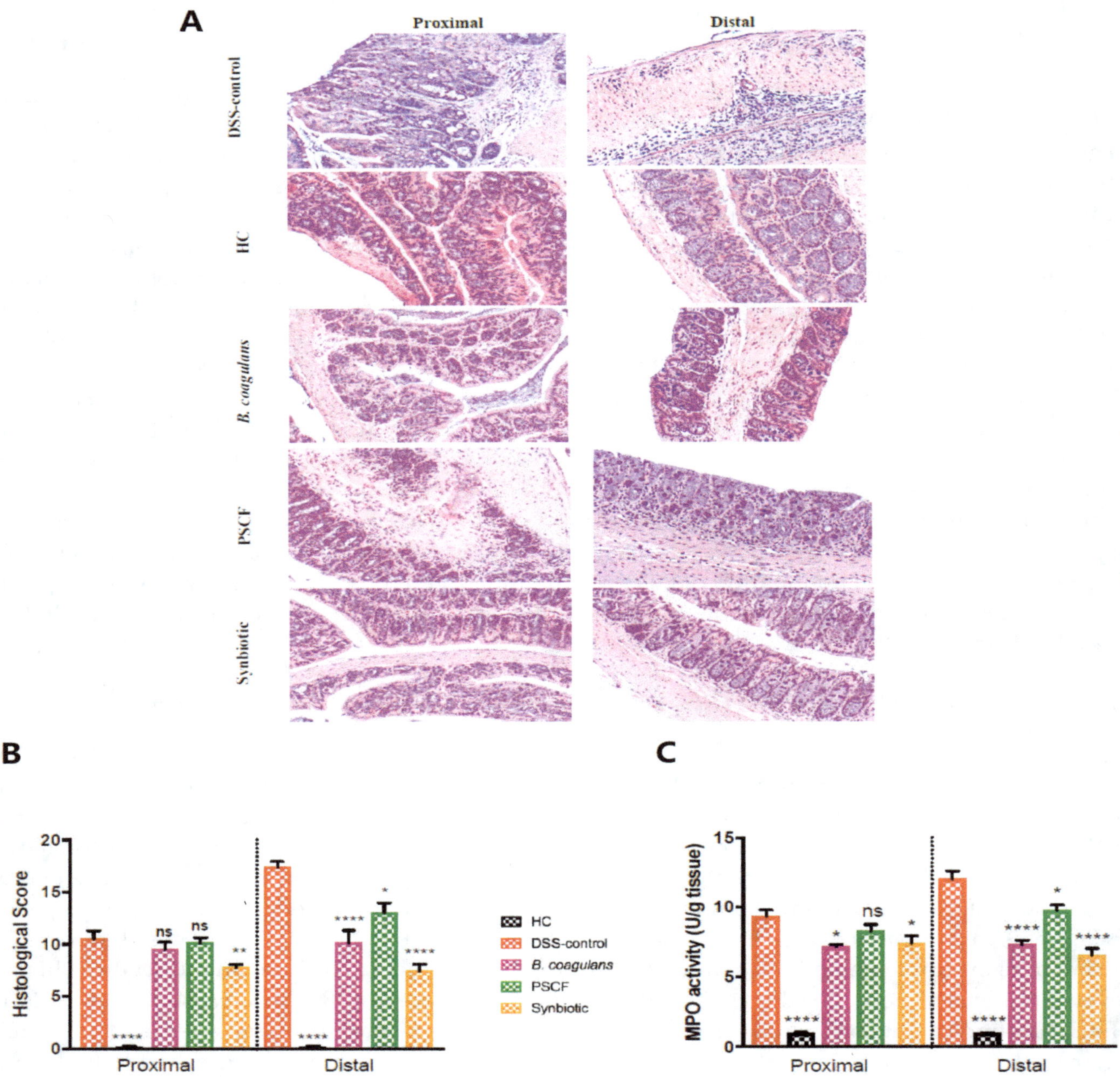

Figure 2. Effect of *B. coagulans* spores, PSCF and synbiotic treatments on DSS-induced colon injury and inflammation. (**A**) Histological images of proximal and distal colonic tissues stained with hematoxylin and eosin at 20× for each experimental group. (**B**) Histological score calculated after microscopic analyses of proximal and distal sections of the colon. (**C**) Myeloperoxidase (MPO) activity in colonic tissues was determined by colorimetric assay. Results expressed as mean ± SEM (n = 8 per group), evaluated by one-way ANOVA followed by Tukey's test (*$p < 0.05$, **$p < 0.01$, ****$p < 0.0001$).

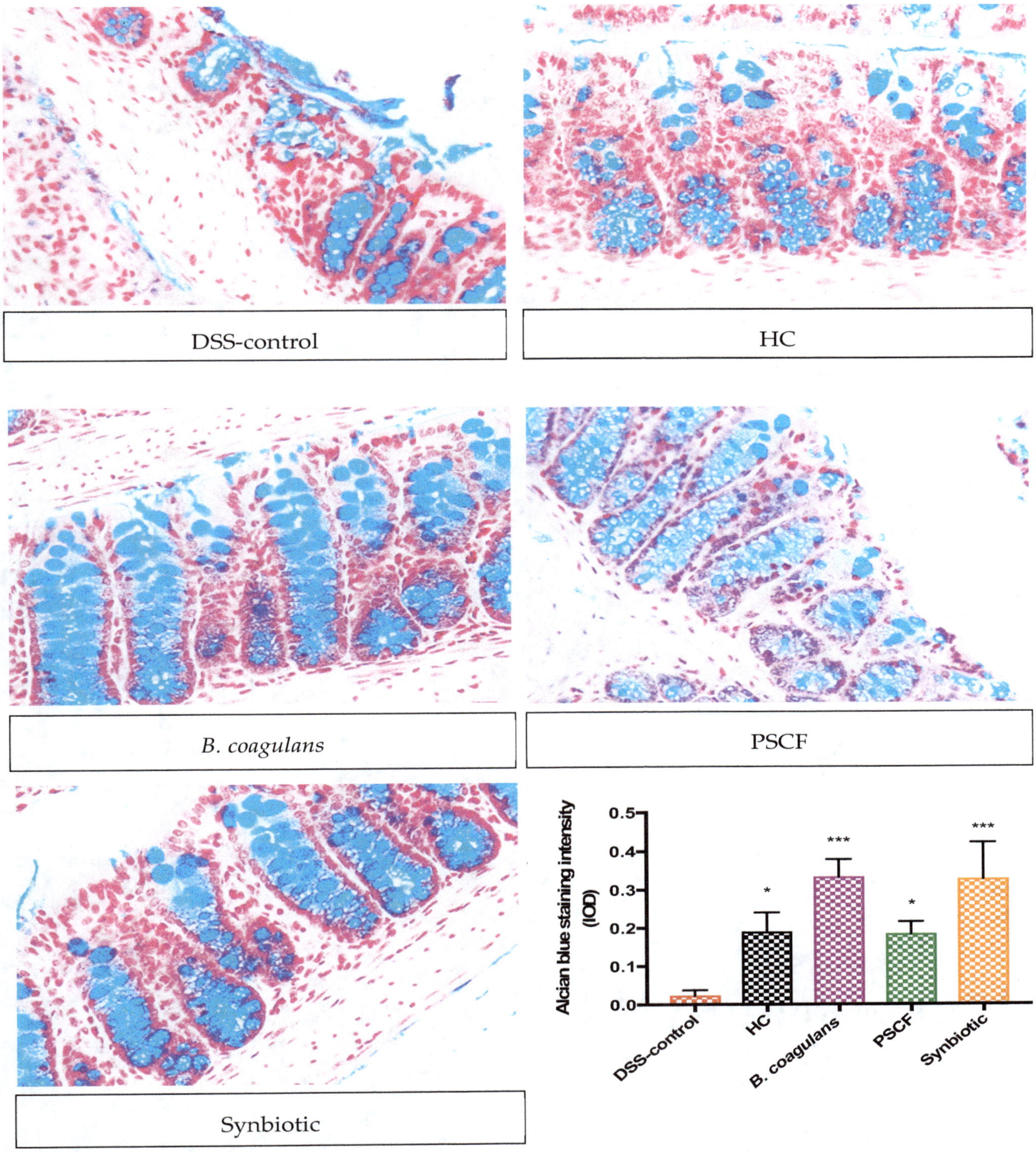

Figure 3. Effect of *B. coagulans* spores, PSCF and synbiotic on goblet cells. The paraffin embedded sections were stained with Alcian Blue to detect changes in goblet cells and in production of mucus in distal colonic tissue in each experimental group (40×) and staining intensity (IOD) of respective group is illustrated in the graph. Results expressed as mean ± SEM (n = 4 per group), evaluated by one-way ANOVA followed by Tukey's test (*$p < 0.05$, ***$p < 0.001$).

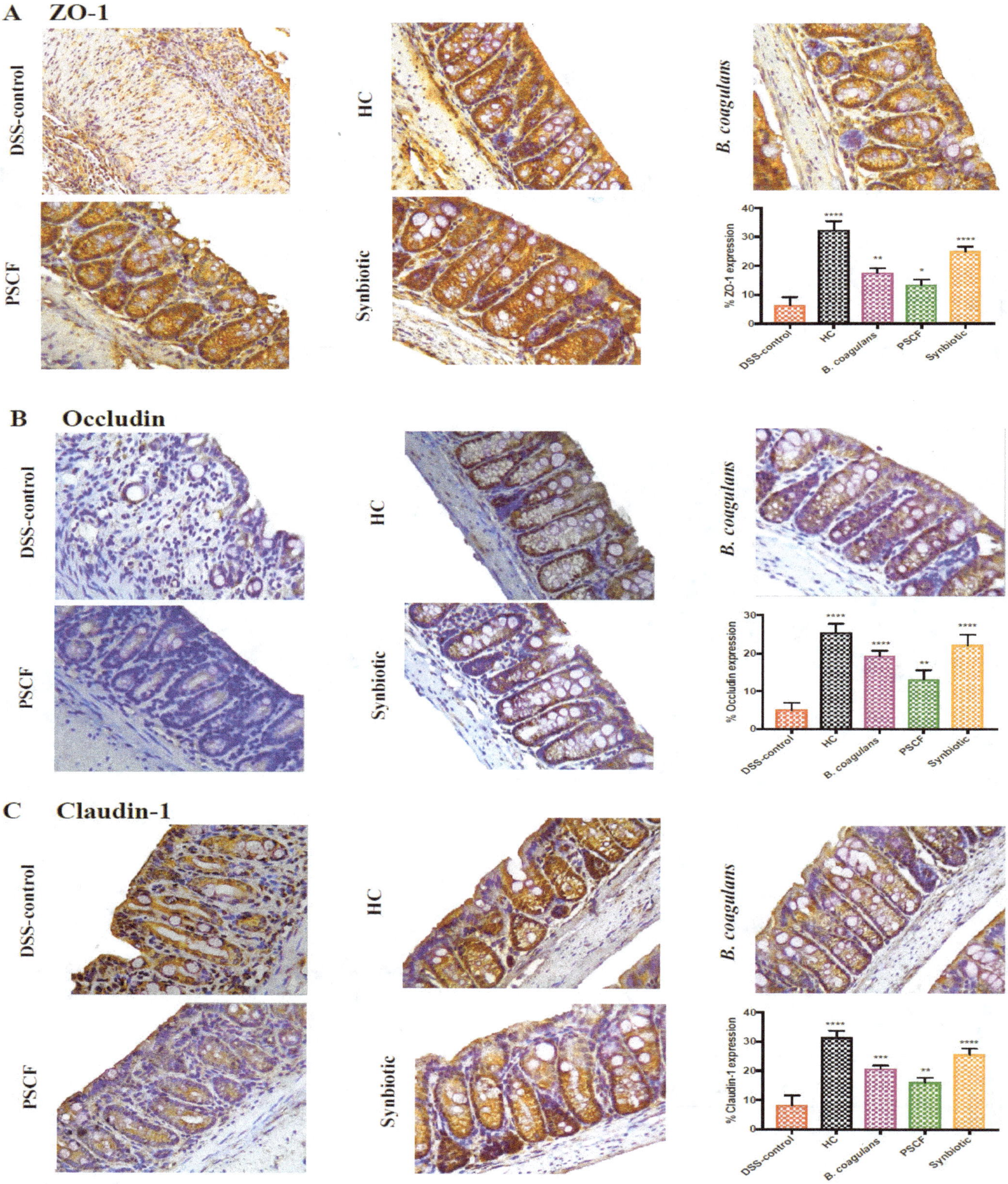

Figure 4. Effects of *B. coagulans* spores, PSCF and synbiotic on expression of epithelial tight junction proteins. Immunohistochemical detection of (**A**) ZO-1, (**B**) Occludin and (**C**) claudin-1 and its respective percentage of expression in colon at 40×. Data expressed as mean ± SEM (n = 4 per group) and statistical significance among groups evaluated by one-way ANOVA followed by Tukey's test *$p < 0.05$, **$p < 0.01$, ***$p < 0.001$, ****$p < 0.0001$ vs. DSS-control group.

3.4. Immunomodulatory Effects of B. Coagulans, PSCF, and Synbiotic Supplementation on Immune Markers in DSS-Induced Mice

The cytokine analysis of the colonic segments and serum measured the intestinal immunomodulatory and anti-inflammatory effects of *B. coagulans*, PSCF and their synbiotic combination. A beneficial impact of ameliorating the altered immune response induced by DSS intake was noted. Overall, probiotic, prebiotic, and synbiotic treatments remarkably reduced the pro-inflammatory cytokine secretions of IL-1α, IL-1β, IL-6, IL-12, TNF-α, and IFN-γ in proximal and distal colon segments compared with that of the DSS-colitic segments (Figure 5), while no significant effect of supplementations was noted on other cytokine levels (Supplementary Figure S1). *B. coagulans* and synbiotic treatments were equally effective in maintaining the levels of these altered cytokines relative to that of non-colitic mice while PSCF did not show significant effective reduction of IL-12 cytokine levels (Figure 5D). Synbiotic treatment was statistically more potent in suppressing the elevated levels of IL-1α (−90.29%) and IL-12 (−67.42%) compared with *B. coagulans* (−85.94%, −52.20%, respectively) in the DC. No positive effect was observed in the PC segment for IL-6 and TNF-α levels by PSCF treatment. However, the excellent immunomodulatory effect in the DC for respective cytokines was confirmed (Figure 5C,E), implicating its differential effects in these colonic segments.

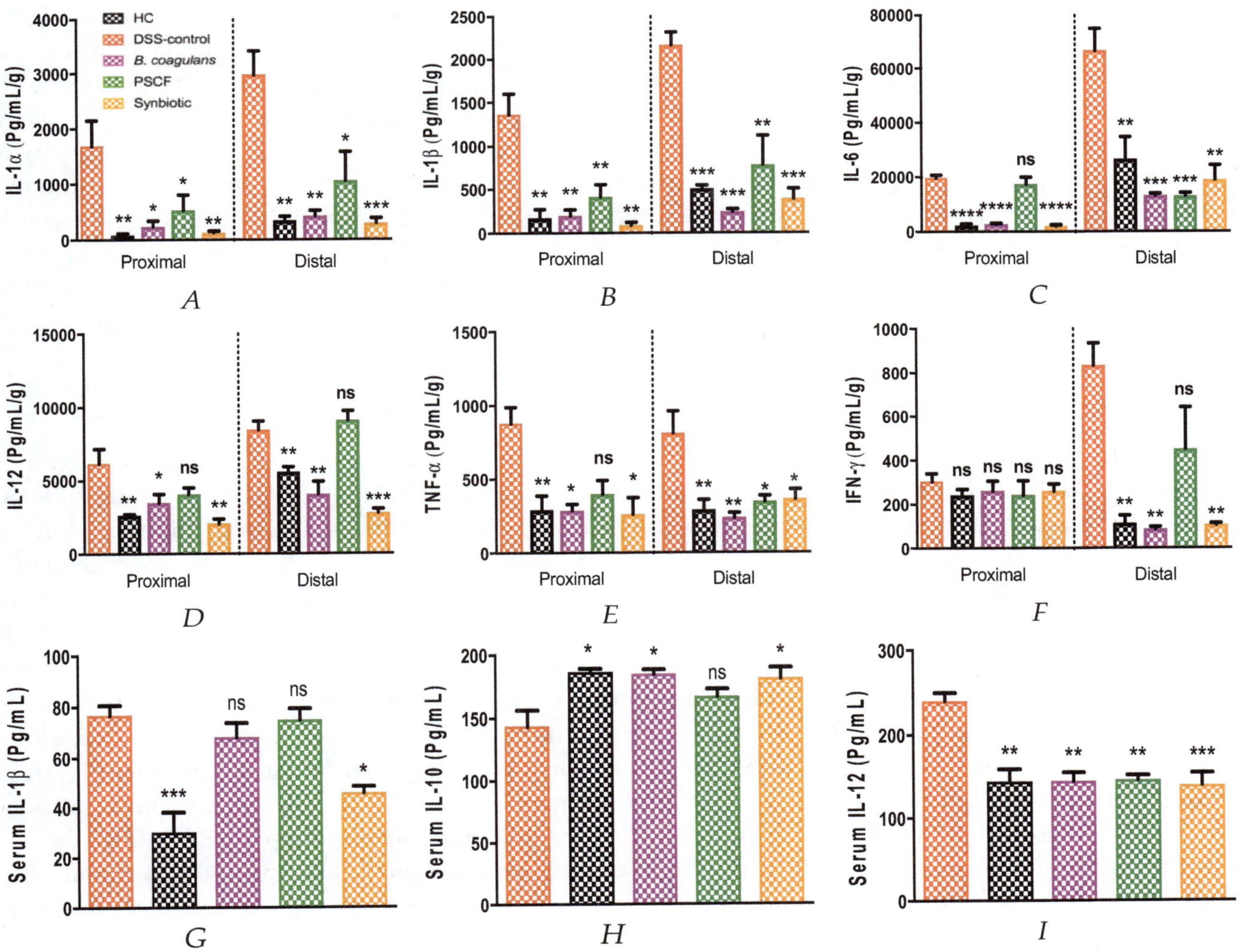

Figure 5. *Cont.*

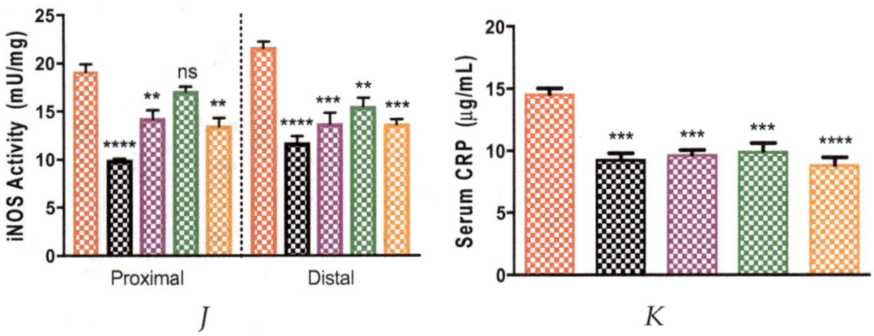

Figure 5. Effect of *B. coagulans* spores, PSCF and synbiotic on immune markers in colon tissues and blood serum. Protein levels of cytokines including (**A**) IL-1α, (**B**) IL-1β, (**C**) IL-6, (**D**) IL-12, (**E**) TNF-α, (**F**) IFN-γ in proximal and distal colon explants as well as cytokine levels of (**G**) IL-1β, (**H**) IL-10, and (**I**) IL-12 in blood serum were analysed by Bio-plex. iNOS activity in colon tissues (**J**) measured by NOS activity assay and CRP levels in serum (**K**) by ELISA. Statistical significance among groups evaluated by one-way ANOVA followed by Tukey's test. *$p < 0.05$, **$p < 0.01$, ***$p < 0.001$, ****$p < 0.0001$ vs. DSS-colitic group and data expressed as mean ± SEM ($n = 3$ per group).

Similar immunomodulatory effects were found on the serum cytokines Il-1β, IL-12, and IL-10 (Figure 5G–I), while no significant effect was observed for other serum cytokines (Supplementary Figure S1). All three treatments substantially restored the IL-12 levels to values similar to HC mice, while synbiotic treatment was significantly more efficacious in reducing pro-inflammatory IL-1β levels in serum. Moreover, *B. coagulans* and synbiotic treatments increased the anti-inflammatory IL-10 levels in serum (181.2 ± 8.70, 184.7 ± 3.81 pg/mL respectively) compared with the DSS-colitic group (143.8 ± 12.80 pg/mL) (Figure 3H). iNOS activity which is known to be high in colitis in response to pro-inflammatory stimuli [33], was significantly suppressed in both colon segments by all treatments (Figure 5J) compared with DSS-colitic levels. Serum CRP level was significantly higher in the DSS-control group (14.58 ± 0.45 µg/mL) in comparison with HC animals (9.32 ± 0.45 µg/mL). Bacillus, PSCF and synbiotic remarkably normalised the CRP levels (9.67 ± 0.34, 9.95 ± 0.65, 8.83 ± 0.59 µg/mL, respectively) to that of the HC group. These results confirmed the notable anti-inflammatory efficacy of probiotic *Bacillus* spores, prebiotic PSCF and synbiotic treatments used in our study.

3.5. Effects of B. coagulans, PSCF and Synbiotic Supplementation on Altered Fecal Metabolic Profile in DSS-Induced Mice

Fecal metabolites were analysed using GC-MS to gain an overview of changes induced by *B. coagulans*, PSCF and synbiotic supplementation in DSS-treated mice. A total of 61 metabolites of different functional groups such as sugars, amino acids, volatile fatty acids, and biogenic amines were detected. A supervised partial least squares-discriminant analysis (PLS-DA) was performed to evaluate metabolic phenotyping of each experimental group as shown in Figure 6A. The samples from HC and DSS-control clusters were clearly divergent indicating marked distinction in metabolic patterns between the two groups. While, clusters of supplemented mice samples overlapped with that of HC and DSS-control, clear demarcation of the synbiotic and *B. coagulans* cluster was noted, with PSCF showing only partial divergence relative to that of DSS-control. This indicates substantial efficacy of *B. coagulans* to metabolise PSCF that, in turn, induced significant biochemical changes potentially owing to their synergistic effects as evidenced from synbiotic samples. Combination of PLS-DA ($R^2Y = 0.810$ ($p = 0.01$), $Q^2 = 0.710$), VIP scores (Figure 6B) and significance analysis for microarrays (SAM) enabled us to identify potential biomarkers. The results showed 61 metabolites with 40 statistically significant compounds contributing to the clustering, with their SAM scores fold changes and International Chemical Identifiers (InChI) and standard InChI hashes (InChIKey IDs) listed in Table S1. Key metabolic markers making a significant contribution were identified by VIP analysis as displayed in Figure 6B. Among these identified metabolites, noticeable differences between DSS-control, and HC samples were noted particularly for succinic acid, stearic acid, and glycerol. Synbiotic supplementation was beneficial in minimising the metabolite alterations induced by DSS (Figure 6B and Table S1).

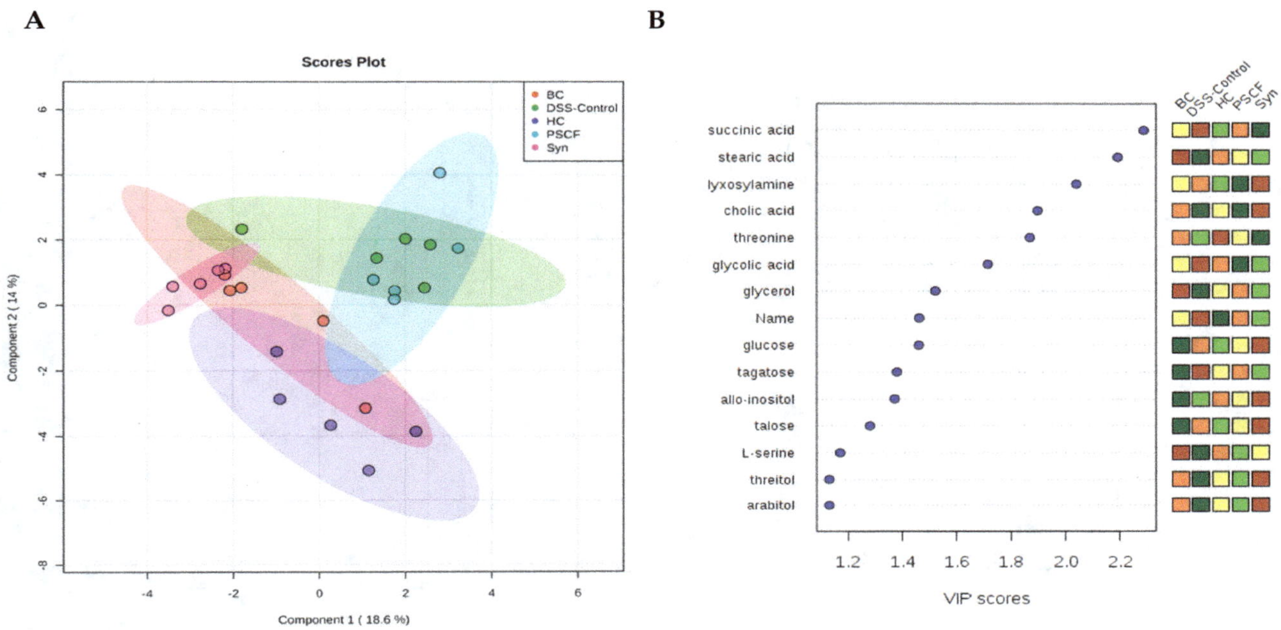

Figure 6. Effect of *B. coagulans* spores, PSCF and synbiotic on metabolic modulations in DSS-induced colitic mice. (**A**) 2D-PLS-DA plot showing spatial division among groups that received different supplementations, DSS-control mice that received no supplementation and HC. (**B**) Key compounds separating the groups based on variable importance projection (VIP) score plot in PLS-DA analysis. (BC-*B. coagulans*, Syn-synbiotic).

3.6. Effects of B. Coagulans, PSCF and Synbiotic Supplementation SCFA Levels in DSS-Induced Mice

As shown in Figure 7, supplementation of DSS-induced mice with *B. coagulans*, PSCF, and synbiotic treatments induced substantial modulations in the SCFA concentrations and their effects varied across cecal, luminal and fecal contents. Overall, the highest concentration of SCFA were noted in cecal contents compared to mucosal and fecal contents. There were no significant differences between the concentration of acetate and propionate in DSS-control and HC mice. PSCF however, induced a significant increase in the acetate levels in cecal and mucosal samples while, Synbiotic treatment was most significant in elevating acetate concentrations in mucosal-associated samples. All three supplementations were significantly effective in improving the propionate concentrations in cecal and mucosal contents while, only synbiotic supplementation increased propionate levels in fecal samples.

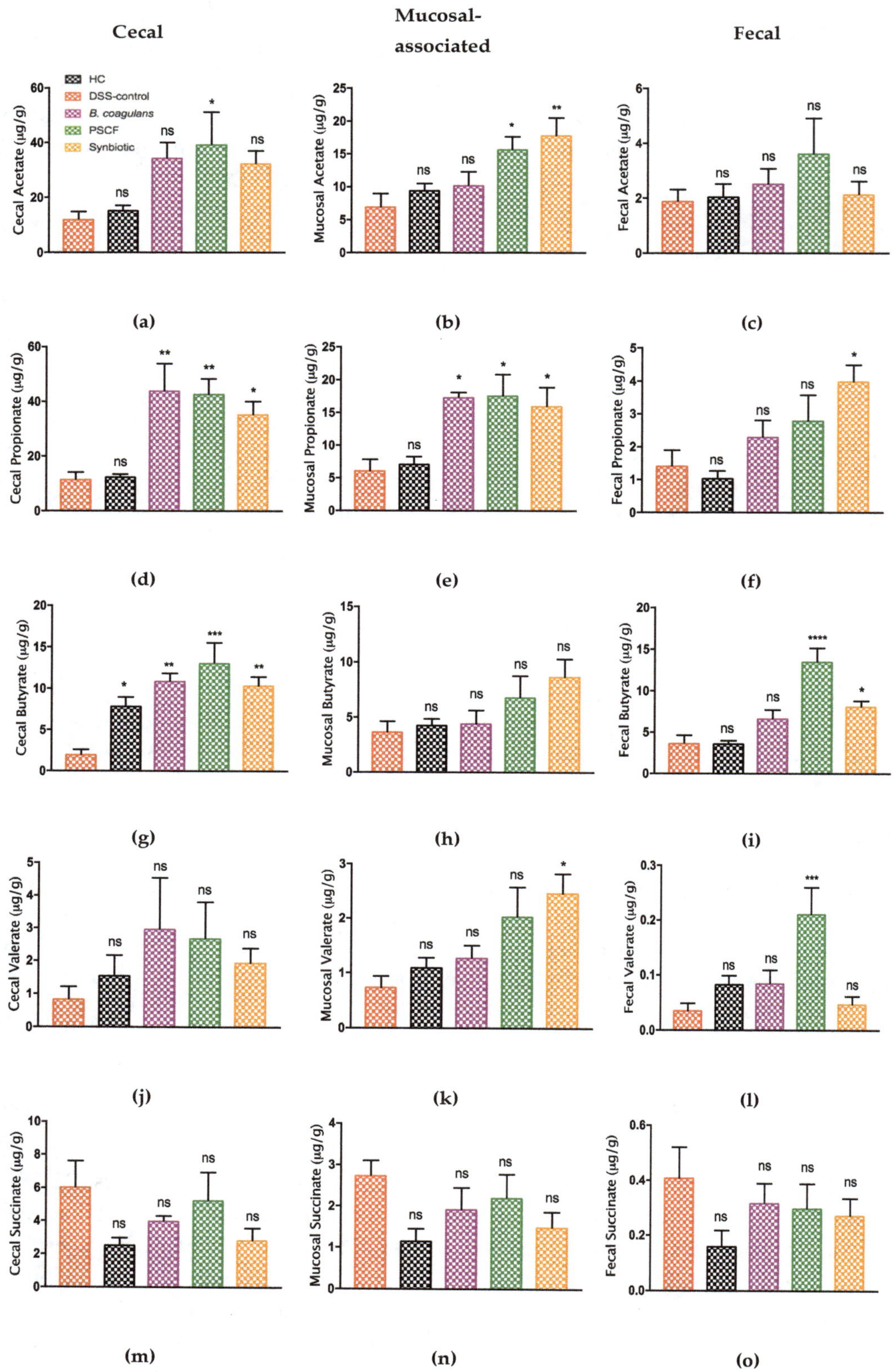

Figure 7. Effects of *B. coagulans* spores, PSCF and synbiotic in modulating SCFA concentrations in cecal, mucosal-associated and fecal contents in DSS-induced colitis. Cecal- acetate (**a**), proionate (**d**), butyrate (**g**), valerate (**j**), succinate (**m**); mucosal-associated acetate (**b**), proionate (**e**), butyrate (**h**), valerate (**k**), succinate (**n**) and fecal- acetate (**c**), propionate (**f**), butyrate (**i**), valerate (**l**), succinate (**o**). -Statistical significance among groups evaluated by one-way ANOVA followed by Tukey's test. $^*p < 0.05$, $^{**}p < 0.01$, $^{***}p < 0.001$, $^{****}p < 0.0001$ vs. DSS-colitic group and data expressed as mean $\pm$ SEM ($n = 5$ per group). ns-non-significant

Butyrate levels were significantly decreased by DSS administration (2.05 ± 0.6 μg/g) compared with that of HC mice (7.91 ± 1.1 μg/g) in the cecum. The decrease in butyrate induced by DSS was maintained at control levels with all three supplements in the cecum with PSCF (13.2 ± 2.4 μg/g) being significantly more effective than *B. coagulans* (11 ± 0.9 μg/g) and synbiotic (10.4 ± 1.0 μg/g). Similarly, in fecal content, PSCF significantly improved butyrate (13.6 ± 1.6 μg/g compared with 3.72 ± 0.1 μg/g for DSS-colitic followed by synbiotic (8.15 ± 0.6 μg/g) while *B. coagulans* (6.69 ± 0.1 μg/g) had no effect. Synbiotic supplementation resulted in marked increase in mucosal-assocaited valerate while, PSCF caused elevation in its concentration in fecal content. Similarly, synbiotic was more efficient in reducing elevated succinate levels.

4. Discussion

Dietary strategies involving probiotic and prebiotic fibre components that function by modulating immune responses, colonic epithelial integrity and microbial composition and related metabolites are being widely investigated for the prevention or reduction of severity of IBD [40,41]. The present study clearly supported the premise that conditioning of the gut with synbiotic supplementation containing compatible probiotic and prebiotic fibre can be greatly beneficial to reducing the symptoms and severity of DSS-induced acute colitis in mice. The observations confirmed substantial anti-inflammatory efficacy by synbiotic supplementation containing *B. coagulans* and PSCF. This was evidenced by the improvement of clinical symptoms, macroscopic, histological, biochemical, metabolic and immune parameters in the DSS-induced colitic mice model.

The addition of 2% (*w*/*v*) DSS to drinking water for seven days without ameliorating treatments resulted in a progressive rise in DAI (Figure 1A), owing to both body weight loss (Figure 1B) and excretion of diarrheic/bleeding feces. However, the supplementation of DSS-induced mice with *B. coagulans*, PSCF, and their synbiotic combination significantly attenuated the severity of the DSS damage and improved DAI and macroscopic markers of inflammation (Figure 1C–F). The ability of PSCF to show early effect on DAI and body weight could be related to its high content of insoluble hemicellulose. This fraction has a large water-holding capacity thus, could appropriately contribute to regulating the fecal water content in colitic mice [42,43]. The anti-diarrheal effect of *B. coagulans* have been previously confirmed [44]. The increased beneficial effects of synbiotic supplementation in reducing the disease severity could be related to the synergistic actions between the probiotic and prebiotic components.

A potentiated synbiotic effect relative to that of *B. coagulans* and PSCF individually was also evident from the histology of the colon compared with DSS-control mice (Figure 2A,B). Synbiotic supplementation showed substantial protection to the colonic epithelial architecture by mitigating crypt disruption, loss of goblet cells, submucosal edema and epithelial structure damage induced by DSS. Synbiotic supplementation also induced suppression of infiltration of activated neutrophils as evidenced by significant reduction in MPO activity in DSS-induced mice (Figure 2C). The infiltration of activated neutrophils is one of the most prominent histological features observed in IBD and is directly proportional to the MPO activity. Superoxide anions and other reactive species produced by neutrophils leads to tissue necrosis and mucosal dysfunction in IBD [39]. The reduction in MPO activity suggests that synbiotic supplementation imparted an anti-inflammatory effect, in addition to histological protection.

Disruption of intestinal epithelial TJs and impaired epithelial barrier function is a central event in the pathogenesis of IBD and may lead to persistent aberrant immune reactions, thus accelerating gut inflammation and the inflammatory circuit [45]. Synbiotic treatment in our study was the most effective followed by *B. coagulans* and PSCF in protecting the expression level of TJ proteins (ZO-1, occludin and claudin-1) in DSS-induced mice (Figure 4). TJs create a semi-permeable barrier against paracellular penetration of harmful substances from the gut lumen [45]. *Bacillus subtilis* intake has been recently confirmed to upregulate the expressions of TJ proteins for improved barrier function in colitic mice [46] and corroborates with our results. Moreover, synbiotic and *B. coagulans* protected the goblet cells and mucin production more effectively than PSCF alone (Figure 3). This indicates the possible ability of these *B. coagulans* MTCC 5856 spores to benefit goblet cell structure and function and needs further investigation to determine the mechanism of this effect. Some *Bacillus* species have been shown to upregulate mucin glycoproteins and protect colonic mucus layer integrity and goblet cell function [47]. Although we could not confirm if synbiotic supplementation had a stimulating effect on TJ proteins and/or localisation or, instead if it avoided TJ degradation by DSS, we observed that synbiotic supplementation significantly maintained the TJ patterns similar to that of animals in HC. This is indicative that synbiotic supplementation significantly preserved the integrity of the epithelium. The synergy between *B. coagulans* and PSCF could have imparted excellent protection and/or maintenance of epithelial integrity on DSS-induced mice, thus supporting its application in IBD to reinforce intestinal barrier integrity.

Alterations in the barrier integrity in IBD also leads to aberrant immune responses resulting in an inflammation cascade and tissue damage [48]. Although *B. coagulans* and PSCF supplementations alone were able to modulate the tested cytokines (IL-1α, IL-1β, IL-6, IL-12, TNF-α, and IFN-γ), a more profound anti-inflammatory effect was observed with synbiotic supplementation in both the colon and serum (Figure 5A–I). A spike in the levels of IL-1β, IL-6, and TNF-α have been implicated in human IBD pathogenesis [49]. Such pro-inflammatory cytokines are secreted at high levels by activated lamina propria antigen presenting cells in response to inflammation. Pro-inflammatory cytokines such as IL-6, TNF-α, and IL-1β are being targeted by therapeutic approaches to curb the aberrant inflammatory response in IBD due to their roles in the pathogenesis of the disease [50–52]. TNF-α is reported to exert its pro-inflammatory effect through elevated production of IL-6 and IL-1β [53]. This is in line with the present study, where DSS-induction caused elevated secretions of these cytokines in DSS-control group relative to that of HC (Figure 5). Upregulation of pro-inflammatory cytokine levels has also been reported to upregulate iNOS expression and secretion of nitric oxide that causes tissue damage in IBD [54]. The anti-inflammatory effects of synbiotic, *B. coagulans* and PSCF in suppressing the levels of these pro-inflammatory cytokines as well as reducing iNOS activity in colonic tissues, indicates their immunomodulatory potentials. *B. coagulans* MTCC 5856 spores in our previous study showed excellent immunomodulatory effect in vitro [22]. Marked reduction in pro-inflammatory cytokines in the colon of DSS-induced mice in the current study further supports its excellent immunomodulatory efficacy in IBD application.

Synbiotic supplementation was the most effective in demonstrating noticeable anti-inflammatory effect by significantly reducing the serum levels of pro-inflammatory IL-1β and IL-12 while concurrently elevating anti-inflammatory IL-10 in the serum. IL-10 plays a prominent role in counterbalancing Th1 and Th17 immune activity in IBD towards a Th2 response by downregulating antigen presentation and subsequent release of proinflammatory cytokines thereby attenuating mucosal inflammation [53]. IL-10 has been reported to play a role in maintaining intestinal barrier integrity possibly owing to effects on zonulin pathway [55]. The ability of *B. coagulans* spores to elicit IL-10 levels in inflammatory condition has been determined in vitro and in human subjects. Thus, the anti-inflammatory efficacy of synbiotic supplementation could be related to major immune-regulating capability of *B. coagulans* MTCC 5856 spores, thereby supporting its application in synbiotic therapies for IBD. Furthermore, synbiotic treatment also reduced the increased CRP levels in the serum of DSS-induced mice. In the inflammatory state, circulating IL-6 promotes CRP production in the liver and its release into the bloodstream [56]. Elevated levels of CRP has been implicated in human IBD patients [57]. The reduction in overall pro-inflammatory mediators by synbiotic supplementation may be due to either direct immune-regulating effect of the *B. coagulans* and PSCF on cytokine secretion or it could be owing to their indirect effect on the protection of intestinal barrier integrity. In either case this leads to reduction in luminal antigens and full activation of the innate immune system.

DNA extracted from cecal, fecal and mucosal-associated contents from DSS-induced mice in the present study, failed amplification before 16s rRNA sequencing owing to the presence of DSS in the samples that inhibited the PCR amplification as known earlier [58]. The microbiota profiling of DSS samples could therefore not be performed and is the limitation of the study. The levels of microbiota-derived untargeted metabolites and SCFAs were therefore alternatively analysed as signatures of the gut microbiota that contribute to modulating the immune activity of the intestinal mucosa [59,60]. The untreated DSS-control mice exhibited distinct fecal metabolic phenotype relative to that of HC. This was reflective of clinical and animal IBD studies that confirmed significant differences in metabolic profiles between healthy and IBD patients [61–63]. The metabolic analysis of supplemented mice in our study resulted in considerable normalization of metabolic profile indicating the positive effects of synergistic combination of *B. coagulans* and PSCF that induced marked improvement in metabolic pattern. Notably for mice supplemented with PSCF there was not much distinction from the DSS-control group was observed but the synbiotic combination with *B. coagulans* resulted in an improved metabolic pattern. This marked synergism could be associated with the acceleration of fermentation of insoluble plant cellular materials, such as hemicellulose in PSCF, by the supplemented *B. coagulans* [18]. The resulting higher levels of fermentation metabolites would thus, in turn, influence other beneficial microbial metabolic activities. This further supports the application of compatible synbiotic components to generate maximum benefits through increased SCFA production.

Increased levels of microbiota-derived SCFAs are inversely associated with dysbiosis in IBD [64]. Of particular interest are higher levels of acetate, propionate and butyrate, which results from fermentation of indigestible carbohydrates from fibre-rich diets. The effects of SCFAs have been studied to in animal models of colitis [42] and clinical UC [65]. Each type of SCFA is likely to contribute to host health [66]. In this study we determined the SCFA profile along the gastro-intestinal tract, analyzing samples across cecal, mucosal-associated, and fecal contents. The concentration of SCFAs varied along the length of the gut, with most abundant levels in the cecum and PC, while it declined towards the DC [66]. In line with a recent study [67], cecum showed the highest levels of all the SCFAs tested in our study irrespective of the supplementation. Cecum is considered the major site for fermentation in the rodent gut and contains the largest pool of microbiota. It therefore generates the most SCFAs. However, some recent studies have also reported changes in the microbiota and associated amounts of metabolites in along different regions of gastro-intestinal (GI) tract [67–69]. Therefore, the overall GI profile is of importance when associating the gut microbiome and metabolites with health outcomes.

All three supplementations caused a substantial increase in concentrations of measured SCFAs compares with that of DSS-control group. However, the potentiated effect of synbiotic supplementation is evidenced by induction of SCFA production along the entire length of the colon compared to *B. coagulans* supplementation alone where the additional SCFA production capacity was absent past the cecum. This effect highlights the advantage of using a compatible prebiotic fibre as synbiotic companion with a particular probiotic that can metabolize it. The high total dietary fibre content of PSCF (87%) [17] would contribute to this effect. PSCF supplementation resulted in increased butyrate levels line with an in-vitro study with human gut microbiota utilizing sugar cane fibre [17]. The effect of additional SCFA production in cecum by *B. coagulans* would not extend to the proximal or distal parts of the colon. In the current study, the elicited extra SCFAs with synbiotic supplementation from cecum to the fecal pellets indicated the ability of *B. coagulans* to utilize the PSCF to also generate SCFAs after the cecum. The ability of *B. coagulans* to metabolize a variety of plant fibers for fermentation, including cranberry fibre [70] and fenugreek seeds [71], to produce SCFAs and hemicellulose [18] for lactic acid production has been previously determined.

PSCF supplementation also resulted in increased butyrate levels, correlating with results of an in-vitro study with human gut microbiota utilizing sugar cane fibre [17]. This ability of synbiotic supplementation for eliciting butyrate levels along the entire length of colon could contribute to the beneficial effect observed in the current study. Butyrate is the preferred energy source for colonocytes and has the ability to regulate cytokines thus showing protection against inflammation in UC and colorectal cancer [66]. Butyrate has been demonstrated in in vitro [72,73] and in vivo [74] studies to increase epithelial integrity and mucus secretion, consistent with the immunohistological and mucus staining analysis in the present study. The substantial increase in butyrate levels in the cecum by *B. coagulans* supplementation may be due to ability to support the growth and activity of butyrate producers probably via cross-feeding of the lactic acid production. *B. coagulans* are known to be efficient at producing lactic acid through fermentation of various plant substrates, including hemicellulose [18,19]. Lactic acid is reported to be utilized by strictly anaerobic butyrate-producing bacteria of clostridial clusters XIVa for the production of high concentrations of butyric acid [75]. Thus, the synbiotic approach with probiotic bacteria and prebiotic fibre that directly or indirectly influence butyrate production may help to restore intestinal barrier integrity in diseased state. This effect was evidenced by the significant reduction in DSS-induced colonic epithelial damage (Figure 2) by synbiotic supplementation in our study.

Acetate and propionate have also been studied to benefit epithelial integrity via binding with certain metabolite-sensing G-protein-coupled receptors (such as GPR43, GPR109A) and modulating immune response [76–78]. Valerate that has been determined to stimulate intestinal growth and attenuate inflammatory pathogenesis in colitis and cancer to metabolic disorders [79] was increased by synbiotic supplementation. Besides its positive effect in colon, SCFAs have also been exhibited to mediate improved host metabolism and modulate the activity of the enteric nervous system [66], thus providing benefits beyond GI tract. The high levels of immuno-modulatory effects observed in the present study could also possibly be correlated to high SCFA levels induced by synbiotic supplementation owing to the synergistic combination. SCFAs by engaging with engage with GPRs are known to induce immune-modulation leading to a direct local and systemic anti-inflammatory effects [76,80]. This further supports the application of synergistic synbiotic combinations to achieve maximum benefits in resolving the inflammatory circuit in IBD.

5. Conclusions

This is a detailed study highlighting the site-specific inflammatory and SCFA changes in a mice model of IBD as a result of synbiotic supplementation of the normal diet with prebiotic whole plant fibre and probiotic spores. The synbiotic pre-supplementation resulted in a substantial anti-inflammatory effect, reducing disease severity, colonic damage, and inflammatory mediators while modulating the metabolite and SCFA profiles of DSS-induced gut damage. The research has clearly demonstrated that the supplementation of whole plant PSCF and *B. coagulans* spores produced a synergistic combination that protected mice against acute damage induced by DSS in mice. The results underscore the significant efficacy of synbiotic applications to increase the beneficial and preventive effects on the host by targeting different mechanistic approaches to resolve inflammation cycle. However, the differences in the evolved biology of humans compared to mice requires caution in translation of the results to impacts on human disease [81]. While mice models do allow the changes in gut microbiota, as a result of pre- and probiotic combinations to be studied in a controlled experiment direct human trials will be needed. The delineation of the synergistic biological actions of probiotic *B. coagulans* spores and prebiotic PSCF in mouse model of IBD provides support for investigating their therapeutic and preventive effects in human IBD. However, the ability to reduce the severity of DSS-induced colitis was demonstrated using pre-supplementation. Human trials should be aimed at proactive prevention or after partial control of inflammatory disease, such as in association with drug treatment.

Patents: The information from this study has been filed as a provisional patent application in Australia titled "Preparation for the Treatment of Inflammatory Bowel Disease using a Whole Plant Fibre Extract from Sugar Cane" with application number 2018902145 and a filing date of 15 June 2018. Information relating to novelty of synergy between probiotic *Bacillus coagulans* and prebiotic whole plant sugar cane fibre in imparting health benefits is the subject of the patented claim.

Supplementary Materials: Figure S1: Effect of B. coagulans spores, PSCF and synbiotic on immune markers in colon tissues and blood serum, Table S1: Most significant compounds identified by OPLS-DA and SAM analysis in HC, DSS-control, B. coagulans (BC), PSCF and synbiotic groups.

Author Contributions: Conceptualization: T.S., R.E., and R.S.; data curation: T.S.; formal analysis: T.S., A.P.P., R.V., S.S., and B.S.; funding acquisition: R.E. and R.S.; investigation: T.S.; methodology: T.S., S.V.G., A.V.K., and D.J.B.; resources: S.V.G., A.V.K., D.J.B., R.E., and R.S.; supervision: R.E. and R.S.; validation: R.S.; visualization: T.S.; writing—original draft: T.S.; writing—review and editing: T.S., S.V.G., A.V.K., D.J.B., R.E., and R.S.

Acknowledgments: The support from Tasmanian Government for Tasmania Graduate Research Scholarship for the PhD study of T.S. is gratefully acknowledged.

References

1. Vindigni, S.M.; Zisman, T.L.; Suskind, D.L.; Damman, C.J. The intestinal microbiome, barrier function, and immune system in inflammatory bowel disease: A tripartite pathophysiological circuit with implications for new therapeutic directions. *Ther. Adv. Gastroenterol.* **2016**, *9*, 606–625. [CrossRef]
2. Ng, S.C.; Shi, H.Y.; Hamidi, N.; Underwood, F.E.; Tang, W.; Benchimol, E.I.; Panaccione, R.; Ghosh, S.; Wu, J.C.; Chan, F.K. Worldwide incidence and prevalence of inflammatory bowel disease in the 21st century: A systematic review of population-based studies. *Lancet* **2017**, *390*, 2769–2778. [CrossRef]
3. Hou, J.K.; Lee, D.; Lewis, J. Diet and inflammatory bowel disease: Review of patient-targeted recommendations. *Clin. Gastroenterol. Hepatol.* **2014**, *12*, 1592–1600. [CrossRef]
4. Palumbo, V.; Romeo, M.; Marino Gammazza, A.; Carini, F.; Damiani, P.; Damiano, G.; Buscemi, S.; Lo Monte, A.; Gerges Geagea, A.; Jurjus, A. The long-term effects of probiotics in the therapy of ulcerative colitis: A clinical study. *Biomed. Pap.* **2016**, *160*, 372–377. [CrossRef]
5. Abruzzo, A.; Damiano, G.; Altomare, R.; Palumbo, V.; Tomasello, G.; Buscemi, S.; Lo Monte, G.; Maione, C.; Buscemi, G.; Lo Monte, A. The influence of some dietary components on intestinal microbiota. *Prog. Nutr.* **2016**, *18*, 205–212.
6. Steed, H.; Macfarlane, G.T.; Blackett, K.L.; Bahrami, B.; Reynolds, N.; Walsh, S.V.; Cummings, J.H.; Macfarlane, S. Clinical trial: The microbiological and immunological effects of synbiotic consumption—A randomized double-blind placebo-controlled study in active crohn's disease. *Aliment. Pharmacol. Ther.* **2010**, *32*, 872–883. [CrossRef]
7. Wasilewski, A.; Zielińska, M.; Storr, M.; Fichna, J. Beneficial effects of probiotics, prebiotics, synbiotics, and psychobiotics in inflammatory bowel disease. *Inflamm. Bowel Dis.* **2015**, *21*, 1674–1682. [CrossRef]
8. Moroeanu, V.I.; Vamanu, E.; Paun, G.; Neagu, E.; Ungureanu, O.R.; Eremia, S.A.; Radu, G.-L.; Ionescu, R.; Pelinescu, D.R. Probiotic strains influence on infant microbiota in the in vitro colonic fermentation model gis1. *Indian J. Microbiol.* **2015**, *55*, 423–429. [CrossRef] [PubMed]
9. Wong, C.; Harris, P.J.; Ferguson, L.R. Potential benefits of dietary fibre intervention in inflammatory bowel disease. *Int. J. Mol. Sci.* **2016**, *17*, 919. [CrossRef]
10. Pituch-Zdanowska, A.; Banaszkiewicz, A.; Albrecht, P. The role of dietary fibre in inflammatory bowel disease. *Prz. Gastroenterol.* **2015**, *10*, 135. [CrossRef]
11. Galvez, J.; Rodríguez-Cabezas, M.E.; Zarzuelo, A. Effects of dietary fiber on inflammatory bowel disease. *Mol. Nutr. Food Res.* **2005**, *49*, 601–608. [CrossRef]
12. Williams, B.A.; Grant, L.J.; Gidley, M.J.; Mikkelsen, D. Gut fermentation of dietary fibres: Physico-chemistry of plant cell walls and implications for health. *Int. J. Mol. Sci.* **2017**, *18*, 2203. [CrossRef]
13. Tuohy, K.M.; Conterno, L.; Gasperotti, M.; Viola, R. Up-regulating the human intestinal microbiome using whole plant foods, polyphenols, and/or fiber. *J. Agric. Food Chem.* **2012**, *60*, 8776–8782. [CrossRef]
14. Liu, R.H. Health benefits of fruit and vegetables are from additive and synergistic combinations of phytochemicals. *Am. J. Clin. Nutr.* **2003**, *78*, 517S–520S. [CrossRef]
15. Edwards, G.; Ball, M. Dietary Supplement for the Treatment of Acid Reflux and Gastro-Oesophageal Reflux Disease (Gord/Gerd). U.S. Patent US20160287657A, 2016.
16. Ball, M.; Edwards, G. Use of Dietary Fibre Supplement in a Food Formulation. U.S. Patent WO2014162303A1, 2016.
17. Gamage, H.K.; Tetu, S.G.; Chong, R.W.; Bucio-Noble, D.; Rosewarne, C.P.; Kautto, L.; Ball, M.S.; Molloy, M.; Packer, N.H.; Paulsen, I.T. Fibre supplements derived from sugarcane stem, wheat dextrin and psyllium husk have different in vitro effects on the human gut microbiota. *Front. Microbiol.* **2018**, *9*, 1618. [CrossRef]
18. Walton, S.L.; Bischoff, K.M.; van Heiningen, A.R.; van Walsum, G.P. Production of lactic acid from hemicellulose extracts by bacillus coagulans mxl-9. *J. Ind. Microbiol. Biotechnol.* **2010**, *37*, 823–830. [CrossRef]
19. Konuray, G.; Erginkaya, Z. Potential use of bacillus coagulans in the food industry. *Foods* **2018**, *7*, 92. [CrossRef]

20. Slavin, J.L.; Brauer, P.M.; Marlett, J.A. Neutral detergent fiber, hemicellulose and cellulose digestibility in human subjects. *J. Nutr.* **1981**, *111*, 287–297. [CrossRef]
21. Leschine, S.B. Cellulose degradation in anaerobic environments. *Annu. Rev. Microbiol.* **1995**, *49*, 399–426. [CrossRef]
22. Shinde, T.; Vemuri, R.; Shastri, M.D.; Perera, A.P.; Tristram, S.; Stanley, R.; Eri, R. Probiotic bacillus coagulans mtcc 5856 spores exhibit excellent in-vitro functional efficacy in simulated gastric survival, mucosal adhesion and immunomodulation. *J. Funct. Foods* **2019**, *52*, 100–108. [CrossRef]
23. Baron, M. Original research: A patented strain of *bacillus coagulans* increased immune response to viral challenge. *Postgrad. Med.* **2009**, *121*, 114–118. [CrossRef]
24. Chassaing, B.; Aitken, J.D.; Malleshappa, M.; Vijay-Kumar, M. Dextran sulfate sodium (dss)-induced colitis in mice. *Curr. Protoc. Immunol.* **2014**, *104*, 15.25. 1–15.25. 14.
25. Murthy, S.; Cooper, H.S.; Shim, H.; Shah, R.S.; Ibrahim, S.A.; Sedergran, D.J. Treatment of dextran sulfate sodium-induced murine colitis by intracolonic cyclosporin. *Dig. Dis. Sci.* **1993**, *38*, 1722–1734. [CrossRef]
26. Perera, A.P.; Fernando, R.; Shinde, T.; Gundamaraju, R.; Southam, B.; Sohal, S.S.; Robertson, A.A.; Schroder, K.; Kunde, D.; Eri, R. Mcc950, a specific small molecule inhibitor of nlrp3 inflammasome attenuates colonic inflammation in spontaneous colitis mice. *Sci. Rep.* **2018**, *8*, 8618. [CrossRef]
27. Demon, D.; Kuchmiy, A.; Fossoul, A.; Zhu, Q.; Kanneganti, T.-D.; Lamkanfi, M. Caspase-11 is expressed in the colonic mucosa and protects against dextran sodium sulfate-induced colitis. *Mucosal Immunol.* **2014**, *7*, 1480. [CrossRef]
28. Eri, R.; McGuckin, M.A.; Wadley, R. T cell transfer model of colitis: A great tool to assess the contribution of t cells in chronic intestinal inflammation. In *Leucocytes*; Springer: Berlin/Heidelberg, Germany, 2012; pp. 261–275.
29. Koelink, P.J.; Wildenberg, M.E.; Stitt, L.W.; Feagan, B.G.; Koldijk, M.; van't Wout, A.B.; Atreya, R.; Vieth, M.; Brandse, J.F.; Duijst, S. Development of reliable, valid and responsive scoring systems for endoscopy and histology in animal models for inflammatory bowel disease. *J. Crohn's Colitis* **2018**, *1*, 10. [CrossRef]
30. Sovran, B.; Lu, P.; Loonen, L.M.; Hugenholtz, F.; Belzer, C.; Stolte, E.H.; Boekschoten, M.V.; Van Baarlen, P.; Smidt, H.; Kleerebezem, M. Identification of commensal species positively correlated with early stress responses to a compromised mucus barrier. *Inflamm. Bowel Dis.* **2016**, *22*, 826–840. [CrossRef]
31. Li, P.; Zhang, R.; Wang, L.; Gan, Y.; Xu, Y.; Song, L.; Luo, L.; Zhao, C.; Zhang, C.; Ouyang, B. Long-term load duration induces n-cadherin down-regulation and loss of cell phenotype of nucleus pulposus cells in a disc bioreactor culture. *Biosci. Rep.* **2017**, *37*, BSR20160582. [CrossRef]
32. Lean, Q.Y.; Eri, R.D.; Randall-Demllo, S.; Sohal, S.S.; Stewart, N.; Peterson, G.M.; Gueven, N.; Patel, R.P. Orally administered enoxaparin ameliorates acute colitis by reducing macrophage-associated inflammatory responses. *PLoS ONE* **2015**, *10*, e0134259. [CrossRef] [PubMed]
33. Mei, Q.; Xu, J.; Xiang, L.; Hu, Y.; Hu, X.; Xu, Z. Change of nitric oxide in experimental colitis and its inhibition by melatonin in vivo and in vitro. *Postgrad. Med. J.* **2005**, *81*, 667–672. [CrossRef] [PubMed]
34. Furuhashi, T.; Sugitate, K.; Nakai, T.; Jikumaru, Y.; Ishihara, G. Rapid profiling method for mammalian feces short chain fatty acids by gc-ms. *Anal. Biochem.* **2018**, *543*, 51–54. [CrossRef] [PubMed]
35. Vemuri, R.; Shinde, T.; Gundamaraju, R.; Gondalia, S.; Karpe, A.; Beale, D.; Martoni, C.; Eri, R. Lactobacillus acidophilus dds-1 modulates the gut microbiota and improves metabolic profiles in aging mice. *Nutrients* **2018**, *10*, 1255. [CrossRef]
36. Sansone, S.-A.; Fan, T.; Goodacre, R.; Griffin, J.L.; Hardy, N.W.; Kaddurah-Daouk, R.; Kristal, B.S.; Lindon, J.; Mendes, P.; Morrison, N. The metabolomics standards initiative. *Nat. Biotechnol.* **2007**, *25*, 846.
37. Smart, K.F.; Aggio, R.B.; Van Houtte, J.R.; Villas-Bôas, S.G. Analytical platform for metabolome analysis of microbial cells using methyl chloroformate derivatization followed by gas chromatography–mass spectrometry. *Nat. Protoc.* **2010**, *5*, 1709. [CrossRef]
38. Srutkova, D.; Schwarzer, M.; Hudcovic, T.; Zakostelska, Z.; Drab, V.; Spanova, A.; Rittich, B.; Kozakova, H.; Schabussova, I. Bifidobacterium longum ccm 7952 promotes epithelial barrier function and prevents acute dss-induced colitis in strictly strain-specific manner. *PLoS ONE* **2015**, *10*, e0134050. [CrossRef]
39. Han, F.; Fan, H.; Yao, M.; Yang, S.; Han, J. Oral administration of yeast β-glucan ameliorates inflammation and intestinal barrier in dextran sodium sulfate-induced acute colitis. *J. Funct. Foods* **2017**, *35*, 115–126. [CrossRef]

40. Al Mijan, M.; Lim, B.O. Diets, functional foods, and nutraceuticals as alternative therapies for inflammatory bowel disease: Present status and future trends. *World J. Gastroenterol.* **2018**, *24*, 2673. [CrossRef]
41. Ferguson, L.R.; Shelling, A.N.; Browning, B.L.; Huebner, C.; Petermann, I. Genes, diet and inflammatory bowel disease. *Mutat. Res. /Fundam. Mol. Mech. Mutagenesis* **2007**, *622*, 70–83. [CrossRef]
42. Kanauchi, O.; Serizawa, I.; Araki, Y.; Suzuki, A.; Andoh, A.; Fujiyama, Y.; Mitsuyama, K.; Takaki, K.; Toyonaga, A.; Sata, M. Germinated barley foodstuff, a prebiotic product, ameliorates inflammation of colitis through modulation of the enteric environment. *J. Gastroenterol.* **2003**, *38*, 134–141. [CrossRef]
43. Mitsuyama, K.; Saiki, T.; Kanauchi, O.; Iwanaga, T.; Tomiyasu, N.; Nishiyama, T.; Tateishi, H.; Shirachi, A.; Ide, M.; Suzuki, A. Treatment of ulcerative colitis with germinated barley foodstuff feeding: A pilot study. *Aliment. Pharmacol. Ther.* **1998**, *12*, 1225–1230. [CrossRef]
44. Majeed, M.; Nagabhushanam, K.; Natarajan, S.; Sivakumar, A.; Ali, F.; Pande, A.; Majeed, S.; Karri, S.K. *Bacillus coagulans* mtcc 5856 supplementation in the management of diarrhea predominant irritable bowel syndrome: A double blind randomized placebo controlled pilot clinical study. *Nutr. J.* **2016**, *15*, 21. [CrossRef]
45. Turner, J.R. Intestinal mucosal barrier function in health and disease. *Nat. Rev. Immunol.* **2009**, *9*, 799. [CrossRef]
46. Gong, Y.; Li, H.; Li, Y. Effects of bacillus subtilis on epithelial tight junctions of mice with inflammatory bowel disease. *J. Interferon Cytokine Res.* **2016**, *36*, 75–85. [CrossRef]
47. Zhang, W.; Zhu, Y.-H.; Zhou, D.; Wu, Q.; Song, D.; Dicksved, J.; Wang, J.-F. Oral administration of a select mixture of bacillus probiotics affects the gut microbiota and goblet cell function following escherichia coli challenge in newly weaned pigs of genotype muc4 that are supposed to be enterotoxigenic e. Coli f4ab/ac receptor negative. *Appl. Environ. Microbiol.* **2017**, *83*, e02747-16. [CrossRef]
48. Xavier, R.; Podolsky, D. Unravelling the pathogenesis of inflammatory bowel disease. *Nature* **2007**, *448*, 427. [CrossRef]
49. Neurath, M.F. Cytokines in inflammatory bowel disease. *Nat. Rev. Immunol.* **2014**, *14*, 329. [CrossRef]
50. Hyams, J.S.; Lerer, T.; Griffiths, A.; Pfefferkorn, M.; Kugathasan, S.; Evans, J.; Otley, A.; Carvalho, R.; Mack, D.; Bousvaros, A. Long-term outcome of maintenance infliximab therapy in children with crohn's disease. *Inflamm. Bowel Dis.* **2008**, *15*, 816–822. [CrossRef]
51. Atreya, R.; Mudter, J.; Finotto, S.; Müllberg, J.; Jostock, T.; Wirtz, S.; Schütz, M.; Bartsch, B.; Holtmann, M.; Becker, C. Blockade of interleukin 6 trans signaling suppresses t-cell resistance against apoptosis in chronic intestinal inflammation: Evidence in crohn disease and experimental colitis in vivo. *Nat. Med.* **2000**, *6*, 583. [CrossRef]
52. Jobin, C.; Sartor, B.R. Nf-κb signaling proteins as therapeutic targets for inflammatory bowel diseases. *Inflamm. Bowel Dis.* **2000**, *6*, 206–213. [CrossRef]
53. Neuman, M.G. Immune dysfunction in inflammatory bowel disease. *Transl. Res.* **2007**, *149*, 173–186. [CrossRef]
54. Soufli, I.; Toumi, R.; Rafa, H.; Touil-Boukoffa, C. Cytokines and nitric oxide in immunopathogenesis of ibd and potential therapeutic approaches. In *New Insights into Inflammatory BOWEL disease*; InTech: Vienna, Austria, 2016.
55. Groschwitz, K.R.; Hogan, S.P. Intestinal barrier function: Molecular regulation and disease pathogenesis. *J. Allergy Clin. Immunol.* **2009**, *124*, 3–20. [CrossRef]
56. Del Giudice, M.; Gangestad, S.W. Rethinking il-6 and crp: Why they are more than inflammatory biomarkers, and why it matters. *Brainbehav. Immun.* **2018**, *70*, 61–75. [CrossRef]
57. Solem, C.A.; Loftus, E.V., Jr.; Tremaine, W.J.; Harmsen, W.S.; Zinsmeister, A.R.; Sandborn, W.J. Correlation of c-reactive protein with clinical, endoscopic, histologic, and radiographic activity in inflammatory bowel disease. *Inflamm. Bowel Dis.* **2005**, *11*, 707–712. [CrossRef]
58. Kerr, T.; Ciorba, M.; Matsumoto, H.; Davis, V.; Luo, J.; Kennedy, S.; Xie, Y.; Shaker, A.; Dieckgraefe, B.; Davidson, N. Dextran sodium sulfate inhibition of real-time polymerase chain reaction amplification: A poly-a purification solution. *Inflamm. Bowel Dis.* **2011**, *18*, 344–348. [CrossRef]
59. Levy, M.; Thaiss, C.A.; Elinav, E. Metabolites: Messengers between the microbiota and the immune system. *Genes Dev.* **2016**, *30*, 1589–1597. [CrossRef]
60. Vernocchi, P.; Del Chierico, F.; Putignani, L. Gut microbiota profiling: Metabolomics based approach to unravel compounds affecting human health. *Front. Microbiol.* **2016**, *7*, 1144. [CrossRef]

61. Martin, F.-P.; Su, M.-M.; Xie, G.-X.; Guiraud, S.P.; Kussmann, M.; Godin, J.-P.; Jia, W.; Nydegger, A. Urinary metabolic insights into host-gut microbial interactions in healthy and ibd children. *World J. Gastroenterol.* **2017**, *23*, 3643. [CrossRef]
62. Marchesi, J.R.; Holmes, E.; Khan, F.; Kochhar, S.; Scanlan, P.; Shanahan, F.; Wilson, I.D.; Wang, Y. Rapid and noninvasive metabonomic characterization of inflammatory bowel disease. *J. Proteome Res.* **2007**, *6*, 546–551. [CrossRef]
63. Robinson, A.M.; Gondalia, S.V.; Karpe, A.V.; Eri, R.; Beale, D.J.; Morrison, P.D.; Palombo, E.A.; Nurgali, K. Fecal microbiota and metabolome in a mouse model of spontaneous chronic colitis: Relevance to human inflammatory bowel disease. *Inflamm. Bowel Dis.* **2016**, *22*, 2767–2787. [CrossRef]
64. Sun, M.; Wu, W.; Liu, Z.; Cong, Y. Microbiota metabolite short chain fatty acids, gpcr, and inflammatory bowel diseases. *J. Gastroenterol.* **2017**, *52*, 1–8. [CrossRef]
65. Breuer, R.I.; Buto, S.K.; Christ, M.L.; Bean, J.; Vernia, P.; Paoluzi, P.; Di Paolo, M.; Caprilli, R. Rectal irrigation with short-chain fatty acids for distal ulcerative colitis. *Dig. Dis. Sci.* **1991**, *36*, 185–187. [CrossRef]
66. Koh, A.; De Vadder, F.; Kovatcheva-Datchary, P.; Bäckhed, F. From dietary fiber to host physiology: Short-chain fatty acids as key bacterial metabolites. *Cell* **2016**, *165*, 1332–1345. [CrossRef]
67. Kaur, A.; Tuncil, Y.E.; Sikaroodi, M.; Gillevet, P.; Patterson, J.A.; Keshavarzian, A.; Hamaker, B.R. Alterations in the amounts of microbial metabolites in different regions of the mouse large intestine using variably fermentable fibres. *Bioact. Carbohydr. Diet. Fibre* **2018**, *13*, 7–13. [CrossRef]
68. Pang, W.; Vogensen, F.K.; Nielsen, D.S.; Hansen, A.K. Faecal and caecal microbiota profiles of mice do not cluster in the same way. *Lab. Anim.* **2012**, *46*, 231–236. [CrossRef]
69. Hirano, A.; Umeno, J.; Okamoto, Y.; Shibata, H.; Ogura, Y.; Moriyama, T.; Torisu, T.; Fujioka, S.; Fuyuno, Y.; Kawarabayasi, Y. Comparison of the microbial community structure between inflamed and non-inflamed sites in patients with ulcerative colitis. *J. Gastroenterol. Hepatol.* **2018**, *33*, 1590–1597. [CrossRef]
70. Majeed, M.; Nagabhushanam, K.; Arumugam, S.; Natarajan, S.; Majeed, S.; Pande, A.; Beede, K.; Ali, F. Cranberry seed fibre: A promising prebiotic fibre and its fermentation by the probiotic bacillus coagulans mtcc 5856. *Int. J. Food Sci. Technol.* **2018**, *53*, 1640–1647. [CrossRef]
71. Majeed, M.; Majeed, S.; Nagabhushanam, K.; Arumugam, S.; Natarajan, S.; Beede, K.; Ali, F. Galactomannan from trigonella foenum-graecum l. Seed: Prebiotic application and its fermentation by the probiotic bacillus coagulans strain mtcc 5856. *Food Sci. Nutr.* **2018**, *6*, 666–673. [CrossRef]
72. Nielsen, D.S.G.; Jensen, B.B.; Theil, P.K.; Nielsen, T.S.; Knudsen, K.E.B.; Purup, S. Effect of butyrate and fermentation products on epithelial integrity in a mucus-secreting human colon cell line. *J. Funct. Foods* **2018**, *40*, 9–17. [CrossRef]
73. Zheng, L.; Kelly, C.J.; Battista, K.D.; Schaefer, R.; Lanis, J.M.; Alexeev, E.E.; Wang, R.X.; Onyiah, J.C.; Kominsky, D.J.; Colgan, S.P. Microbial-derived butyrate promotes epithelial barrier function through il-10 receptor–dependent repression of claudin-2. *J. Immunol.* **2017**, *199*, 2976–2984. [CrossRef]
74. Simeoli, R.; Mattace Raso, G.; Pirozzi, C.; Lama, A.; Santoro, A.; Russo, R.; Montero-Melendez, T.; Berni Canani, R.; Calignano, A.; Perretti, M. An orally administered butyrate-releasing derivative reduces neutrophil recruitment and inflammation in dextran sulphate sodium-induced murine colitis. *Br. J. Pharmacol.* **2017**, *174*, 1484–1496. [CrossRef]
75. Van Immerseel, F.; Ducatelle, R.; De Vos, M.; Boon, N.; Van De Wiele, T.; Verbeke, K.; Rutgeerts, P.; Sas, B.; Louis, P.; Flint, H.J. Butyric acid-producing anaerobic bacteria as a novel probiotic treatment approach for inflammatory bowel disease. *J. Med. Microbiol.* **2010**, *59*, 141–143. [CrossRef]
76. Tedelind, S.; Westberg, F.; Kjerrulf, M.; Vidal, A. Anti-inflammatory properties of the short-chain fatty acids acetate and propionate: A study with relevance to inflammatory bowel disease. *World J. Gastroenterol. WJG* **2007**, *13*, 2826. [CrossRef]
77. Maslowski, K.M.; Vieira, A.T.; Ng, A.; Kranich, J.; Sierro, F.; Yu, D.; Schilter, H.C.; Rolph, M.S.; Mackay, F.; Artis, D. Regulation of inflammatory responses by gut microbiota and chemoattractant receptor gpr43. *Nature* **2009**, *461*, 1282. [CrossRef]
78. Macia, L.; Tan, J.; Vieira, A.T.; Leach, K.; Stanley, D.; Luong, S.; Maruya, M.; McKenzie, C.I.; Hijikata, A.; Wong, C. Metabolite-sensing receptors gpr43 and gpr109a facilitate dietary fibre-induced gut homeostasis through regulation of the inflammasome. *Nat. Commun.* **2015**, *6*, 6734. [CrossRef]

79. Yuille, S.; Reichardt, N.; Panda, S.; Dunbar, H.; Mulder, I.E. Human gut bacteria as potent class i histone deacetylase inhibitors in vitro through production of butyric acid and valeric acid. *PLoS ONE* **2018**, *13*, e0201073. [CrossRef]
80. Thorburn, A.N.; Macia, L.; Mackay, C.R. Diet, metabolites, and "western-lifestyle" inflammatory diseases. *Immunity* **2014**, *40*, 833–842. [CrossRef]
81. Nguyen, T.L.A.; Vieira-Silva, S.; Liston, A.; Raes, J. How informative is the mouse for human gut microbiota research? *Dis. Models Mech.* **2015**, *8*, 1–16. [CrossRef]

6

Combination of *Lactobacillus acidophilus* and *Bifidobacterium animalis* subsp. *lactis* Shows a Stronger Anti-Inflammatory Effect than Individual Strains in HT-29 Cells

Sing-Chung Li [1], Wei-Fang Hsu [1], Jung-Su Chang [1,2] and Chun-Kuang Shih [1,3,4,*]

1 School of Nutrition and Health Sciences, College of Nutrition, Taipei Medical University, Taipei 11031, Taiwan; sinchung@tmu.edu.tw (S.-C.L.); greg_hsu@hotmail.com (W.-F.H.); susanchang@tmu.edu.tw (J.-S.C.)
2 Graduate Institute of Metabolism and Obesity Sciences, College of Nutrition, Taipei Medical University, Taipei 11031, Taiwan
3 School of Food Safety, College of Nutrition, Taipei Medical University, Taipei 11031, Taiwan
4 Master Program in Food Safety, College of Nutrition, Taipei Medical University, Taipei 11031, Taiwan
* Correspondence: ckshih@tmu.edu.tw

Abstract: Inflammatory bowel disease (IBD) is an emerging health problem associated with the dysregulation of the intestinal immune system and microbiome. Probiotics are able to reduce inflammatory responses in intestinal epithelial cells (IECs). However, entire signaling pathways and the interaction between different probiotics have not been well-documented. This study was designed to investigate the anti-inflammatory effects and mechanisms of single and combined probiotics. HT-29 cells were induced by lipopolysaccharide (LPS) and tumor necrosis factor (TNF)-α, treated with *Lactobacillus acidophilus*, *Bifidobacterium animalis* subsp. *lactis* or their combination and analyzed for inflammation-related molecules. Both *L. acidophilus* and *B. animalis* subsp. *lactis* reduced interleukin (IL)-8 secretion and the expressions of phosphorylated p65 nuclear factor-kappa B (*p*-p65 NF-κB), phosphorylated p38 mitogen-activated protein kinase (*p*-p38 MAPK), vascular cell adhesion molecule-1 (VCAM-1) and cyclooxygenase-2 (COX-2), while they increased toll-like receptor 2 (TLR2) expression. *L. acidophilus* did not decrease intercellular adhesion molecule-1 (ICAM-1) but enhanced the inhibitory efficacy of *B. animalis* subsp. *lactis*. Combined probiotics showed the best anti-inflammatory activity. These results suggest that *L. acidophilus* and *B. animalis* subsp. *lactis* may exert a potent anti-inflammatory effect through modulating TLR2-mediated NF-κB and MAPK signaling pathways in inflammatory IECs. Both strains, especially their combination, may be novel adjuvants for IBD therapy.

Keywords: intestinal epithelial cells; inflammation; probiotics; *Lactobacillus acidophilus*; *Bifidobacterium animalis* subsp. *lactis*

---

1. Introduction

Inflammatory bowel disease (IBD), including ulcerative colitis (UC) and Crohn's disease (CD), is traditionally a common chronic gastrointestinal disease in several Western countries. The highest reported prevalence rates of IBD are in Europe (505/100,000 for UC in Norway and 322/100,000 for CD in Germany) and North America (286/100,000 for UC in the USA and 319/100,000 for CD in Canada) [1]. The overall prevalence of IBD has exceeded 0.3% in North America and many European countries [1]. However, IBD has become a global disease with accelerating incidence in newly industrialized countries in Asia, Africa and South America [1]. According to a recent study of Yen et al. [2], both the incidence and prevalence of IBD increased continuously in Taiwan from 2001 to 2015. Improved hygiene, civilization and Westernization may be possible causes [2]. Several studies suggest that IBD is an emerging health problem in the world [1–3]. The reason for the global increase in this initially Western-prevalent disease is still unknown, but it may be closely associated with environmental and social changes, such as the adoption of Western lifestyle and diet [1,2]. The rise of IBD in adults and children has been observed in Western developed countries, while gut microbiota and dietary fiber-rich diet of rural African individuals may protect them from the threat of IBD [4].

The etiology of IBD is thought to relate to a complex interaction of genetic and environmental factors, including the dysregulation of the enteric immune system and alterations in the intestinal microbiome [5]. Patients with IBD have typical dysbiosis characterized by an increase in pro-inflammatory bacteria, a decrease in anti-inflammatory bacteria and a reduction in bacterial diversity compared to the healthy population [5]. A reduced diversity of the gut microbiota in IBD patients is largely due to a low abundance of probiotics belonging to the *Lactobacillus* and *Bifidobacterium* genera [6]. IBD is characterized by mucosal and systemic inflammatory responses to the gut microbiome, which is the outcome of a lack of mucosal immune tolerance [6]. It is well-known that chronic inflammation is related to carcinogenesis and thus long-standing IBD is considered as a risk factor of colorectal cancer (CRC), especially colitis-associated colorectal cancer (CAC). In recent years, high incidence rates of CRC have been observed in Taiwan and other countries where the rates were historically low [7]. This increasing trend of CRC is similar to that of IBD in many countries. Both CRC and IBD are now global health issues that cannot be ignored.

The mucosal tissue of the intestine contains the largest part of the immune system in humans. It is estimated that 70% of immune cells are present in the gut [8]. Intestinal epithelial cells (IECs) provide a physical and chemical barrier between the intestinal lumen and the lamina propria [8]. They represent the first contact point for bacteria within the gut and thus prevent microbial penetration and induce communication for immune recognition of intestinal bacteria [9]. The activation of the pro-inflammatory genes in IECs in response to challenges by bacterial products such as lipopolysaccharide (LPS) or pro-inflammatory cytokines such as tumor necrosis factor (TNF)-α is associated with acute and chronic intestinal inflammation [10]. However, bacterial ligands may not directly alter the inflammation of IECs, although bacterial cell wall components, such as LPS and lipoteichoic acid (LTA), contribute to toll-like receptor (TLR)-mediated inflammation [11]. Ligands from pathogenic bacteria efficiently activate monocytes and macrophages through the secretion of pro-inflammatory cytokines such as TNF-α, interleukin (IL)-1β, IL-6 and IL-8 [11]. In contrast, ligands from probiotic bacteria only minimally induce TNF-α production [11]. These studies suggest that it is reasonable to simulate the inflammatory environment of the intestine using a combination of bacterial ligands and pro-inflammatory cytokines.

Probiotics have beneficial effects on the host through their ability to modulate the mucosal immune system. They have been shown to both augment/modulate homeostatic immune defenses and to ameliorate infection, inflammation and allergy by modulating gut function [12]. Treatment with probiotics has been considered to be potentially effective and safe in patients with IBD. It has been reported that individual probiotic species have variable potential to stimulate the mucosal immune system [13]. Probiotics differentially modulate IECs' responses via the activation or suppression of distinct signaling pathways, such as TLR, nuclear factor-kappa B (NF-κB) and mitogen-activated protein kinase (MAPK) signaling pathways, in a strain-dependent manner, including strains of the same species [12,14].

The majority of probiotic microorganisms belong to the genera *Lactobacillus* and *Bifidobacterium*, and most *Lactobacillus* and *Bifidobacterium* species belong to probiotics [15]. *Lactobacillus* and *Bifidobacterium* species have been shown to reduce inflammatory responses, including NF-κB activation and IL-8 production, in inflammatory IECs, rodent colitis models and patients with IBD [9,16]. However, not all probiotics exert constant anti-inflammatory effects in experimental models of intestinal inflammation. For example, *L. acidophilus*, *B. lactis* and *L. casei* have an anti-inflammatory activity in the 2,4,6-trinitrobenzene sulfonic acid (TNBS) model of rat colitis but each probiotic shows its own anti-inflammatory profile [17]. It would be interesting to compare different probiotics in the same experimental model, in order to establish the best profile in a given setting and to further apply this new concept for IBD therapy [17]. A recent meta-analysis study demonstrated that results from clinical trials of probiotics on IBD were inconsistent [5]. Among all trials included in this meta-analysis, some showed an improvement in the maintenance or induction of remission by probiotics, while others failed to show any benefit [5]. This could be due to the species or strains of probiotics used, or the methodological differences among studies. Some studies found that probiotics may be as effective as 5-aminosalicylates (5-ASAs), a common drug for the treatment of IBD, in preventing relapse of quiescent UC but other studies showed that there was no benefit of probiotics over placebo in inducing remission of active UC [5]. However, when only trials of VSL#3—a mixed preparation of probiotics—were considered, there appeared to be a benefit. VSL#3 may be effective in inducing remission in patients with active UC [5]. These findings suggest that combination of probiotics seems to be more effective in anti-inflammation than single strains. However, the detailed anti-inflammatory mechanism of each probiotic and their interactions are still unclear.

Although some strains of probiotics belonging to the *Lactobacillus* and *Bifidobacterium* genera have been shown to possess anti-inflammatory and immunomodulatory activities, their entire signaling pathways have not been well-documented. There are only limited studies that have examined the inflammation-associated signaling pathways of *L. acidophilus* and *B. animalis* subsp. *lactis*, two common strains of probiotics used in fermented dairy products, especially the comparison and interaction between these probiotics. The aim of the present study was to investigate the anti-inflammatory effects and associated mechanisms of *L. acidophilus*, *B. animalis* subsp. *lactis* and their combination in LPS- and TNF-α-induced inflammatory IECs.

2. Materials and Methods

2.1. Cell Culture

Human colon cancer cell line HT-29 cells were purchased from the Food Industry Research and Development Institute (Hsinchu, Taiwan) and incubated in 9-cm culture dishes as a monolayer in Roswell Park Memorial Institute (RPMI) 1640 medium supplemented with 10% fetal bovine serum (FBS), 1% L-glutamine (*v*/*v*) and 1% penicillin/streptomycin and maintained at 37 °C in a humidified atmosphere of 5% CO_2. Cells were sub-cultured following enzymatic digestion using 1% trypsin solution.

2.2. Bacterial Strains

L. acidophilus and *B. animalis* subsp. *lactis* (Chr. Hansen, Denmark) were grown in the Man-Rogosa-Sharpe (MRS) broth overnight at 37 °C in anaerobic conditions. Viable bacteria were counted by plating serial dilutions on MRS agar. Both strains of probiotics were heat-inactivated by water-bath at 60 °C for 30 min, then collected by centrifugation at 500× *g* for 10 min at 4 °C and washed in phosphate-buffered saline (PBS), as described in previous studies [18,19].

2.3. Treatments of Cells

HT-29 cells were seeded in a 24-well microtiter plate at a density of 3×10^5 cells/well in volume of 400 μL medium for one day. Cells as an inflammatory group were treated with non-FBS medium containing LPS (1 μg/mL) and TNF-α (20 ng/mL) from *Escherichia coli* O58:B5 (L6529 Sigma-Aldrich,

St. Louis, MO, USA) for 24 h [20]. Cells as intervention groups were added to probiotics at the designated multiplicity of infection (MOI) of 0.1, 1, 10 [21], and incubated in 5% CO_2 at 37 °C with non-FBS medium containing LPS and TNF-α. The culture medium was harvested and analyzed for IL-8 secretion by enzyme-linked immunosorbent assay (ELISA). We chose the doses of probiotics with an inhibitory effect on IL-8 secretion for comparing the anti-inflammatory effects of single and combined probiotics. Cells were incubated with or without probiotics (*L. acidophilus*, *B. animalis* subsp. *lactis* or both), then medium and cells were collected and analyzed by ELISA and Western blot, respectively.

2.4. Cell Viability Assay

HT-29 cells were seeded in a 96-well microtiter plate at a density of 1×10^4 cells/well in volume of 100 μL medium. Cells were treated with *L. acidophilus*, *B. animalis* subsp. *lactis* or both and with LPS and TNF-α for 24 h. After the above treatments, cells were incubated with 3-(4,5-dimethylthiazol-2-yl)-2,5-diphenyltetrazolium bromide (MTT) dye (0.5 μg/μL) at 37 °C for 4 h. Absorbance of the product was read at 570 nm by ELISA reader.

2.5. Analysis of IL-8 Secretion by ELISA

IL-8 levels in HT-29 conditioned media were measured by a commercially available ELISA kit (BioLegend, San Diego, CA, USA).

2.6. Analysis of Protein Expression by Western Blot

The analytical procedures were modified from previous studies [22,23]. Cells were sonicated for 20 min and then lysed cells were centrifuged at 10,000× *g* for 10 min at 4 °C. Supernatants were collected and the protein concentration was determined using the Bio-Rad Bradford assay (Bio-Rad, Hercules, CA, USA). Samples (each containing 30 μg of supernatant protein) were mixed with NuPAGE LDS sample buffer and β-mercaptoethanol (Invitrogen, Carlsbad, CA, USA), heated at 95 °C for 10 min, cooled to room temperature and electrophoretically resolved on 10% NuPAGE Bis-Tris gels (Invitrogen, Carlsbad, CA, USA). Proteins were then transferred to polyvinylidene difluoride (PVDF) membrane, which was then blocked with blocking buffer (TBST containing 5% albumin) at room temperature for 1 h. The blot was probed with TLR2 (1:1000 dilution, BioVision, Milpitas, CA, USA), phosphorylated p65 NF-κB (*p*-p65 NF-κB, 1:1000 dilution, Bioworld, Dublin, OH, USA), phosphorylated p38 MAPK (*p*-p38 MAPK, 1:1000 dilution, BioVision, Milpitas, CA, USA), cyclooxygenase-2 (COX-2, 1:1000 dilution, Santa Cruz Biotechnology, Santa Cruz, CA, USA), intercellular adhesion molecule-1 (ICAM-1, 1:1000 dilution, BioVision, Milpitas, CA, USA) or vascular cell adhesion molecule-1 (VCAM-1, 1:1000 dilution, Abbiotec, San Diego, CA, USA) polyclonal antibody at 4 °C for 16 h. After being washed extensively to eliminate nonspecific binding, the membrane was incubated with the secondary alkaline phosphatase-labeled antibody at room temperature for 1 h and incubated with 5-bromo-4-chloro-3-indolyl-phosphate/nitroblue tetrazolium (BCIP/NBT) substrate solution (Sigma-Aldrich Inc., St. Louis, MO, USA) for 20 min in the dark. The reactive solution was removed, and the reaction was stopped using 50% methanol. Blot intensities were quantified using Bio-Rad Quantity One software (Bio-Rad Laboratories, Hercules, CA, USA). All experimental data are triplicates.

2.7. Statistical Analysis

Data are expressed as means and standard deviations. The difference among groups was analyzed by one-way analysis of variance (ANOVA) and Duncan's multiple range test using SAS software (SAS Institute, Cary, NC, USA). The significant difference was set at $p < 0.05$.

3. Results

3.1. *Effects of Different Doses of Single Probiotics on IL-8 Secretion in Inflammatory HT-29 Cells*

HT-29 cells stimulated with LPS and TNF-α secreted significantly higher IL-8 levels than did unstimulated cells (Figure 1A,B). *L. acidophilus* at MOI of 1 and 10 significantly decreased IL-8 secretion in inflammatory HT-29 cells (Figure 1A). *B. animalis* subsp. *lactis* at MOI of 10 showed an inhibitory effect on IL-8 secretion (Figure 1B). As a result, we chose *L. acidophilus* at MOI of 1 as group A, *B. animalis* subsp. *lactis* at MOI of 10 as group B, and combination of *L. acidophilus* at MOI of 1 and *B. animalis* subsp. *lactis* at MOI of 10 as group AB for further studies.

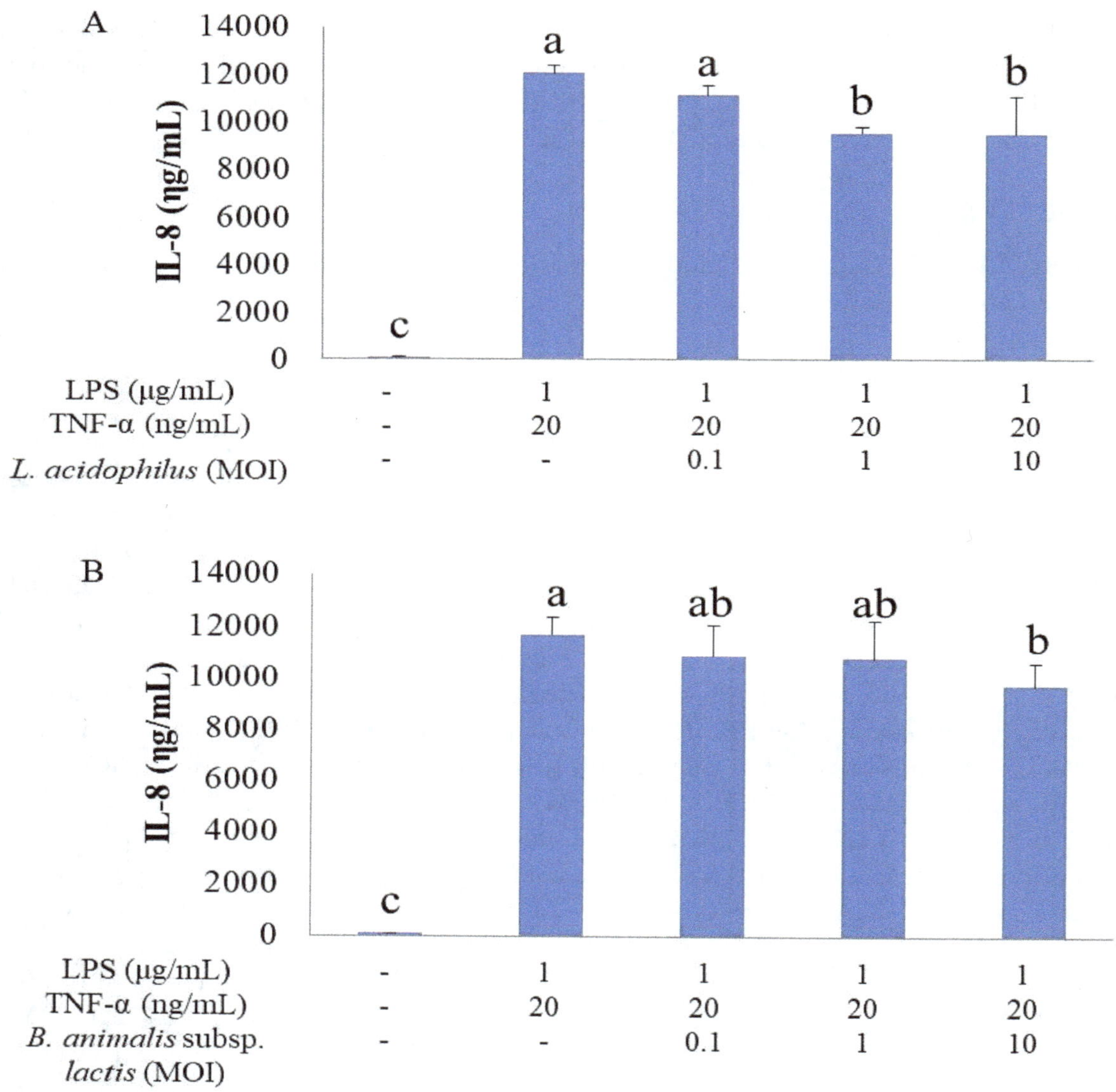

Figure 1. Effects of different doses of single probiotics on IL-8 secretion in inflammatory HT-29 cells. All values except for control are mean ± SD (n = 3). Bars with the same letter are not significantly different from one another determined by Duncan's multiple range test, $p < 0.05$. (**A**) The inhibitory effect of *L. acidophilus* on IL-8 secretion; (**B**) the inhibitory effect of *B. animalis* subsp. *lactis* on IL-8 secretion.

3.2. *Effects of Pro-Inflammatory Factors and Probiotics on Cell Viability*

The viabilities of HT-29 cells were not different among groups after 24 h of incubation (Figure 2), showing that pro-inflammatory factors (LPS and TNF-α) and probiotics (alone or in combination) did not affect the growth of HT-29 cells.

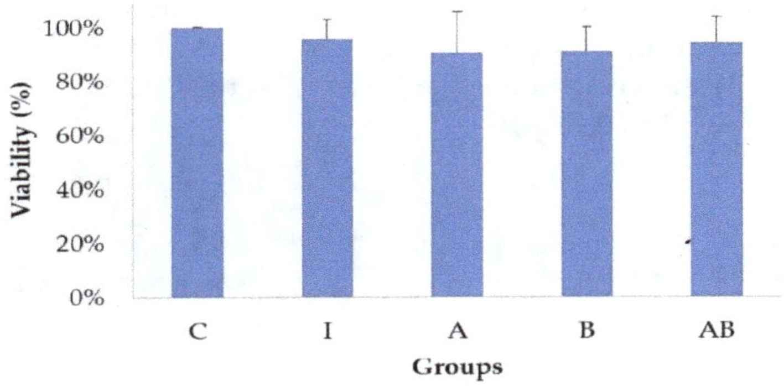

Figure 2. Effects of pro-inflammatory factors and probiotics on viability of HT-29 cells. All values except for control are mean ± SD (n = 3). There is no significant difference among groups determined by Duncan's multiple range test, $p < 0.05$. C, control; I, TNF-α (20 ng/mL) with LPS (1 μg/mL); A, *L. acidophilus* at MOI of 1 with TNF-α (20 ng/mL) and LPS (1 μg/mL); B, *B. animalis* subsp. *lactis* at MOI of 10 with TNF-α (20 ng/mL) and LPS (1 μg/mL); AB, *L. acidophilus* at MOI of 1 and *B. animalis* subsp. *lactis* at MOI of 10 with TNF-α (20 ng/mL) and LPS (1 μg/mL). Control group is used as the reference.

3.3. *Effects of Probiotics on IL-8 Secretion in Inflammatory HT-29 Cells*

A shown in Figure 3, all probiotics-treated inflammatory HT-29 cells (groups A, B and AB) had significantly lower IL-8 levels than did cells stimulated with LPS and TNF-α (group I). In addition, the IL-8 level was significantly lower in group AB than in either group A or B.

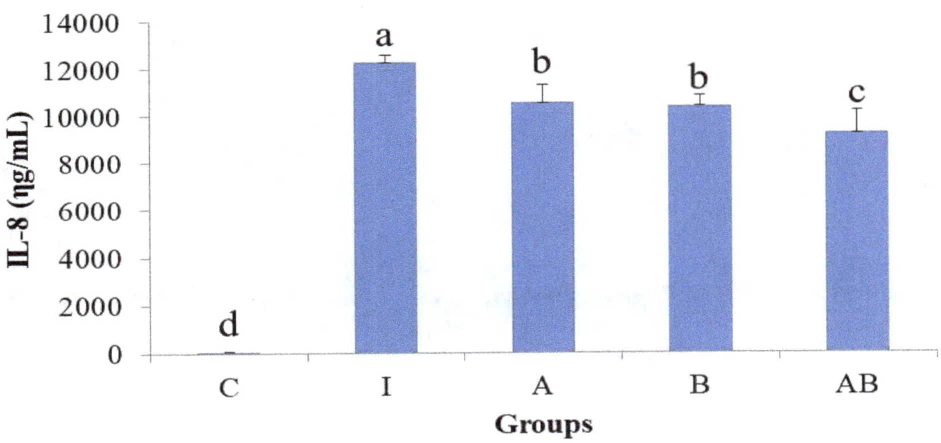

Figure 3. Effects of probiotics on IL-8 secretion in inflammatory HT-29 cells. All values except for control are mean ± SD (n = 3). Bars with the same letter are not significantly different from one another determined by Duncan's multiple range test, $p < 0.05$. C, control; I, TNF-α (20 ng/mL) with lipopolysaccharide (LPS) (1 μg/mL); A, *L. acidophilus* at MOI of 1 with TNF-α (20 ng/mL) and LPS (1 μg/mL); B, *B. animalis* subsp. *lactis* at MOI of 10 with TNF-α (20 ng/mL) and LPS (1 μg/mL); AB, *L. acidophilus* at MOI of 1 and *B. animalis* subsp. *lactis* at MOI of 10 with TNF-α (20 ng/mL) and LPS (1 μg/mL).

3.4. *Effects of Probiotics on the Expression of Inflammation-Related Proteins in Inflammatory HT-29 Cells*

Groups A, B and AB had significantly higher expression of TLR2 (Figure 4A) and lower expressions of *p*-p65 NF-κB (Figure 4B), *p*-p38 MAPK (Figure 4C) and COX-2 (Figure 4D) than did group I. Group AB showed the best inhibitory effect on the expressions of inflammation-related proteins, including *p*-p65 NF-κB (Figure 4B), *p*-p38 MAPK (Figure 4C) and COX-2 (Figure 4D). *B. animalis* subsp. *lactis* treatment (groups B and AB) significantly decreased ICAM-1 expression compared with group I, and this inhibitory effect was more potent in group AB than in group B (Figure 4E). *L. acidophilus* alone (group A) had no inhibitory effect on ICAM-1 expression but it enhanced the efficacy of *B. animalis* subsp. *lactis* when they were used in combination (group AB, Figure 4E). All probiotics-treated groups (groups A, B and AB) had significantly lower VCAM-1 expressions than did group I, while *L. acidophilus* treatment (groups A and AB) showed a better inhibitory effect on VCAM-1 than did *B. animalis* subsp. *lactis* alone (group B), as shown in Figure 4F.

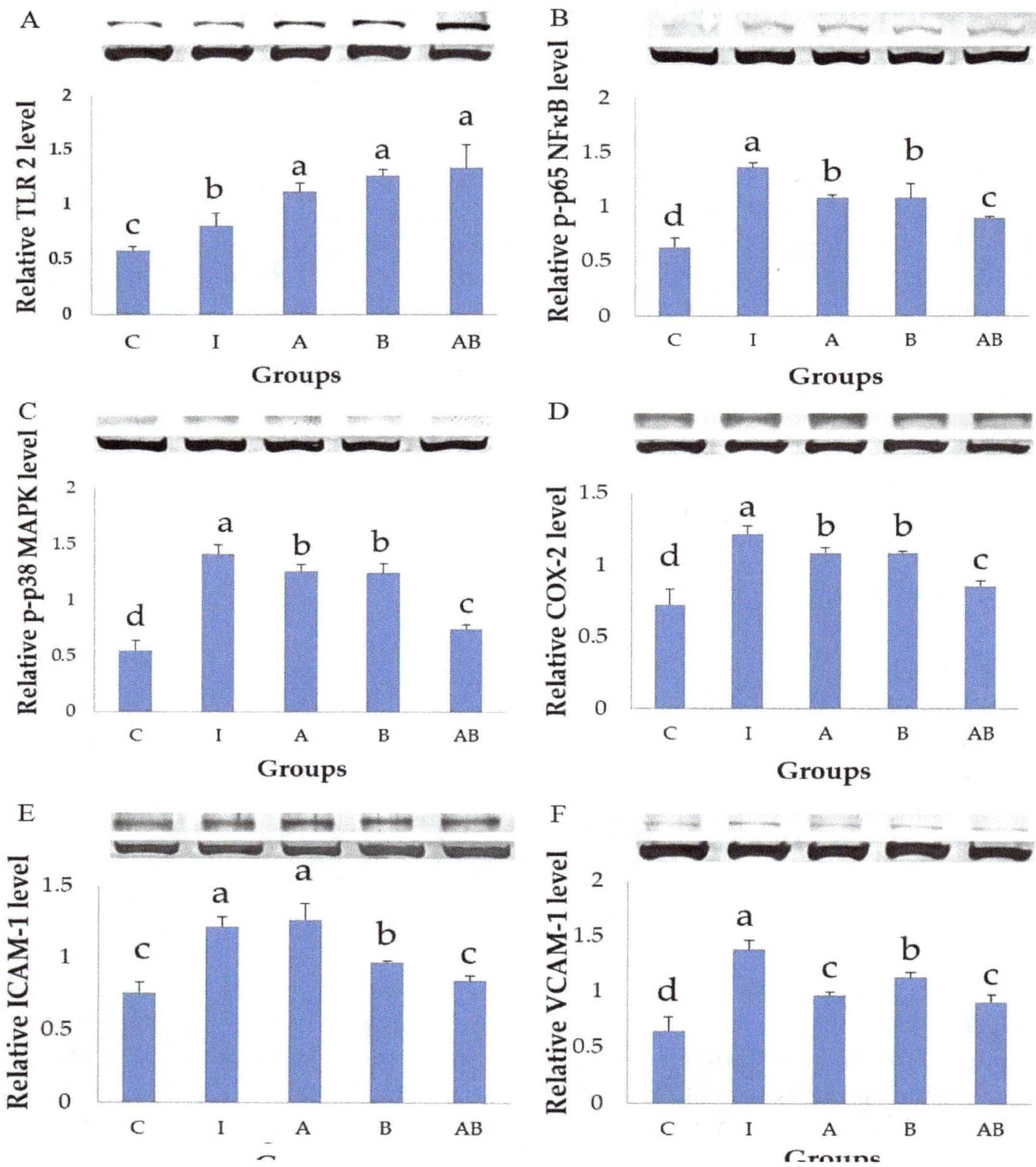

Figure 4. Effects of probiotics on the expression of inflammation-related proteins in inflammatory HT-29 cells. All values are mean ± SD (n = 3). Bars with the same letter are not significantly different from one another determined by Duncan's multiple range test, $p < 0.05$. C, control; I, TNF-α (20 ng/mL) with LPS (1 μg/mL); A, *L. acidophilus* at MOI of 1 with TNF-α (20 ng/mL) and LPS (1 μg/mL); B, *B. animalis* subsp. *lactis* at MOI of 10 with TNF-α (20 ng/mL) and LPS (1 μg/mL); AB, *L. acidophilus* at MOI of 1 and *B. animalis* subsp. *lactis* at MOI of 10 with TNF-α (20 ng/mL) and LPS (1 μg/mL). (**A**), expression of toll-like receptor 2 (TLR2); (**B**), expression of phosphorylated p65 nuclear factor kappa B (*p*-p65 NFκB); (**C**), expression of phosphorylated p38 mitogen-activated protein kinase (*p*-p38 MAPK); (**D**), expression of cyclooxygenase-2 (COX-2); (**E**), expression of intercellular adhesion molecule-1 (ICAM-1); (**F**), expression of vascular cell adhesion molecule-1 (VCAM-1).

4. Discussion

The present study demonstrated that both *L. acidophilus* and *B. animalis* subsp. *lactis* significantly reduced the secretion of IL-8 and the expressions of *p*-p65 NF-κB, *p*-p38 MAPK, VCAM-1 and COX-2, as well as increased the expression of TLR2 in LPS- and TNF-α-induced inflammatory IECs. *B. animalis* subsp. *lactis* significantly reduced the expression of ICAM-1 and this inhibitory effect was enhanced by *L. acidophilus,* which did not affect ICAM-1 expression directly. The combination of two strains showed the best anti-inflammatory activity. These results suggest that both *L. acidophilus* and *B. animalis* subsp. *lactis* possess a potent anti-inflammatory activity in inflammatory IECs and there is an interaction between these two strains of probiotics.

Lactobacillus is an important genus of probiotics, which plays an essential role of immunomodulation in the intestinal mucosa. For example, *L. acidophilus* DDS-1 demonstrated a superior survival rate, good adhesion capacity and strong immunomodulatory effect under experimental conditions with or without LPS stimulation [24]. Most *L. acidophilus* species can be well adapted and are able to survive during harsh conditions of digestion [24]. Due to this stability, *L. acidophilus* has been considered an ideal vehicle for mucosal-targeted delivery of drugs [24]. The amount of *L. acidophilus* remained almost unchanged in the gut for a long time [25].

The modulatory effects of *L. acidophilus* on intestinal inflammation and the immune system are dependent on the stimulation in IECs. *L. acidophilus* significantly increased COX-2 expression and prostaglandin E_2 (PGE_2) secretion in unstimulated Colo320 cells, but not in TNF-α-induced cells [26]. *L. acidophilus* NCFM could rapidly but transiently induce the production of pro-inflammatory cytokines and chemokines in unstimulated Caco-2 cells [21]. In addition, *L. acidophilus* NCFM activated the pathogen-associated molecular pattern (PAMP) receptor TLR2 and enhanced the phosphorylation of p65 NF-κB and p38 MAPK in unstimulated Caco-2 cells [21]. The activation of TLR2-mediated NF-κB and MAPK signaling pathways played a key role in the production of cytokines and chemokines in IECs [21].

In contrast, *L. acidophilus* showed an anti-inflammatory effect in IECs stimulated by bacterial ligands or pro-inflammatory cytokines. *L. acidophilus* Bar13 were effective in inhibiting IL-8 production in HT-29 cells stimulated by TNF-α, IL-1β or LPS [27]. *L. acidophilus* DDS-1 significantly upregulated anti-inflammatory IL-10 and downregulated pro-inflammatory TNF-α production and IL-8 levels in LPS-treated HT-29 cells [24]. *L. acidophilus* LAB20 increased the transepithelial electrical resistance (TER) of enterocyte monolayers and thus strengthened intestinal barrier function [16]. *L. acidophilus* LAB20 also showed anti-inflammatory capacity by attenuating the LPS-induced IL-8 production in HT-29 cells [16]. The results suggest that this strain may balance the IL-8 expression of IECs in response to stimulation by LPS from Gram-negative bacteria in the intestine. Our study used LPS and TNF-α to induce inflammatory responses of HT-29 cells and the results were in agreement with the above studies, showing an anti-inflammatory effect of *L. acidophilus*. Some animal studies also demonstrated an anti-inflammatory activity of *L. acidophilus* in the intestinal tract. *L. acidophilus* administration reduced colonic leukotriene B_4 (LTB_4) production, inducible nitrogen oxide synthase (iNOS) expression and myeloperoxidase (MPO) activity in the TNBS model of rat colitis [17]. *L. acidophilus* inhibited colitis by inducing goblet cell differentiation, interfering with endoplasmic reticulum stress and suppressing NF-κB activation in dextran sulfate sodium (DSS)-treated mice [28]. These findings suggest that *L. acidophilus* can be used as a potent immunomodulator for IBD treatment.

Probiotics modulate immune- and inflammation-associated signaling pathways by gastrointestinal digested products of probiotics and bacterial metabolites. The active compounds of *L. acidophilus* for the anti-inflammatory effect may include either cell components or secretory factors. Cell wall components play a critical role in modulating intestinal inflammation and immune function. Some components of *L. acidophilus,* such as cell wall-associated polysaccharides, proteins and LTAs, could directly inhibit NF-κB activation in HT-29 cells [28]. The surface-layer protein (SLP) from *L. acidophilus* is closely related to a human health-promoting effect via modulation of the immune system. For example, SLP extracted from *L. acidophilus* NCFM was found to inhibit the production of reactive oxygen species (ROS), nitrogen oxide (NO), PGE_2, TNF-α and IL-1β through attenuating the activation of MAPK and NF-κB in LPS-induced RAW264.7 cells [29]. This SLP inhibited NO and PGE_2 production by downregulating the protein expression levels of iNOS and COX-2 [29]. On the other hand, the cell-free supernatant of *L. acidophilus* was able to downregulate IL-8 expression in HT-29 cells stimulated by LPS [30]. Otte et al. (2009) indicated that distinct probiotics could specifically and significantly decrease the induced COX-2 expression in IECs, most likely mediated by released factors such as protein, butyrate and propionate and in part by bacterial DNA [26]. A preliminary study of Kainulainen et al. (2015) suggested that exopolysaccharide (EPS) of *L. acidophilus* LAB20 may have a role in its immunomodulatory activity [16].

Bifidobacteria make up 3–5% of adult microflora and thus constitute one of the predominant species of the human colonic microflora [31]. They are more abundant in human gut microbiota than *Lactobacilli* [32] and showed a moderate to low adhesion capacity of IECs [24]. *B. animalis* subsp. *lactis* has well-established probiotic characteristics and proven beneficial health effects for gastrointestinal health and immune function [33]. This strain also has potent anti-inflammatory and anti-proliferative effects [10]. The capacity of *Bifidobacteria* to inhibit LPS-induced NF-κB activation is strain-dependent in IECs. For example, *B. bifidum* was reported as a promising candidate for probiotic intervention in inflammatory diseases of the gastrointestinal tract [31]. A recent study screened new probiotic strains for IBD management by combining in vitro and in vivo methods and found that the best anti-inflammatory capacity in peripheral blood mononuclear cells (PBMCs) from healthy donors were observed for *Bifidobacteria*, while the anti-inflammatory profile of *Lactobacilli* was strain-dependent [6]. *B. bifidum* PI22, the strain that exhibited the most protective capacity against acute colitis, was only slightly efficacious against chronic colitis in TNBS-treated mice. This strain inhibited the expression of genes encoding chemokine C-X-C motif ligand 2 (CXCL2), IL-1β, TNF-α, IL-6 and IL-17 [6]. In contrast, *B. lactis* LA804 which was less efficacious in the acute model was the most protective against chronic colitis by downregulating the expression of genes for CXCL2, IL-1β and TNF-α in TNBS-treated mice [6].

Similar to *L. acidophilus*, the modulatory effects of *B. animalis* subsp. *lactis* on intestinal inflammation and the immune system are also dependent on the stimulation used in IECs and animal models. *B. lactis* BB12 transiently triggered the phosphorylation of p65 NF-κB and p38 MAPK in unstimulated native epithelium after the initial monoassociation of rats and in unstimulated Mode-K IECs [34]. TLR2 played an important role in mediating the initial interaction of *B. lactis* BB12 with the intestinal epithelium [34]. This study suggested that probiotics could transiently trigger innate signal transduction and pro-inflammatory gene expression in the intestinal epithelium in the early stages of bacterial colonization [34].

In contrast, *B. animalis* subsp. *lactis* showed an anti-inflammatory effect in IECs stimulated by bacterial ligands or pro-inflammatory cytokines and in animals treated with pro-inflammatory compounds. *B. lactis* inhibited NF-κB and its regulated genes for COX-2, matrix metalloproteinase-9 (MMP-9) and vascular endothelial growth factor (VEGF) in HT-29 cells stimulated with IL-1β, TNF-α or LPS [10]. Another study showed that *B. animalis* ssp. *lactis* UABla-12 was able to downregulate IL-8 levels in LPS-treated HT-29 cells [24]. Our study used LPS and TNF-α to induce inflammatory responses of HT-29 cells and showed an anti-inflammatory effect of *B. animalis* subsp. *lactis*, in agreement with previous studies. Animal studies also confirmed the anti-inflammatory activity of this strain of probiotics. For example, *B. lactis* treatment reduced colonic TNF-α production and the expressions of iNOS and COX-2 in TNBS model of rat colitis [17]. *B. lactis* prevented DSS-induced acute colitis and CAC in mice and could be a therapeutic agent for IBD as well as a potential preventive agent for CAC [10].

Previous studies found that *Bifidobacterium* strains' DNA was effective in limiting epithelial pro-inflammatory responses in IL-10-deficient mice and in HT-29 cells challenged with TNF-α; however, the pro-inflammatory response to LPS in HT-29 cells was not inhibited by probiotic DNA [31]. These authors indicated that the anti-inflammatory compound is neither actively secreted by *Bifidobacteria* nor released from lysed cells. The mechanisms by which whole cells of *Bifidobacteria* inhibit inflammatory responses are distinct from their DNA [31]. Recent studies have focused on the surface-associated structural components of *Bifidobacteria*, such as EPS, peptidoglycan, LTA and lipoglycans [35]. The biosynthesis of EPS has been described in several species of *Bifdobacterium* and it seems that these molecules play a relevant role in their immunomodulatory and anti-inflammatory capabilities [36].

The synergistic effect of different probiotic strains may have a higher impact on host cells compared to single probiotic strains. Some studies on the anti-inflammatory effects of probiotics were performed using mixtures of different probiotic strains, mainly probiotics belonging to *Lactobacillus* and *Bifidobacterium* genera [31]. Clinical reports have found that administration of mixed probiotics exhibits a combinatorial effect in the host [35]. The enhanced efficacy of multi-strain/combinatorial therapy may arise due to a combination of several probiotic mechanisms, with each strain making their own contributions [35]. Some combined probiotics have been shown to possess a good anti-inflammatory activity in vivo and in vitro. A combination of *Streptococcus thermophilus* ATCC19258 and *L. acidophilus* ATCC4356 had a pronounced effect on the phosphorylation of p38 MAPK and extracellular signal regulated kinase (ERK)1/2 in HT-29 cells with or without the stimulation of interferon-γ (IFN-γ) or TNF-α [30]. In addition, this probiotic combination reduced the phosphorylation of the nuclear factor of kappa light polypeptide gene enhancer in B-cells inhibitor α (IκB-α) [37]. These results suggest that the probiotic combination may activate the MAPK signaling pathway but inhibit the NF-κB signaling pathway in IECs challenged by pro-inflammatory cytokines. VSL#3 probiotics significantly ameliorated the disease activity index (DAI), prevented the decrease of tight junction proteins including occludin and zonula occludens (ZO)-1 and increased the expression of *p*-p38 MAPK and phosphorylated ERK (*p*-ERK) in DSS-treated rats [38]. Furthermore, tight junction proteins (occludin and ZO-1), *p*-p38 MAPK and *p*-ERK in the VSL#3 group were significantly higher than those in either the control or TNF-α group in TNF-α-induced HT-29 cells [38]. This study suggests that VSL#3 probiotics may enhance the tight junction and protect the epithelial barrier in vivo and in vitro by activating the p38 MAPK and ERK signaling pathways. Ultrabletique, a probiotic cocktail, exerted an anti-inflammatory effect and contributed to the rapid recovery of DSS-induced acute colitis in mice [39]. The results were associated with reduced expressions of TLR4, iNOS and NF-κB in colonic tissues [39].

There are limited studies investigating the interaction between different probiotics. *L. acidophilus* Bar13 and *B. longum* Bar33 were effective in inhibiting IL-8 secretion in HT-29 cells stimulated by TNF-α, IL-1β or LPS, and *B. longum* Bar33 presented the highest effect [27]. Both strains showed the potential to protect enterocytes against an acute inflammatory response [27]. However, a combination of these two strains did not show an additive effect. Another study demonstrated that each of *L. acidophilus*, *B. lactis* or their combination had an individual modulatory impact on the immune system, including regulatory T (Treg) cells and effector T helper (Th) cells, of UC patients [13]. However, there is no synergistic effect between these two strains. *B. lactis* had a more stimulatory effect on the Treg cells of UC patients, although it also stimulated the effector Th cells [13]. Based on the IL-10 and transforming growth factor-β (TGF-β) levels of PBMCs stimulated by probiotics, the authors supposed that *B. lactis* could be a better candidate for Treg cells stimulation compared with *L. acidophilus* and mixed probiotics in UC patients. Our study found that both *L. acidophilus* and *B. animalis* subsp. *lactis* significantly suppressed inflammation in LPS- and TNF-α-stimulated HT-29 cells and that the combination of these two strains showed the best anti-inflammatory effect. Our results also indicated that TLR, NF-κB and MAPK signaling pathways and their associated factors, such as adhesion molecules and inflammatory mediators, played important roles in the observed anti-inflammatory activity. The two strains may have an interaction through these pathways.

TLRs are pattern recognition receptors (PRR) expressed by various cells in the gastrointestinal tract, including IECs [8]. TLRs represent the first point of contact between environment and organism and are powerful molecular regulators by which the immune system may sense the environment and protect the host from pathogens or endogenous threats [40]. TLRs are membrane bound and provide pathogen surveillance, which upon ligand binding, activate NF-κB signaling and lead to the production of pro-inflammatory cytokines, chemokines and antimicrobial peptides [12]. TLR signaling in IECs plays several crucial roles in maintaining healthy gut epithelial barrier that includes proliferation of epithelial cells, production of antimicrobials, maintenance of tight junction and modulation of immune system [36]. TLR signaling in the gut is involved in either maintaining intestinal homeostasis or inducing an inflammatory response [8]. Under normal conditions, IECs show low expression of TLRs and are therefore unresponsive to TLR stimuli; under inflammatory conditions, epithelial TLR expression is increased, which contributes to both inflammation and immune tolerance [8]. Epithelial TLR2 activation has been described to protect against barrier disruption in IECs [8].

TLR2 recognizes a wide range of ligands, among which the best characterized are lipoproteins highly expressed on the outer membrane of Gram-positive bacteria [40]. The cell wall of probiotic bacteria contains peptidoglycan, lipoproteins and lipopeptides, described as TLR2 ligands, and thus TLR2 plays an important role in the recognition of anti-inflammatory probiotic bacteria [36]. The immunomodulatory role of LTA in probiotic *Lactobacillus* through TLR2 recognition is well established. Although these biopolymers have long been identified in *Bifidobacterium*, their roles in PRR-mediated interaction in host have not yet been well studied [35]. In contrast, the activation of TLR4 by LPS from Gram-negative bacteria leads to the secretion of pro-inflammatory mediators in the intestinal mucosa, mainly through the activation of the transcription factor NF-κB [39]. TLR2 ligation may induce a suppressive effect on TLR4-mediated inflammatory responses via the expression or activation of TLR negative regulators [12]. The present study showed that *L. acidophilus* and *B. animalis* subsp. *lactis*, either alone or in combination, significantly enhanced TLR2 expression in HT-29 cells stimulated with LPS and TNF-α, suggesting the potential of these probiotics in protecting IECs against bacteria- and cytokine-mediated inflammation.

NF-κB transcriptional system in IEC plays an essential role in the regulation of inflammation in patients with various intestinal disorders [10]. It regulates the transcription of a series of genes involved in acute responses to injury and in chronic intestinal inflammation including the genes for IL-1β, TNF-α, IL-6, IL-8, COX-2, ICAM-1, and so on [31]. NF-κB is activated through a wide range of stimuli such as TNF-α, IL-1β and LPS [31] and acts as a central regulator of the IEC innate immune response and as an essential transcription factor for integrating the pro-inflammatory response to infection with enteroinvasive bacteria [41]. In addition, NF-κB, as an important downstream pathway in LPS-mediated signal responses, is also closely related to tumor growth, inflammation and apoptosis [29]. Probiotics can alter the NF-κB pathway at many different levels including degradation, ubiquitination and inhibition of proteasome function [39]. Induction of the nuclear export of complexes formed by nuclear factor NF-κB and peroxisome proliferator-activated receptor-γ (PPAR-γ) is another anti-inflammatory mechanism induced by probiotics [39].

MAPK proteins, including ERK, c-Jun N-terminal kinase (JNK), and p38 protein kinases, are activated to act on their respective substrates to regulate the inflammatory response in LPS-stimulated cells [29]. Activation of the MAPK signaling pathway by LPS can indirectly activate the downstream NF-κB pathway, initiate protein expression and stimulate complex physiological responses [29]. Probiotics can affect the MAPK signaling pathway independent of NF-κB signaling. Suppression of p38 phosphorylation has been associated with the inhibition of IL-8 secretion without impacting on IL-8 mRNA levels or the activation of NF-κB [14]. Probiotic-induced changes in phosphorylation levels of p38, JNK and ERK1/2 MAPKs can affect cytokine secretion and apoptosis [14].

The present study showed that LPS and TNF-α stimulation significantly increased the phosphorylated forms of p65 NF-κB and p38 MAPK in HT-29 cells, suggesting the activation of NF-κB and MAPK signaling pathways. Inflammatory cells treated with either *L. acidophilus* or *B. animalis* subsp. *lactis* had significantly lower expression of phosphorylated p65 NF-κB and p38 MAPK proteins compared with untreated cells. Furthermore, the combination of *L. acidophilus* and *B. animalis* subsp. *lactis* showed the best inhibitory effect on the activation of NF-κB and MAPK. These results suggest that the two strains of probiotics may exert an anti-inflammatory effect by modulating NF-κB and MAPK signaling pathways in IECs.

IL-8 is a chemokine produced by many types of cells, including IECs [11]. IL-8 is responsible for the initiation of inflammatory cascades and the recruitment of neutrophils into the mucosa of lesions [16]. It also plays important roles in angiogenesis and the metastasis of tumors [11]. In response to enteropathogens infection the IECs release IL-8 and other pro-inflammatory molecules that initiate an acute inflammatory response [27]. A prolonged infection can result in a massive and long-lasting IL-8 release by IECs [27]. LPS, IL-1α, IL-1β, IL-10, IFN-γ and TNF-α regulate IL-8 production in various cell types [11]. HT-29 cells produce IL-8 after stimulation by TNF-α and IL-1β, but not by IFN-γ, IL-10 or IL-13 [11]. TNF-α plays a guiding role in the production of IL-8, and NF-κB establishes a feedback mechanism via autocrine/paracrine factors to regulate the expression and activation of IL-8 [42].

COX-2 plays an important role in inflammation. A variety of extracellular and intracellular stimuli, including LPS and TNF-α, rapidly induce the expression of COX-2 [43]. There are strain- and stimulation-specific effects of probiotics on COX-2 expression in IECs. Both probiotic *E. coli* Nissle and mixed probiotics VSL#3 had no effect on basal COX-2 expression but decreased stimulated COX-2 activity, protein expression and PGE_2 secretion, while *L. acidophilus* increased COX-2 expression and PGE_2 secretion in unstimulated Colo320 and SW480 IECs and in gastrin-induced Colo320 cells but not in TNF-α-induced Colo320 cells [26]. Although the precise mechanisms regulating COX-2 expression in IECs have not been fully clarified, activator protein-1 (AP-1) and p38 MAPK are the only regulatory elements identified in IECs so far [26].

The present study found that stimulation by LPS and TNF-α significantly increased the secretory level of IL-8 and the expression of COX-2 in HT-29 cells, showing a typical inflammatory response. In contrast, the inflammatory cells treated with either *L. acidophilus* or *B. animalis* subsp. *lactis* had significantly lower IL-8 level and COX-2 expression compared to those without probiotics treatment. Additionally, combination of *L. acidophilus* and *B. animalis* subsp. *lactis* showed the best inhibitory effect on IL-8 secretion and COX-2 expression. These effects are in agreement with those on NF-κB and MAPK and suggest that these two strains of probiotics are able to suppress inflammation by modulating IL-8 secretion and COX-2 expression in IECs.

Cell adhesion molecules (CAMs) are categorized as cadherins, selectins, integrins and immunoglobulin-like adhesion molecules (IgCAMs) such as mucosal addressin cell adhesion molecule 1 (MAdCAM-1), ICAM-1 and VCAM-1. They are required for the binding of leukocytes to tissue components and the directional movement of leukocytes toward inflamed sites [44]. Human IECs are normally lack of ICAM-1 and VCAM-1 expressions but induction of their expressions has been reported in response to pro-inflammatory cytokines such as IL-1β, IL-6 and IFN-γ [45]. Our study also induced the expressions of ICAM-1 and VCAM-1 by LPS and TNF-α. ICAM-1 and VCAM-1 are closely related to NF-κB and MAPK signaling pathways. The binding sites for NF-κB have been identified in the promoter regions of the genes for ICAM-1 and VCAM-1 [46]. Another study has indicated that there is a possible relationship between inhibition of MAPKs and decreased expression of ICAM-1 and VCAM-1 [45].

ICAM-1 is constitutively expressed by several types of cells, including leukocytes, endothelial cells and IECs [47,48]. The major agonists for ICAM-1 expression are bacterial products (such as LPS) and pro-inflammatory cytokines (such as TNF-α, IL-1 and IFN-γ) released at inflammatory sites [47]. Expression of ICAM-1 in human IECs is upregulated following infection with invasive bacteria and stimulation with TNF-α and IFN-γ [47]. Transcription of ICAM-1 is under regulation by cytokines such as IL-1β, TNF-α and IFN-γ as well as by growth factors and stress oxidants through various signaling pathways, including NF-κB and AP-1 pathways [44]. ICAM-1 plays an important role in both innate and adaptive immune responses. It is involved in the transendothelial migration of leukocytes to inflammatory sites, as well as interactions between antigen presenting cells (APC) and T cells [48]. ICAM-1 on IECs is involved in the immune defense, including attraction of neutrophils to the surface defect, adhesion of transmigrated neutrophils to face the luminal content and binding of microbial surface molecules [44]. Both active UC and CD are associated with marked infiltration of inflammatory cells, while ICAM-1 is involved in leukocyte infiltration [49]. ICAM-1 plays a specific role in the pathogenesis of IBD, so loss of ICAM-1 function may be effective in controlling IBD [44].

VCAM-1 is inducible and predominantly expressed in endothelial cells and also on the surface of other cells, including macrophages and cancer cells [50]. The expression of VCAM-1 is activated by pro-inflammatory cytokines, including TNF-α, and also by ROS, oxidized low-density lipoprotein (oLDL), high glucose concentration, TLR agonists (such as LPS) and shear stress [50]. VCAM-1 is an important modulator of lymphocyte and monocyte trafficking [46]. VCAM-1 was originally identified as a cell adhesion molecule that helps regulate inflammation-associated vascular adhesion and the transendothelial migration of leukocytes such as macrophages and T cells [50]. Recent evidence suggests that VCAM-1 is closely associated with the progression of various immunological disorders and cancers, so it is a potential therapeutic target in these diseases [50]. Experimental studies have shown that blockade of VCAM-1 results in a higher inhibition of leukocyte adhesion in colonic venules and a potent effect on preventing or reversing established inflammation in various animal models [51–53].

In human intestinal microvascular endothelial cells, ICAM-1 is constitutively expressed and VCAM-1 is not detectable in basal conditions but a marked increase in both adhesion molecules is observed after challenges of these cells with IL-1β, TNF-α or LPS [46]. In the murine intestine, the constitutive level of VCAM-1 expression is substantially lower than that of ICAM-1; however, a significant increase in the endothelial cell surface density of VCAM-1 is noted by cytokine stimulation [46]. Remarkable increases in VCAM-1 expression have also been documented in rodent models of chemically induced colitis, as well as in colitis of IL-10 knockout mice [46,51,52]. In these animal models, the expression of ICAM-1 was not increased or was only slightly elevated, whereas increased expressions of MAdCAM-1 and VCAM-1 were observed. VCAM-1, in contrast with ICAM-1, is not involved in physiological leukocyte recirculation and selective blockade of its function might attenuate the inflammatory response without altering physiological immune mechanisms [46]. Specific blockade of the adhesion molecules such as ICAM-1 involved in leukocyte recruitment to the inflamed intestine is considered to be one of the most promising therapeutic targets for IBD [53,54].

Limited studies have investigated the effect of probiotics on adhesion molecules. Riedel et al. (2006) reported that *B. bifidum* S17 decreased mRNA level of ICAM-1 in LPS-induced HT-29 cells [31]. Angulo et al. (2006) demonstrated that *L. casei* attenuated leukocyte recruitment in experimental colitis induced by TNBS in rats [55]. This effect was possibly related to the suppression of ICAM-1 upregulation, although VCAM-1 expression was unaffected. Chu et al. (2010) indicated that *L. plantarum* treatment improved the histological damage score and interfered with the upregulation of adhesion molecules such as ICAM-1 in IL-10 knockout mice [49]. In addition to whole probiotics, the cell wall components of probiotics also play an important role in regulation of adhesion molecules and other inflammatory-related factors. Kim et al. (2012) showed that LTA from *L. plantarum* inhibited TNF-α-induced inflammatory responses, including increased IL-8, iNOS, NO and ICAM-1, in HT-29 cells through inhibition of the NF-κB and MAPK signaling pathways [11].

Our study successfully induced strong expressions of ICAM-1 and VCAM-1 in HT-29 cells stimulated with LPS and TNF-α. Interestingly, *L. acidophilus* and *B. animalis* subsp. *lactis* showed a different impact on ICAM-1 and VCAM-1. *L. acidophilus* and *B. animalis* subsp. *lactis*, either alone or in combination, significantly decreased VCAM-1 expression in inflammatory HT-29 cells compared with those untreated with probiotics. *L. acidophilus* showed higher efficacy on VCAM-1 inhibition than did *B. animalis* subsp. *lactis*. However, *L. acidophilus* alone did not inhibit ICAM-1 expression but enhanced the efficacy of *B. animalis* subsp. *lactis* which significantly decreased ICAM-1 expression in inflammatory HT-29 cells. It shows a synergistic effect between two strains of probiotics. ICAM-1, associated with the recruitment and adhesion of neutrophils, is known to play a determining role in acute inflammatory conditions, while VCAM-1 is more relevant as a mediator of chronic inflammatory diseases in which the recruitment of lymphocytes is the main cellular event [44,55]. Blocking ICAM-1 and VCAM-1 may have therapeutic benefits for the acute inflammatory component of IBD in SAMP-1/Yi adoptive transfer model mice [56]. These findings suggest that *B. animalis* subsp. *lactis* may have the potential to alleviate acute inflammation in the gut, while *L. acidophilus* may be a candidate for remission of chronic intestinal inflammation. Combination of two strains seems to have the best anti-inflammatory activity in the intestinal tract and may be a candidate adjuvant for IBD treatment.

5. Conclusions

In conclusion, the present study showed that *L. acidophilus* and *B. animalis* subsp. *lactis* exerted a potent anti-inflammatory effect through modulating TLR2-mediated NF-κB and MAPK signaling pathways in inflammatory IECs. Both strains, especially their combination, may have the potential to be developed as a novel adjuvant for IBD therapy.

Author Contributions: Conceptualization, S.-C.L., W.-F.H., J.-S.C. and C.-K.S.; Methodology, S.-C.L., W.-F.H., J.-S.C. and C.-K.S.; Data Analysis, S.-C.L. and W.-F.H.; Original Draft Preparation, S.-C.L., W.-F.H., J.-S.C. and C.-K.S.; Review, Editing & Final approval of the manuscript, C.-K.S.

Acknowledgments: This study was supported by the grants from the Ministry of Science and Technology, Taiwan (NSC102-2313-B-038-006, MOST103-2313-B-038-004 & MOST104-2320-B-038-024).

References

1. Ng, S.C.; Shi, H.Y.; Hamidi, N.; Underwood, F.E.; Tang, W.; Benchimol, E.I.; Panaccione, R.; Ghosh, S.; Wu, J.C.Y.; Chan, F.K.L.; et al. Worldwide incidence and prevalence of inflammatory bowel disease in the 21st century: A systematic review of population-based studies. *Lancet* **2018**, *390*, 2769–2778. [CrossRef]
2. Yen, H.H.; Weng, M.T.; Tung, C.C.; Wang, Y.T.; Chang, Y.T.; Chang, C.H.; Shieh, M.J.; Wong, J.M.; Wei, S.C. Epidemiological trend in inflammatory bowel disease in Taiwan from 2001 to 2015: A nationwide populationbased study. *Intest. Res.* **2019**, *17*, 54–62. [CrossRef] [PubMed]
3. Molodecky, N.A.; Soon, I.S.; Rabi, D.M.; Ghali, W.A.; Ferris, M.; Chernoff, G.; Benchimol, E.I.; Panaccione, R.; Ghosh, S.; Barkema, H.W.; et al. Increasing incidence and prevalence of the inflammatory bowel diseases with time, based on systematic review. *Gastroenterology* **2012**, *142*, 46–54. [CrossRef]
4. De Filippo, C.; Cavalieri, D.; Di Paola, M.; Ramazzotti, M.; Poullet, J.B.; Massart, S.; Collini, S.; Pieraccini, G.; Lionetti, P. Impact of diet in shaping gut microbiota revealed by a comparative study in children from Europe and rural Africa. *Proc. Natl. Acad. Sci. USA* **2010**, *107*, 14691–14696. [CrossRef] [PubMed]
5. Derwa, Y.; Gracie, D.J.; Hamlin, P.J.; Ford, A.C. Systematic review with meta-analysis: The efficacy of probiotics in inflammatory bowel disease. *Aliment. Pharm.* **2017**, *46*, 389–400. [CrossRef]
6. Alard, J.; Peucelle, V.; Boutillier, D.; Breton, J.; Kuylle, S.; Pot, B.; Holowacz, S.; Grangette, C. New probiotic strains for inflammatory bowel disease management identified by combining in vitro and in vivo approaches. *Benef. Microbes* **2018**, *9*, 317–331. [CrossRef] [PubMed]
7. Torre, L.A.; Siegel, R.L.; Ward, E.M.; Jemal, A. Global cancer incidence and mortality rates and trends—An update. *Cancer Epidemiol. Biomark. Prev.* **2016**, *25*, 16–27. [CrossRef]
8. De Kivit, S.; Tobin, M.C.; Forsyth, C.B.; Keshavarzian, A.; Landay, A.L. Regulation of intestinal immune responses through tlr activation: Implications for pro-and prebiotics. *Front Immunol.* **2014**, *5*, 60. [CrossRef] [PubMed]
9. Kaci, G.; Lakhdari, O.; Dore, J.; Ehrlich, S.D.; Renault, P.; Blottiere, H.M.; Delorme, C. Inhibition of the NF-kappaB pathway in human intestinal epithelial cells by commensal *Streptococcus salivarius*. *Appl. Environ. Microbiol.* **2011**, *77*, 4681–4684. [CrossRef] [PubMed]
10. Kim, S.W.; Kim, H.M.; Yang, K.M.; Kim, S.A.; Kim, S.K.; An, M.J.; Park, J.J.; Lee, S.K.; Kim, T.I.; Kim, W.H.; et al. *Bifidobacterium lactis* inhibits NF-kappaB in intestinal epithelial cells and prevents acute colitis and colitis-associated colon cancer in mice. *Inflamm. Bowel Dis.* **2010**, *16*, 1514–1525. [CrossRef]
11. Kim, H.; Jung, B.J.; Jung, J.H.; Kim, J.Y.; Chung, S.K.; Chung, D.K. *Lactobacillus plantarum* lipoteichoic acid alleviates TNF-alpha-induced inflammation in the HT-29 intestinal epithelial cell line. *Mol. Cells* **2012**, *33*, 479–486. [CrossRef] [PubMed]
12. Llewellyn, A.; Foey, A. Probiotic modulation of innate cell pathogen sensing and signaling events. *Nutrients* **2017**, *9*, 1156. [CrossRef] [PubMed]

13. Sheikhi, A.; Shakerian, M.; Giti, H.; Baghaeifar, M.; Jafarzadeh, A.; Ghaed, V.; Heibor, M.R.; Baharifar, N.; Dadafarin, Z.; Bashirpour, G. Probiotic yogurt culture *Bifidobacterium animalis* subsp. *lactis* BB-12 and *Lactobacillus acidophilus* LA-5 modulate the cytokine secretion by peripheral blood mononuclear cells from patients with ulcerative colitis. *Drug Res.* **2016**, *66*, 300–305. [CrossRef]
14. Thomas, C.M.; Versalovic, J. Probiotics-host communication: Modulation of signaling pathways in the intestine. *Gut Microbes* **2010**, *1*, 148–163. [CrossRef]
15. De Vrese, M.; Schrezenmeir, J. Probiotics, prebiotics, and synbiotics. *Adv. Biochem. Eng. Biotechnol.* **2008**, *111*, 1–66. [PubMed]
16. Kainulainen, V.; Tang, Y.; Spillmann, T.; Kilpinen, S.; Reunanen, J.; Saris, P.E.; Satokari, R. The canine isolate *Lactobacillus acidophilus* LAB20 adheres to intestinal epithelium and attenuates LPS-induced IL-8 secretion of enterocytes in vitro. *BMC Microbiol.* **2015**, *15*, 4. [CrossRef]
17. Peran, L.; Camuesco, D.; Comalada, M.; Bailon, E.; Henriksson, A.; Xaus, J.; Zarzuelo, A.; Galvez, J. A comparative study of the preventative effects exerted by three probiotics, *Bifidobacterium lactis*, *Lactobacillus casei* and *Lactobacillus acidophilus*, in the TNBS model of rat colitis. *J. Appl. Microbiol.* **2007**, *103*, 836–844. [CrossRef] [PubMed]
18. Ostad, S.; Salarian, A.; Ghahramani, M.; Fazeli, M.; Samadi, N.; Jamalifar, H. Live and heat-inactivated lactobacilli from feces inhibit *Salmonella typhi* and *Escherichia coli* adherence to Caco-2 cells. *Folia Microbiol.* **2009**, *54*, 157–160. [CrossRef]
19. Bevilacqua, A.; Cagnazzo, M.T.; Caldarola, C.; Ciuffreda, E.; Dragano, A.R.; Franchino, S.; Lauriola, R.; Pacifico, A.; Corbo, M.R.; Sinigaglia, M. Bifidobacteria as potential functional starter cultures: A case study by msc students in food science and technology (University of Foggia, Southern Italy). *Food Nutr. Sci.* **2012**, *3*, 55. [CrossRef]
20. Lee, S.K.; Kim, T.I.; Kim, Y.K.; Choi, C.H.; Yang, K.M.; Chae, B.; Kim, W.H. Cellular differentiation-induced attenuation of LPS response in HT-29 cells is related to the down-regulation of TLR4 expression. *Biochem. Biophys. Res. Commun.* **2005**, *337*, 457–463. [CrossRef]
21. Jiang, Y.; Lü, X.; Man, C.; Han, L.; Shan, Y.; Qu, X.; Liu, Y.; Yang, S.; Xue, Y.; Zhang, Y. *Lactobacillus acidophilus* induces cytokine and chemokine production via NF-κB and p38 mitogen-activated protein kinase signaling pathways in intestinal epithelial cells. *Clin. Vaccine Immunol.* **2012**, *19*, 603–608. [CrossRef]
22. Bradford, M.M. A rapid and sensitive method for the quantitation of microgram quantities of protein utilizing the principle of protein-dye binding. *Anal. Biochem.* **1976**, *72*, 248–254. [CrossRef]
23. Jeong, C.H.; Seok, J.S.; Petriello, M.C.; Han, S.G. Arsenic downregulates tight junction claudin proteins through p38 and NF-κB in intestinal epithelial cell line, HT-29. *Toxicology* **2017**, *379*, 31–39. [CrossRef]
24. Vemuri, R.; Shinde, T.; Shastri, M.D.; Perera, A.P.; Tristram, S.; Martoni, C.J.; Gundamaraju, R.; Ahuja, K.D.K.; Ball, M.; Eri, R. A human origin strain *Lactobacillus acidophilus* DDS-1 exhibits superior in vitro probiotic efficacy in comparison to plant or dairy origin probiotics. *Int. J. Med. Sci.* **2018**, *15*, 840–848. [CrossRef] [PubMed]
25. Agah, S.; Alizadeh, A.M.; Mosavi, M.; Ranji, P.; Khavari-Daneshvar, H.; Ghasemian, F.; Bahmani, S.; Tavassoli, A. More protection of *Lactobacillus acidophilus* than *Bifidobacterium bifidum* probiotics on azoxymethane-induced mouse colon cancer. *Probiotics Antimicrob. Proteins* **2018**. [CrossRef]
26. Otte, J.M.; Mahjurian-Namari, R.; Brand, S.; Werner, I.; Schmidt, W.E.; Schmitz, F. Probiotics regulate the expression of COX-2 in intestinal epithelial cells. *Nutr. Cancer* **2009**, *61*, 103–113. [CrossRef]
27. Candela, M.; Perna, F.; Carnevali, P.; Vitali, B.; Ciati, R.; Gionchetti, P.; Rizzello, F.; Campieri, M.; Brigidi, P. Interaction of probiotic lactobacillus and bifidobacterium strains with human intestinal epithelial cells: Adhesion properties, competition against enteropathogens and modulation of il-8 production. *Int. J. Food Microbiol.* **2008**, *125*, 286–292. [CrossRef]
28. Kim, D.H.; Kim, S.; Lee, J.H.; Kim, J.H.; Che, X.; Ma, H.W.; Seo, D.H.; Kim, T.I.; Kim, W.H.; Kim, S.W.; et al. *Lactobacillus acidophilus* suppresses intestinal inflammation by inhibiting endoplasmic reticulum stress. *J. Gastroenterol. Hepatol.* **2019**, *34*, 178–185. [CrossRef]
29. Wang, H.; Zhang, L.; Xu, S.; Pan, J.; Zhang, Q.; Lu, R. Surface-layer protein from *Lactobacillus acidophilus* NCFM inhibits lipopolysaccharide-induced inflammation through MAPK and NF-κB signaling pathways in RAW264. 7 cells. *J. Agric. Food Chem.* **2018**, *66*, 7655–7662. [CrossRef]

30. De Marco, S.; Sichetti, M.; Muradyan, D.; Piccioni, M.; Traina, G.; Pagiotti, R.; Pietrella, D. Probiotic cell-free supernatants exhibited anti-inflammatory and antioxidant activity on human gut epithelial cells and macrophages stimulated with LPS. *Evid. Based Complement. Altern. Med.* **2018**, *2018*, 1756308. [CrossRef] [PubMed]
31. Riedel, C.U.; Foata, F.; Philippe, D.; Adolfsson, O.; Eikmanns, B.J.; Blum, S. Anti-inflammatory effects of bifidobacteria by inhibition of LPS-induced NF-kappaB activation. *World J. Gastroenterol.* **2006**, *12*, 3729–3735. [CrossRef]
32. Pham, T.; Teoh, K.T.; Savary, B.J.; Chen, M.H.; McClung, A.; Lee, S.O. In vitro fermentation patterns of rice bran components by human gut microbiota. *Nutrients* **2017**, *9*, 1237. [CrossRef] [PubMed]
33. Jungersen, M.; Wind, A.; Johansen, E.; Christensen, J.E.; Stuer-Lauridsen, B.; Eskesen, D. The science behind the probiotic strain *Bifidobacterium animalis* subsp. *lactis* BB-12. *Microorganisms* **2014**, *2*, 92–110. [CrossRef] [PubMed]
34. Ruiz, P.A.; Hoffmann, M.; Szcesny, S.; Blaut, M.; Haller, D. Innate mechanisms for bifidobacterium lactis to activate transient pro-inflammatory host responses in intestinal epithelial cells after the colonization of germ-free rats. *Immunology* **2005**, *115*, 441–450. [CrossRef] [PubMed]
35. Sarkar, A.; Mandal, S. Bifidobacteria—Insight into clinical outcomes and mechanisms of its probiotic action. *Microbiol. Res.* **2016**, *192*, 159–171. [CrossRef]
36. Wachi, S.; Kanmani, P.; Tomosada, Y.; Kobayashi, H.; Yuri, T.; Egusa, S.; Shimazu, T.; Suda, Y.; Aso, H.; Sugawara, M. *Lactobacillus delbrueckii* TUA 4408 L and its extracellular polysaccharides attenuate enterotoxigenic *Escherichia coli*-induced inflammatory response in porcine intestinal epitheliocytes via toll-like receptor-2 and 4. *Mol. Nutr. Food Res.* **2014**, *58*, 2080–2093. [CrossRef]
37. Resta-Lenert, S.; Barrett, K.E. Probiotics and commensals reverse TNF-alpha- and IFN-gamma-induced dysfunction in human intestinal epithelial cells. *Gastroenterology* **2006**, *130*, 731–746. [CrossRef] [PubMed]
38. Dai, C.; Zhao, D.-H.; Jiang, M. VSL#3 probiotics regulate the intestinal epithelial barrier in vivo and in vitro via the p38 and erk signaling pathways. *Int. J. Mol. Med.* **2012**, *29*, 202–208.
39. Toumi, R.; Soufli, I.; Rafa, H.; Belkhelfa, M.; Biad, A.; Touil-Boukoffa, C. Probiotic bacteria lactobacillus and bifidobacterium attenuate inflammation in dextran sulfate sodium-induced experimental colitis in mice. *Int. J. Immunopathol. Pharm.* **2014**, *27*, 615–627. [CrossRef]
40. Hug, H.; Mohajeri, M.H.; La Fata, G. Toll-like receptors: Regulators of the immune response in the human gut. *Nutrients* **2018**, *10*, 203. [CrossRef]
41. Elewaut, D.; DiDonato, J.A.; Kim, J.M.; Truong, F.; Eckmann, L.; Kagnoff, M.F. NF-κB is a central regulator of the intestinal epithelial cell innate immune response induced by infection with enteroinvasive bacteria. *J. Immunol.* **1999**, *163*, 1457–1466.
42. Zhang, J.; Yi, R.; Qian, Y.; Sun, P.; Zhao, X.; Yang, Z. *Lactobacillus plantarum* CQPC06 activity prevents dextran sulfate sodium-induced colitis by regulating the IL-8 pathway. *J. Food Sci.* **2018**, *83*, 2653–2661. [CrossRef] [PubMed]
43. Williams, C.S.; Mann, M.; DuBois, R.N. The role of cyclooxygenases in inflammation, cancer, and development. *Oncogene* **1999**, *18*, 7908–7916. [CrossRef]
44. Vainer, B. Intercellular adhesion molecule-1 (ICAM-1) in ulcerative colitis: Presence, visualization, and significance. *Apmis* **2010**, *118*, 1–43. [CrossRef]
45. Gallicchio, M.; Rosa, A.C.; Dianzani, C.; Brucato, L.; Benetti, E.; Collino, M.; Fantozzi, R. Celecoxib decreases expression of the adhesion molecules ICAM-1 and VCAM-1 in a colon cancer cell line (HT29). *Br. J. Pharm.* **2008**, *153*, 870–878. [CrossRef] [PubMed]
46. Panés, J.; Peñalva, M.; Piqué, J. New therapeutic targets in inflammatory bowel disease (IBD): Cell adhesion molecules. *Inmunología* **2003**, *22*, 1–12.
47. Huang, G.T.; Eckmann, L.; Savidge, T.C.; Kagnoff, M.F. Infection of human intestinal epithelial cells with invasive bacteria upregulates apical intercellular adhesion molecule-1 (ICAM-1) expression and neutrophil adhesion. *J. Clin. Investig.* **1996**, *98*, 572–583. [CrossRef]
48. Lawson, C.; Wolf, S. ICAM-1 signaling in endothelial cells. *Pharm. Rep.* **2009**, *61*, 22–32. [CrossRef]
49. Chu, Z.X.; Chen, H.Q.; Ma, Y.L.; Zhou, Y.K.; Zhang, M.; Zhang, P.; Qin, H.L. *Lactobacillus plantarum* prevents the upregulation of adhesion molecule expression in an experimental colitis model. *Dig. Dis. Sci.* **2010**, *55*, 2505–2513. [CrossRef]

50. Kong, D.H.; Kim, Y.K.; Kim, M.R.; Jang, J.H.; Lee, S. Emerging roles of vascular cell adhesion molecule-1 (VCAM-1) in immunological disorders and cancer. *Int. J. Mol. Sci.* **2018**, *19*, 1057. [CrossRef]
51. Sans, M.; Panes, J.; Ardite, E.; Elizalde, J.I.; Arce, Y.; Elena, M.; Palacin, A.; Fernandez-Checa, J.C.; Anderson, D.C.; Lobb, R.; et al. VCAM-1 and ICAM-1 mediate leukocyte-endothelial cell adhesion in rat experimental colitis. *Gastroenterology* **1999**, *116*, 874–883. [CrossRef]
52. Soriano, A.; Salas, A.; Salas, A.; Sans, M.; Gironella, M.; Elena, M.; Anderson, D.C.; Piqué, J.M.; Panés, J. VCAM-1, but not ICAM-1 or MadCAM-1, immunoblockade ameliorates DSS-induced colitis in mice. *Lab. Investig.* **2000**, *80*, 1541. [CrossRef] [PubMed]
53. Danese, S.; Panés, J. Development of drugs to target interactions between leukocytes and endothelial cells and treatment algorithms for inflammatory bowel diseases. *Gastroenterology* **2014**, *147*, 981–989. [CrossRef] [PubMed]
54. Reinisch, W.; Hung, K.; Hassan-Zahraee, M.; Cataldi, F. Targeting endothelial ligands: ICAM-1/alicaforsen, MadCAM-1. *J. Crohns Colitis* **2018**, *12*, S669–S677. [CrossRef]
55. Angulo, S.; Llopis, M.; Antolin, M.; Gironella, M.; Sans, M.; Malagelada, J.R.; Pique, J.M.; Guarner, F.; Panes, J. *Lactobacillus casei* prevents the upregulation of ICAM-1 expression and leukocyte recruitment in experimental colitis. *Am. J. Physiol. Gastrointest. Liver Physiol.* **2006**, *291*, G1155–G1162. [CrossRef]
56. Burns, R.C.; Rivera-Nieves, J.; Moskaluk, C.A.; Matsumoto, S.; Cominelli, F.; Ley, K. Antibody blockade of ICAM-1 and VCAM-1 ameliorates inflammation in the SMAP-1/Yit adoptive transfer model of Crohn's disease in mice. *Gastroenterology* **2001**, *121*, 1428–1436. [CrossRef]

7

Towards a Food Pharmacy: Immunologic Modulation through Diet

Ilse Molendijk [1], Sander van der Marel [2] and P.W. Jeroen Maljaars [1,*]

1 Department of Gastroenterology and Hepatology, Leiden University Medical Center, 2313 ZA Leiden, The Netherlands; i.molendijk@lumc.nl
2 Department of Gastroenterology and Hepatology, Haaglanden Medical Center, 2512 VA The Hague, The Netherlands; s.van.der.marel@haaglandenmc.nl
* Correspondence: p.w.j.maljaars@lumc.nl

Abstract: Patients frequently wonder whether their dietary pattern influences the course of inflammatory bowel disease (IBD). Many patients even avoid certain foods that aggravate their symptoms. Although interest in nutritional interventions is rising among physicians, the current application of nutritional interventions in the IBD population is limited due to the lack of scientific evidence from clinical trials. Several studies, however, have identified associations between diet, gut microbiota, intestinal epithelial integrity, and mucosal immune responses. In patients consuming predominantly a Western diet high in n-6 poly-unsaturated fatty acids (PUFAs), sugars, and meat, and low in fruits and vegetables, an impaired gut epithelial barrier and disturbances in the intestinal microbiota have been observed, resulting in a chronic mucosal inflammation. An anti-inflammatory diet may restore this disbalance. In this review, we discuss the effects of diet on the composition of the microbiota, the gut epithelial barrier function, and the mucosal immune system.

Keywords: inflammatory bowel disease; dietary modification; exclusive enteral nutrition; lifestyle modification; Mediterranean diet

---

1. Introduction

Inflammatory bowel diseases (IBDs), consisting of Crohn's disease (CD) and ulcerative colitis (UC), are chronic immune-mediated disorders that can have a large impact on the wellbeing and quality of life of patients worldwide [1,2]. More than 1.5 million Americans are affected by IBDs, as are over 2.2 million Europeans [3], and the incidence of IBDs is increasing in newly industrialized countries in Africa, Asia, and South America [4]. Both diseases are characterized by a relapsing-remitting disease course, necessitating aggressive medical therapies in some cases [1,2].

Diet is important for patients with IBD. Patients often ask their physician whether the food they eat can influence the course of their inflammatory bowel disease. Very little data is available to answer this question. Data from studies in oncology show that eating or avoiding certain foods can increase or decrease the risk for developing colorectal cancer and other digestive cancers, and that this is probably related to the pro-inflammatory aspects of certain foods. This would suggest that nutrition may also affect both the pathogenesis and the disease course of IBD.

Additionally, it appears that dietary patterns in the decades before the onset of CD have been associated with the development of this disease. Patients who followed a healthy diet characterized by high fruit, vegetable, and fish intake during high school were 50% less likely to develop CD [5]. High intake of sugar and soft drinks combined with a low intake of vegetables was associated with UC risk [6].

These observations appear to be corroborated by observations in developing countries and among immigrants from developing countries: adaptation to a Western lifestyle with a Western diet increases both the incidence and prevalence of IBD in these populations [7,8]. The Western diet is high in fat (animal and milk fats, n-6 polyunsaturated fatty acids (PUFAs)) and refined sugars, and contains little fiber and healthy fats (n-3 PUFA). Apart from increasing the risk of developing IBD, the disease course may also be influenced by dietary patterns. Intake of a diet with a high fat content or a low ratio of pro-inflammatory n-6 to anti-inflammatory n-3 fats was associated with a higher level of disease activity [9–11].

This suggests that a Western diet is an environmental risk factor for developing IBD.

2. Diet, Symptoms, and Food Avoidance

A number of studies have assessed CD patients' perception of the role of food and nutrients in gastrointestinal symptoms. Kinsey and Burden [12] found that 42% of IBD patients reported that food affected their symptoms "a lot" or "severely", and 51% of the respondents indicated that diet was important or extremely important as a means of controlling symptoms. Another study found that an even higher percentage, around 70% of patients, thought that diet could trigger a disease flare [13]. Spicy foods are often considered a potential culprit: in a study by Limdi et al., 80% of the patients thought that eating food that was too spicy could result in a disease [14]. Specific items in the diet may aggravate symptoms such as abdominal pain, bloating, and diarrhea, whereas other dietary products alleviate these complaints. For instance, eating products with a high fat content, raw vegetables, and fruits and drinking carbonated beverages were perceived to increase the risk of a relapse by 40–50% of the patients [14]. The perceived relationship between specific foods and IBD complaints and disease activity leads to a high level of food avoidance. Casanova et al. [13] found that during remission, 77% of patients avoid certain foods, and this increased to 86% in patients with active disease. The avoidance of certain products increases the risk of vitamin and other biochemical deficiencies, and also increases the risk of malnutrition, which was estimated to occur in around 14% of the IBD population [13]. Currently, only a diet low in fermentable oligosaccharides, disaccharides, monosaccharides, and polyols (FODMAPS) has been shown to reduce complaints in a substantial part of the IBD population [15].

3. Exclusive Enteral Nutrition

Although certain dietary patterns may be related to a higher risk of developing IBD or a higher risk of disease activity, this does not show that dietary adjustments can influence the disease course or induce remission in patients with active disease. High quality studies in this area are lacking, and this is reflected in the results of a recent meta-analysis on the efficacy of the most studied dietary intervention, exclusive enteral nutrition (EEN), in which all conclusions were based on "very low quality evidence" [16]. EEN is a completely liquid formula containing all macro- and micronutrients a patient needs. EEN formulas can be classified as elemental (monomeric—free amino acids, glucose, oligosaccharides, and small amounts of essential fatty acids), semi-elemental (oligomeric—dipeptides, tripeptides, disaccharides, and medium chain triglycerides) or polymeric (whole protein, oligosaccharides, and long-chain triglycerides). Interventional studies have shown that clinical remission and mucosal healing can be achieved when a patient's diet is replaced by exclusive enteral nutrition. However, the most successful studies have been performed in pediatric patients (Table 1). In a prospective trial, 34 children with newly diagnosed CD received EEN. Twenty-six patients completed at least 6 weeks of EEN. Early clinical remission at week 8 was achieved in 84% of the patients and 76% of the patients had early biochemical remission [17]. Early complete or nearly complete endoscopic mucosal healing was associated with a reduction in endoscopic relapse, anti-TNF (tumor necrosis factor) use, and hospitalization 1 year after EEN. In a 10-week prospective open label study on 37 children who had recently been diagnosed with active CD, 19 children received polymeric EEN to induce remission while 18 children received corticosteroids to induce remission. [18]. At week 10, clinical remission was comparable between both groups, but the number of patients with mucosal healing was significantly higher in the polymeric EEN group than the corticosteroid group

($p < 0.05$). A recent meta-analysis of studies in pediatric patients (consisting of the Borrelli [18] and Terrin [19] papers—see Table 1) found that 83% of pediatric patients achieved remission with EEN, compared to 61% on steroids, but this reached statistical significance only in the per-protocol analysis (Relative risk (RR) 1.43, 95% CI 1.03 to 1.97) [16]. EEN is currently the first-line treatment to induce remission in children with active CD [20,21]. No placebo-controlled trials have been performed in adults with active CD. However, in the controlled studies performed in adults comparing EEN with steroids, steroids appeared to be more effective in inducing remission than EEN [22–24], and a recent meta-analysis confirmed this: steroids were more effective in inducing remission than placebo (Table 1; RR 0.65, 95% CI 0.52 to 0.82; $p < 0.05$) [16]. There was no difference in efficacy between elemental, semi-elemental, and polymeric diets; however, a non-significant trend favoring very low fat and low long-chain triglycerides was observed. The lack of efficacy in adults may be due to non-compliance. Adults more often stop the EEN due to intolerance, and this may be related to the taste or to the method of delivery (a nasogastric tube) or unpalatability when the EEN is ingested orally [16]. Based on these studies, European Crohn and Colitis Organisation (ECCO) guidelines state that enteral therapy is only appropriate as an add-on treatment to support nutrition and not as a primary therapy in adults with active CD [25].

Table 1. Details of papers on EEN referenced in the manuscript.

Reference	Population	Intervention	Control	Duration	Outcome
		Induction of remission			
Narula [16]	Meta-analysis of six studies, 352 adults	Enteral nutrition (EN)	Corticosteroids (CS)		Clinical remission EN: 45% vs. CS: 73%, $p < 0.05$
Grover [17]	34 children	Nutrison	No control	8 weeks	Clinical remission 84%; mucosal healing 42%
Borrelli [18]	37 children	Polymeric diet (PD)	Corticosteroids (CS)	10 weeks	Clinical remission PD: 79% vs. CS: 67%, p = ns. Mucosal healing PD: 74% vs. CS: 33%, $p < 0.05$
Terrin [19]	20 children	Semi-elemental diet (SED)	Corticosteroids (CS)	8 weeks	Clinical remission SED: 90% vs. CS: 50%, $p < 0.01$
		Maintenance of remission			
Takagi [26]	51 adults	Half-elemental diet (HED)	Regular Diet (RD)	1 year	Relapse rate 1 year 35% in HED vs. 64% in RD
Hanai [27]	95 adults	Elemental diet (ED)	6-Mercaptopurin (6-MP), no intervention	2 years	Relapse rate: ED 53%, 6-MP 40%, control 73% ($p < 0.05$ ED vs. control; 6-MP vs. control)
		EEN as co-medication			
Nguyen [28]	Meta-analysis of four studies, 342 adults	Specialized enteral nutrition combined with infliximab (combo)	Infliximab monotherapy	1 year	Induction: 69.4 in combo vs. 45.4 in mono ($p < 0.01$); Maintenance: Combo 74.5%, mono 49.4% ($p < 0.01$)

CD: Crohn's disease; EEN: exclusive enteral nutrition. For a full review of the efficacy of EEN in inducing remission in active Crohn's disease, please see Narula et al. [16].

EEN has also been successful in preventing relapse in children with quiescent disease [29]. In adults, a prospective study randomly assigning 26 patients to a "half elemental" diet and 25 patients to a free diet resulted in a significantly lower relapse rate in the "half elemental" diet group after a mean follow-up of nearly 1 year compared to the patients who continued their own diet [26]. The compliance to the assigned intervention was similar in the two groups. In a study on 95 patients with CD in remission, 6-mercaptopurine (6-MP) was compared to an elemental diet and to a control group [27]. After 24 months, both the elemental diet and the 6-MP were significantly more effective in maintaining quiescent disease compared to patients in the control group ($p < 0.05$). No significant difference in the number of patients in remission was observed between the 6-MP and elemental diet group, suggesting that both interventions were equally able to maintain remission, although this may also be related to the relatively small sample size. A meta-analysis on EEN as an add-on treatment to anti-tumor necrosis factor (TNF) therapy found that the combination improved outcomes compared to anti-TNF without a dietary prescription [28]. Both the number of patients that reached remission as well as the number of patients that were in remission after a year increased significantly when the anti-TNF treatment was combined with the enteral nutrition ($p < 0.01$).

Together, this shows that enteral nutrition can induce remission, maintain remission, and improve the efficacy of other treatments. However, limited palatability and tolerability limit the applicability of this intervention.

4. Anti-Inflammatory Diet

Although EEN seems to reduce patients' abdominal symptoms and inflammation [16–18], it is not completely clear how treatment with EEN results in these beneficial effects. However, in general, three mechanisms have been identified through which a diet could affect an inflamed bowel, although these mechanisms will undoubtedly interact. The current understanding of CD pathogenesis points to a continuum of interactions between the intestinal microbiota, the immune system, and the epithelial barrier function, and all three are amenable to specific environmental factors, such as diet [30,31]. We will discuss these three factors below.

5. Intestinal Barrier Function

Patients with active Crohn's disease (CD) have an increased intestinal permeability. Even when little inflammation is present, intestinal integrity may still be reduced. This is associated with an elevated risk of a disease flare [32] and gastrointestinal complaints [33]. Intestinal permeability is controlled via tight junctions (TJs). TJs seal the paracellular space between the epithelial cells, thereby separating luminal content such as bacterial products and food antigens from the interstitium. TJs are selectively permeable for water, ions, and small molecules, however, a small proportion of luminal pathogens can cross the TJs. Patients that are susceptible to this translocated content develop an exaggerated mucosal immune response, resulting in an increased gut permeability—a "leaky gut" [34,35]. An increased intestinal permeability is also linked to the development of several diseases, including cardiovascular disease, diabetes, and non-alcoholic fatty liver disease (NAFLD) [35–38]. Improving intestinal barrier function may reduce gastrointestinal complaints and decrease the risk of a flare and the rise of metabolic diseases. The gut is continuously exposed to antigens in the food we consume. These dietary antigens may interact with the gut microbiota, changing its composition. This can result in an increased intestinal permeability, leading to an exaggerated immune response. Pathogens such as *Escherichia coli* O127:H6 (EPEC) and O157:H7 (EHEC), and bacterial toxins from, for instance, *Clostridium difficile* interfere with TJs between the epithelial cells, leading to an increased permeability. Also, the non-pathogenic *E. coli* strain C25 induces defects in the TJ complexes [39]. On the other hand, in a mouse model of necrotizing enterocolitis, *Bifidobacteria* preserved TJs and thereby intestinal barrier function [40]. The non-pathogenic yeast *Saccharomyces boulardii* supports barrier integrity and stimulates regeneration of damaged intestinal tissue in different diseases [41]. Dietary interventions such as EEN may be able to influence intestinal permeability [42,43]. In vitro, TNF-alpha decreased the TJ integrity of a monolayer culture. A polymeric formula completely restored the intestinal integrity of these monolayers [44]. Interleukin-10 knockout mice with colitis treated with EEN had an increased expression of TJs at a correct location and reduced epithelial apoptosis [45]. However, as discussed above, the lack of efficacy of EEN in adults may be due to the fact that EEN is unpalatable and/or that EEN is administered via a nasogastric tube. More palatable oral diets may be a solution for this problem. The Mediterranean diet (MD), rich in fresh vegetables, fruits, legumes, minimally processed whole-grains, nuts, fish, and olive oil, reduces systemic inflammation and is associated with increased diversity in gut microbiota and intestinal integrity [37,46,47].

6. Gut Microbiota

Our intestines are colonized with large numbers of bacteria, archaea, viruses, and eukaryotic microbes that form the gut microbiota [48]. The microbiota protects us against pathogens, regulates local immune responses, and has an important impact on host metabolic functions. In the first three years of life, the microbiota is shaped [49]. Next to antibiotic therapy and severe illness in these years, diet influences the composition of the microbiota. The composition of the microbiota depends on our dietary patterns, which can have both short-term and long-term effects on the variety of the gut microbiota [50]. There is a wide variation in the gut microbiota composition in the elderly [51]. These variations are associated with specific food patterns of these people and separate healthy elderly from those in long-term residential care [50]. The microbiota of the latter has been shown to be significantly less diverse than that of healthy elderly, resulting in increased frailty [50]. Changes in the diversity of the microbiota have been correlated with an increased incidence of chronic inflammatory diseases such as obesity [52], type 2 diabetes [53], cardiovascular disease [54,55], asthma [56], rheumatoid arthritis [57], colorectal cancer [58], and IBD [59,60].

There is growing evidence that a predominantly Western diet, high in fat and refined sugars, influences the composition of the microbiota. Consumption of high-fat milk and sugar-sweetened soda is linked to a lower diversity, whereas buttermilk and high polyphenol content beverages are associated with high microbiota diversity [61]. De Filippo et al., compared the gut microbiota of children aged 1–6 years living in Florence (Italy), where they consume a typical diet of the developed world, with children in Boulpon, a village in Burkina Faso, where they eat a traditional rural African diet high in fibers [62]. The microbiota of the children from Boulpon comprised less Firmicutes and Enterobacteriaceae (*Shigella* and *Escherichia*) compared to the children from Florence. *Prevotella*, *Xylanibacter* (Bacteroidetes), and *Treponema* (Spirochaetes) were exclusively present in the microbiota of the children from Boulpon, possibly as a result of high fiber intake. These bacteria can ferment xylan and cellulose, resulting in the production of short-chain fatty acids (SCFAs). SCFAs are an important source of energy for the mucosa, regulate homeostasis in the colon, and maintain an anti-inflammatory state [63]. Marchesi et al. [64] demonstrated that CD patients have decreased levels of butyrate, an abundant bioactive SCFA, and reduced levels of SCFAs in general in comparison to healthy subjects. A plant-based diet rich in polysaccharides and low in fat and sugars may select for SCFAs-producing bacteria and may be used in the maintenance of remission in patients with inflammatory diseases such as IBD. Microbial structures can rapidly be altered by a change in diet. In a two-week food exchange trial, African Americans consumed a high-fiber/low-fat African diet and rural Africans consumed a high-fat/low-fiber Western diet [65]. "Africanization" of the diet led to a 2.5-fold increase of butyrate in the colon as a result of fermentation of fibers by changes in microbiota, whereas in Africans consuming a Western diet, the amounts of butyrate were reduced by 50%. In concordance, a study among 14 obese men showed that diet-driven changes occurred within 3–4 days but were also reversed within the same time frame [66].

7. Immune Responses

The consumption of processed foods in developed countries has led to an excess of salt intake. Increased dietary salt intake is a risk factor for the development of cardiovascular diseases and autoimmune diseases through the induction of pathogenic T helper 17 (Th17) cells [67], a cell type which plays a pivotal role in the pathogenesis of CD [30]. Mutations in the nucleotide-binding oligomerization domain-containing protein 2 (NOD2) gene is associated with CD. NOD-like receptors (NLRs) sense muramyl dipeptide (MDP), present in all Gram-negative and -positive bacteria, leading to bacterial clearance. Mutations in the NOD2 gene, as seen in patients with IBD, are linked to less clearance of bacteria and suppression of the anti-inflammatory cytokine interleukin (IL)-10 [68]. Another family of innate immune receptors associated with IBD are the Toll-like receptors (TLRs). TLRs are expressed by dendritic cells, and TLR2 and TLR4 are upregulated under inflammatory conditions [2]. TLR2 and TLR4 are increased in the mucosa of patients with IBD compared to healthy controls, resulting in the loss of mucosal homeostasis [68]. Specific dietary patterns can influence the expression of both families of innate immune receptors. For instance, a diet high in fat and carbohydrates increased the expression of TLR2 and TLR4 [69]. Plasma concentrations of lipopolysaccharide (LPS) were also increased [69]. The consumption of orange juice during this meal, however, prevented the enhanced expression of both TLRs and LPS. This was probably due to the reactive oxygen species (ROS)-suppressive effect of flavonoids (naringenin and hesperidin) in the orange juice. A meal high in fibers did not result in an increased concentration of LPS and the induction of TLR2 and TLR4. The authors concluded that, although the content of LPS in a high-fiber meal is comparable to a meal high in fat and carbohydrates, the inflammatory nature of the latter possibly reduced the integrity of the mucosal barrier that normally prevents the translocation of bacterial products from the gut. In a mouse model of CD, a Western diet induced gene transcription of NOD2 and increased gut permeability, allowing the adherent-invasive *E. coli* to colonize, which resulted in an inflammatory state [70]. Together, these data suggest that a Western diet, high in salt, fat, and carbohydrates, may contribute to the development of IBD in predisposed patients, and to the loss of remission in patients with quiescent disease.

8. A Mediterranean Diet as an Anti-Inflammatory Diet

A Mediterranean diet (MD) is able to promote a healthy microbiota, reduce systemic inflammation, and reduce intestinal permeability. Two clinical trials evaluating the effect of a MD have been performed in patients with rheumatoid arthritis (RA) and were systematically reviewed by Forsyth et al. [71]. McKellar et al. [72] assigned patients with RA aged 30–70 years to either a 6-week hands-on cooking workshop (2 h per week delivered by nutritionists and teaching staff from local colleges), whereas the control group received a hand out with the general principles of a healthy diet. In this study, the MD reduced symptoms and improved physical functioning. The second study was a randomized controlled trial by Sköldstam et al. [73]. In this study, patients were randomized between a Cretan diet versus an ordinary Western diet. Symptoms, physical functioning, and biomarkers of inflammation (i.e., C-reactive protein (CRP)) improved in the intervention arm. The authors of the systematic review concluded that joint pain could be reduced and joint function could be improved using a MD. In addition, the risk of cardiovascular disease, which is substantially elevated in RA patients, could also be reduced by a MD. Our group recently performed a trial in 38 IBD patients using a group-based Mediterranean diet intervention (Molendijk et al., ECCO 2019) [74]. Patients with quiescent IBD that were willing to change their lifestyle, including dietary habits, were enrolled. Support was provided during three instruction and feedback days, and patients were able to use an online peer support platform. In this study, we found that 70% of patients were able to alter their dietary habits toward a more Mediterranean pattern. Second, we found that quality of life, as assessed with the short-IBD questionnaire, was increased and CRP was decreased in the active group. The magnitude of the changes in CRP and quality of life was correlated to the magnitude of the dietary change.

Together, these data suggest that a MD can increase the wellbeing of patients with inflammatory disorders. Whether a MD can alter the disease course or reduce inflammation is uncertain. However, the fact that the CRP was reduced in the Mediterranean arm is in this respect encouraging.

9. Conclusions

Recent studies have shown promising results of dietary alterations, such as the introduction of a MD, on the three most important players in the pathogenesis of IBD: intestinal permeability, gut microbiota composition, and inflammatory responses. Although patients are interested in lifestyle advice and a subset of physicians is eager to employ lifestyle-related interventions, the current application of lifestyle interventions in clinical practice is limited. This has a number of causes, such as lack of evidence-based interventions (which intervention works) and evidence-based practices (how to apply the intervention in clinical practice). What is clear is that networks have to be established, with physicians of different backgrounds, dieticians, physical therapists, and (physician-)scientists as participants. These collaborations will facilitate the development and implementation of these interventions.

Author Contributions: I.M. performed literature search and wrote the manuscript. S.v.d.M. critically reviewed the manuscript. P.W.J.M. and I.M. designed the study. P.W.J.M. critically reviewed the manuscript. All authors approved the final version of the manuscript.

References

1. Ungaro, R.; Mehandru, S.; Allen, P.B.; Peyrin-Biroulet, L.; Colombel, J.F. Ulcerative colitis. *Lancet* **2017**, *389*, 1756–1770. [CrossRef]
2. Torres, J.; Mehandru, S.; Colombel, J.F.; Peyrin-Biroulet, L. Crohn's disease. *Lancet* **2017**, *389*, 1741–1755. [CrossRef]
3. Ananthakrishnan, A.N. Epidemiology and risk factors for IBD. *Nat. Rev. Gastroenterol. Hepatol.* **2015**, *12*, 205–217. [CrossRef] [PubMed]
4. Ng, S.C.; Shi, H.Y.; Hamidi, N.; Underwood, F.E.; Tang, W.; Benchimol, E.I.; Panaccione, R.; Ghosh, S.; Wu, J.C.Y.; Chan, F.K.L.; et al. Worldwide incidence and prevalence of inflammatory bowel disease in the 21st century: A systematic review of population-based studies. *Lancet* **2018**, *390*, 2769–2778. [CrossRef]
5. Ananthakrishnan, A.N.; Khalili, H.; Song, M.; Higuchi, L.M.; Richter, J.M.; Nimptsch, K.; Kana Wu, K.; Chan, A. High school diet and risk of crohn's disease and ulcerative colitis. *Inflamm. Bowel Dis.* **2015**, *21*, 2311–2319.
6. Racine, A.; Carbonnel, F.; Chan, S.S.; Hart, A.R.; Bueno-de-Mesquita, H.B.; Oldenburg, B.; van Schaik, F.D.M.; Tjonneland, A.; Olsen, A.; Dahm, C.C.; et al. Dietary patterns and risk of inflammatory bowel disease in Europe: Results from the EPIC study. *Inflamm. Bowel Dis.* **2016**, *22*, 345–354. [CrossRef] [PubMed]
7. Molodecky, N.A.; Soon, I.S.; Rabi, D.M.; Ghali, W.A.; Ferris, M.; Chernoff, G.; Benchimol, E.I.; Panaccione, R.; Ghosh, S.; Barkema, H.W.; et al. Increasing incidence and prevalence of the inflammatory bowel diseases with time, based on systematic review. *Gastroenterology* **2012**, *142*, 46–54.e42, quiz e30. [CrossRef] [PubMed]
8. Lewis, J.D.; Abreu, M.T. Diet as a trigger or therapy for inflammatory bowel diseases. *Gastroenterology* **2017**, *152*, 398–414 e6. [CrossRef]
9. Guerreiro, C.S.; Ferreira, P.; Tavares, L.; Santos, P.M.; Neves, M.; Brito, M.; Cravo, M. Fatty acids, IL6, and TNFalpha polymorphisms: An example of nutrigenetics in Crohn's disease. *Am. J. Gastroenterol.* **2009**, *104*, 2241–2249. [CrossRef]
10. Tanaka, M.; Iwao, Y.; Sasaki, S.; Okamoto, S.; Ogata, H.; Hibi, T.; Kazuma, K. Moderate dietary temperance effectively prevents relapse of Crohn disease: A prospective study of patients in remission. *Gastroenterol. Nurs.* **2007**, *30*, 202–210. [CrossRef]
11. Calder, P.C. n-3 polyunsaturated fatty acids, inflammation, and inflammatory diseases. *Am. J. Clin. Nutr.* **2006**, *83* (Suppl. 6), 1505s–1519s. [CrossRef]
12. Kinsey, L.; Burden, S. A survey of people with inflammatory bowel disease to investigate their views of food and nutritional issues. *Eur. J. Clin. Nutr.* **2016**, *70*, 852–854. [CrossRef]
13. Casanova, M.J.; Chaparro, M.; Molina, B.; Merino, O.; Batanero, R.; Duenas-Sadornil, C.; Robledo, P.; Garcia-Albert, A.M.; Gómez-Sánchez, M.B.; Calvet, X.; et al. Prevalence of malnutrition and nutritional characteristics of patients with inflammatory bowel disease. *J. Crohns Colitis* **2017**, *11*, 1430–1439. [CrossRef]
14. Limdi, J.K.; Aggarwal, D.; McLaughlin, J.T. Dietary practices and beliefs in patients with inflammatory bowel disease. *Inflamm. Bowel Dis.* **2016**, *22*, 164–170. [CrossRef]
15. Zhan, Y.L.; Zhan, Y.A.; Dai, S.X. Is a low FODMAP diet beneficial for patients with inflammatory bowel disease? A meta-analysis and systematic review. *Clin. Nutr.* **2018**, *37*, 123–129. [CrossRef] [PubMed]
16. Narula, N.; Dhillon, A.; Zhang, D.; Sherlock, M.E.; Tondeur, M.; Zachos, M. Enteral nutritional therapy for induction of remission in Crohn's disease. *Cochrane Database Syst. Rev.* **2018**, *4*, CD000542. [CrossRef] [PubMed]
17. Grover, Z.; Muir, R.; Lewindon, P. Exclusive enteral nutrition induces early clinical, mucosal and transmural remission in paediatric Crohn's disease. *J. Gastroenterol.* **2014**, *49*, 638–645. [CrossRef]
18. Borrelli, O.; Cordischi, L.; Cirulli, M.; Paganelli, M.; Labalestra, V.; Uccini, S.; Russo, P.M.; Cucchiara, S. Polymeric diet alone versus corticosteroids in the treatment of active pediatric Crohn's disease: A randomized controlled open-label trial. *Clin. Gastroenterol. Hepatol.* **2006**, *4*, 744–753. [CrossRef]

19. Terrin, G.; Berni Canani, R.; Ambrosini, A.; Viola, F.; Bueno de Mesquita, M.; Di Nardo, G.; Cucchiara, S. A semielemental diet (Pregomin) as primary therapy for inducing remission in children with active Crohn's disease. *Ital. J. Pediatr.* **2002**, *28*, 401–405.
20. Forbes, A.; Escher, J.; Hebuterne, X.; Klek, S.; Krznaric, Z.; Schneider, S.; Shamir, R.; Stardelova, K.; Wierdsma, N.; Wiskin, A.E.; et al. ESPEN guideline: Clinical nutrition in inflammatory bowel disease. *Clin. Nutr.* **2017**, *36*, 321–347. [CrossRef]
21. Ruemmele, F.M.; Veres, G.; Kolho, K.L.; Griffiths, A.; Levine, A.; Escher, J.C.; Amil Dias, J.; Barabino, A.; Braegger, C.P.; Bronsky, J.; et al. Consensus guidelines of ECCO/ESPGHAN on the medical management of pediatric Crohn's disease. *J. Crohns Colitis* **2014**, *8*, 1179–1207. [CrossRef]
22. Griffiths, A.M.; Ohlsson, A.; Sherman, P.M.; Sutherland, L.R. Meta-analysis of enteral nutrition as a primary treatment of active Crohn's disease. *Gastroenterology* **1995**, *108*, 1056–1067. [CrossRef]
23. Messori, A.; Trallori, G.; D'Albasio, G.; Milla, M.; Vannozzi, G.; Pacini, F. Defined-formula diets versus steroids in the treatment of active Crohn's disease: A meta-analysis. *Scand. J. Gastroenterol.* **1996**, *31*, 267–272. [CrossRef]
24. Fernandez-Banares, F.; Cabre, E.; Esteve-Comas, M.; Gassull, M.A. How effective is enteral nutrition in inducing clinical remission in active Crohn's disease? A meta-analysis of the randomized clinical trials. *JPEN J. Parenter. Enteral. Nutr.* **1995**, *19*, 356–364. [CrossRef]
25. Gomollon, F.; Dignass, A.; Annese, V.; Tilg, H.; Van Assche, G.; Lindsay, J.O.; Peyrin-Biroulet, L.; Cullen, G.J.; Daperno, M.; Rieder, T.K.F.; et al. 3rd European Evidence-based Consensus on the Diagnosis and Management of Crohn's Disease 2016: Part 1: Diagnosis and Medical Management. *J. Crohns Colitis* **2017**, *11*, 3–25. [CrossRef]
26. Takagi, S.; Utsunomiya, K.; Kuriyama, S.; Yokoyama, H.; Takahashi, S.; Iwabuchi, M.; Takahashi, H.; Takahashi, S.; Kinouchi, Y.; Hiwatashi, Y.; et al. Effectiveness of an 'half elemental diet' as maintenance therapy for Crohn's disease: A randomized-controlled trial. *Aliment. Pharmacol. Ther.* **2006**, *24*, 1333–1340. [CrossRef]
27. Hanai, H.; Iida, T.; Takeuchi, K.; Arai, H.; Arai, O.; Abe, J.; Tanaka, T.; Maruyama, Y.; Ikeya, K.; Sugimoto, K.; et al. Nutritional therapy versus 6-mercaptopurine as maintenance therapy in patients with Crohn's disease. *Dig. Liver Dis.* **2012**, *44*, 649–654. [CrossRef]
28. Nguyen, D.L.; Palmer, L.B.; Nguyen, E.T.; McClave, S.A.; Martindale, R.G.; Bechtold, M.L. Specialized enteral nutrition therapy in Crohn's disease patients on maintenance infliximab therapy: A meta-analysis. *Ther. Adv. Gastroenterol.* **2015**, *8*, 168–175. [CrossRef]
29. Cabre, E.; Gassull, M.A. Nutrition in inflammatory bowel disease: Impact on disease and therapy. *Curr. Opin. Gastroenterol.* **2001**, *17*, 342–349. [CrossRef]
30. Kaser, A.; Zeissig, S.; Blumberg, R.S. Inflammatory bowel disease. *Annu. Rev. Immunol.* **2010**, *28*, 573–621. [CrossRef]
31. Zeissig, S.; Burgel, N.; Gunzel, D.; Richter, J.; Mankertz, J.; Wahnschaffe, U.; Kroesen, A.; Zeitz, M.; Fromm, M.; Schulzke, J.D. Changes in expression and distribution of claudin 2, 5 and 8 lead to discontinuous tight junctions and barrier dysfunction in active Crohn's disease. *Gut* **2007**, *56*, 61–72. [CrossRef]
32. Gutierrez, A.; Zapater, P.; Juanola, O.; Sempere, L.; Garcia, M.; Laveda, R.; Martínez, A.; Scharl, M.; González-Navajas, J.M.; Such, J.; et al. Gut bacterial DNA translocation is an independent risk factor of flare at short term in patients with Crohn's disease. *Am. J. Gastroenterol.* **2016**, *111*, 529–540. [CrossRef]
33. Chang, J.; Leong, R.W.; Wasinger, V.C.; Ip, M.; Yang, M.; Phan, T.G. Impaired intestinal permeability contributes to ongoing bowel symptoms in patients with inflammatory bowel disease and mucosal healing. *Gastroenterology* **2017**, *153*, 723–731 e1. [CrossRef]
34. Landy, J.; Ronde, E.; English, N.; Clark, S.K.; Hart, A.L.; Knight, S.C.; Ciclitira, P.J.; Al-Hassi, H.O. Tight junctions in inflammatory bowel diseases and inflammatory bowel disease associated colorectal cancer. *World J. Gastroenterol.* **2016**, *22*, 3117–3126. [CrossRef]
35. Odenwald, M.A.; Turner, J.R. Intestinal permeability defects: Is it time to treat? *Clin. Gastroenterol. Hepatol.* **2013**, *11*, 1075–1083. [CrossRef]
36. Odenwald, M.A.; Turner, J.R. The intestinal epithelial barrier: A therapeutic target? *Nat. Rev. Gastroenterol. Hepatol.* **2017**, *14*, 9–21. [CrossRef]
37. Casas, R.; Sacanella, E.; Urpi-Sarda, M.; Corella, D.; Castaner, O.; Lamuela-Raventos, R.M.; Salas-Salvadó, J.; Martínez-González, M.-A.; Ros, E.; Estruch, R. Long-term immunomodulatory effects of a mediterranean

diet in adults at high risk of cardiovascular disease in the PREvencion con DIeta MEDiterranea (PREDIMED) randomized controlled trial. *J. Nutr.* **2016**, *146*, 1684–1693. [CrossRef]
38. Mu, Q.; Kirby, J.; Reilly, C.M.; Luo, X.M. Leaky gut as a danger signal for autoimmune diseases. *Front. Immunol.* **2017**, *8*, 598. [CrossRef]
39. Zareie, M.; Riff, J.; Donato, K.; McKay, D.M.; Perdue, M.H.; Soderholm, J.D.; Karmali, M.; Cohen, M.B.; Hawkins, J.; Sherman, P.M. Novel effects of the prototype translocating Escherichia coli, strain C25 on intestinal epithelial structure and barrier function. *Cell. Microbiol.* **2005**, *7*, 1782–1797. [CrossRef]
40. Bergmann, K.R.; Liu, S.X.L.; Tian, R.L.; Kushnir, A.; Turner, J.R.; Li, H.L.; Chou, P.M.; Weber, C.R.; De Plaen, I.G. Bifidobacteria stabilize claudins at tight junctions and prevent intestinal barrier dysfunction in mouse necrotizing enterocolitis. *Am. J. Pathol.* **2013**, *182*, 1595–1606. [CrossRef]
41. Terciolo, C.; Dapoigny, M.; Andre, F. Beneficial effects of Saccharomyces boulardii CNCM I-745 on clinical disorders associated with intestinal barrier disruption. *Clin. Exp. Gastroenterol.* **2019**, *12*, 67–82. [CrossRef]
42. Araujo, J.R.; Tomas, J.; Brenner, C.; Sansonetti, P.J. Impact of high-fat diet on the intestinal microbiota and small intestinal physiology before and after the onset of obesity. *Biochimie* **2017**, *141*, 97–106. [CrossRef] [PubMed]
43. Ma, N.; Tian, Y.; Wu, Y.; Ma, X. Contributions of the Interaction Between Dietary Protein and Gut Microbiota to Intestinal Health. *Curr. Protein Pept. Sci.* **2017**, *18*, 795–808. [CrossRef]
44. Nahidi, L.; Day, A.S.; Lemberg, D.A.; Leach, S.T. Differential effects of nutritional and non-nutritional therapies on intestinal barrier function in an in vitro model. *J. Gastroenterol.* **2012**, *47*, 107–117. [CrossRef]
45. Wang, H.; Shi, P.; Zuo, L.; Dong, J.; Zhao, J.; Liu, Q.; Zhu, W. Dietary non-digestible polysaccharides ameliorate intestinal epithelial barrier dysfunction in IL-10 knockout mice. *J. Crohns Colitis* **2016**, *10*, 1076–1086. [CrossRef]
46. Casas, R.; Sacanella, E.; Estruch, R. The immune protective effect of the Mediterranean diet against chronic low-grade inflammatory diseases. *Endocr. Metab. Immune Disord. Drug Targets* **2014**, *14*, 245–254. [CrossRef]
47. Mitsou, E.K.; Kakali, A.; Antonopoulou, S.; Mountzouris, K.C.; Yannakoulia, M.; Panagiotakos, D.B.; Kyriacou, A. Adherence to the Mediterranean diet is associated with the gut microbiota pattern and gastrointestinal characteristics in an adult population. *Br. J. Nutr.* **2017**, *117*, 1645–1655. [CrossRef]
48. Shreiner, A.B.; Kao, J.Y.; Young, V.B. The gut microbiome in health and in disease. *Curr. Opin. Gastroen.* **2015**, *31*, 69–75. [CrossRef]
49. Yatsunenko, T.; Rey, F.E.; Manary, M.J.; Trehan, I.; Dominguez-Bello, M.G.; Contreras, M.; Magris, M.; Hidalgo, G.; Baldassano, R.N.; Anokhin, A.P.; et al. Human gut microbiome viewed across age and geography. *Nature* **2012**, *486*, 222–227. [CrossRef]
50. Claesson, M.J.; Jeffery, I.B.; Conde, S.; Power, S.E.; O'Connor, E.M.; Cusack, S.; Harris, H.M.B.; Coakley, M.; Lakshminarayanan, B.; O'Sullivan, O.; et al. Gut microbiota composition correlates with diet and health in the elderly. *Nature* **2012**, *488*, 178–184. [CrossRef]
51. Claesson, M.J.; Cusack, S.; O'Sullivan, O.; Greene-Diniz, R.; de Weerd, H.; Flannery, E.; Marchesi, J.R.; Falush, D.; Dinan, T.; Fitzgerald, G.; et al. Composition, variability, and temporal stability of the intestinal microbiota of the elderly. *Proc. Natl. Acad. Sci. USA* **2011**, *108* (Suppl. 1), 4586–4591. [CrossRef]
52. Le Chatelier, E.; Nielsen, T.; Qin, J.; Prifti, E.; Hildebrand, F.; Falony, G.; Almeida, M.; Arumugam, M.; Batto, J.-M.; Kennedy, S.; et al. Richness of human gut microbiome correlates with metabolic markers. *Nature* **2013**, *500*, 541–546. [CrossRef]
53. Karlsson, F.H.; Tremaroli, V.; Nookaew, I.; Bergstrom, G.; Behre, C.J.; Fagerberg, B.; Nielsen, J.; Bäckhed, F. Gut metagenome in European women with normal, impaired and diabetic glucose control. *Nature* **2013**, *498*, 99–103. [CrossRef]
54. Wang, Z.; Klipfell, E.; Bennett, B.J.; Koeth, R.; Levison, B.S.; Dugar, B.; Feldstein, A.E.; Britt, E.B.; Fu, X.; Chung, Y.-M.; et al. Gut flora metabolism of phosphatidylcholine promotes cardiovascular disease. *Nature* **2011**, *472*, 57–63. [CrossRef]
55. Koeth, R.A.; Wang, Z.; Levison, B.S.; Buffa, J.A.; Org, E.; Sheehy, B.T.; Britt, E.B.; Fu, X.; Wu, Y.; Li, L.; et al. Intestinal microbiota metabolism of L-carnitine, a nutrient in red meat, promotes atherosclerosis. *Nat. Med.* **2013**, *19*, 576–585. [CrossRef]
56. Devereux, G. The increase in the prevalence of asthma and allergy: Food for thought. *Nat. Rev. Immunol.* **2006**, *6*, 869–874. [CrossRef]

57. Scher, J.U.; Sczesnak, A.; Longman, R.S.; Segata, N.; Ubeda, C.; Bielski, C.; Rostron, T.; Cerundolo, V.; Pamer, E.G.; Abramson, S.B.; et al. Expansion of intestinal Prevotella copri correlates with enhanced susceptibility to arthritis. *Elife* **2013**, *2*, e01202. [CrossRef]
58. Kostic, A.D.; Chun, E.; Robertson, L.; Glickman, J.N.; Gallini, C.A.; Michaud, M.; Clancy, T.E.; Chung, D.C.; Lochhead, P.; Hold, G.L.; et al. Fusobacterium nucleatum potentiates intestinal tumorigenesis and modulates the tumor-immune microenvironment. *Cell Host Microbe* **2013**, *14*, 207–215. [CrossRef]
59. Gevers, D.; Kugathasan, S.; Denson, L.A.; Vazquez-Baeza, Y.; Van Treuren, W.; Ren, B.; Schwager, E.; Knights, D.; Song, S.J.; Yassour, M.; et al. The treatment-naive microbiome in new-onset Crohn's disease. *Cell Host Microbe* **2014**, *15*, 382–392. [CrossRef]
60. Kostic, A.D.; Xavier, R.J.; Gevers, D. The microbiome in inflammatory bowel disease: Current status and the future ahead. *Gastroenterology* **2014**, *146*, 1489–1499. [CrossRef]
61. Zhernakova, A.; Kurilshikov, A.; Bonder, M.J.; Tigchelaar, E.F.; Schirmer, M.; Vatanen, T.; Mujagic, Z.; Vila, A.V.; Falony, G.; Vieira-Silva, S.; et al. Population-based metagenomics analysis reveals markers for gut microbiome composition and diversity. *Science* **2016**, *352*, 565–569. [CrossRef]
62. De Filippo, C.; Cavalieri, D.; Di Paola, M.; Ramazzotti, M.; Poullet, J.B.; Massart, S.; Collini, S.; Pieraccini, G.; Lionetti, P. Impact of diet in shaping gut microbiota revealed by a comparative study in children from Europe and rural Africa. *Proc. Natl. Acad. Sci. USA* **2010**, *107*, 14691–14696. [CrossRef]
63. Scheppach, W.; Weiler, F. The butyrate story: Old wine in new bottles? *Curr. Opin. Clin. Nutr. Metab. Care* **2004**, *7*, 563–567. [CrossRef]
64. Marchesi, J.R.; Holmes, E.; Khan, F.; Kochhar, S.; Scanlan, P.; Shanahan, F.; Shanahan, F.; Wilson, I.D.; Wang, Y. Rapid and noninvasive metabonomic characterization of inflammatory bowel disease. *J. Proteome Res.* **2007**, *6*, 546–551. [CrossRef]
65. O'Keefe, S.J.; Li, J.V.; Lahti, L.; Ou, J.; Carbonero, F.; Mohammed, K.; Posma, J.M.; Kinross, J.; Wahl, E.; Ruder, E.; et al. Fat, fibre and cancer risk in African Americans and rural Africans. *Nat. Commun.* **2015**, *6*, 6342. [CrossRef]
66. Walker, A.W.; Ince, J.; Duncan, S.H.; Webster, L.M.; Holtrop, G.; Ze, X.; Brown, D.; Stares, M.D.; Scott, P.; Bergerat, A.; et al. Dominant and diet-responsive groups of bacteria within the human colonic microbiota. *ISME J.* **2011**, *5*, 220–230. [CrossRef]
67. Kleinewietfeld, M.; Manzel, A.; Titze, J.; Kvakan, H.; Yosef, N.; Linker, R.A.; Muller, A.N.; Hafler, D.A. Sodium chloride drives autoimmune disease by the induction of pathogenic TH17 cells. *Nature* **2013**, *496*, 518–522. [CrossRef]
68. De Souza, H.S.; Fiocchi, C. Immunopathogenesis of IBD: Current state of the art. *Nat. Rev. Gastroenterol. Hepatol.* **2016**, *13*, 13–27. [CrossRef]
69. Ghanim, H.; Sia, C.L.; Upadhyay, M.; Korzeniewski, K.; Viswanathan, P.; Abuaysheh, S.; Mohanty, P.; Dandona, P. Orange juice neutralizes the proinflammatory effect of a high-fat, high-carbohydrate meal and prevents endotoxin increase and Toll-like receptor expression. *Am. J. Clin. Nutr.* **2010**, *91*, 940–949. [CrossRef]
70. Martinez-Medina, M.; Denizot, J.; Dreux, N.; Robin, F.; Billard, E.; Bonnet, R.; Darfeuille-Michaud, A.; Barnich, N. Western diet induces dysbiosis with increased E coli in CEABAC10 mice, alters host barrier function favouring AIEC colonisation. *Gut* **2014**, *63*, 116–124. [CrossRef]
71. Forsyth, C.; Kouvari, M.; D'Cunha, N.M.; Georgousopoulou, E.N.; Panagiotakos, D.B.; Mellor, D.D.; Kellett, J.; Naumovski, N. The effects of the Mediterranean diet on rheumatoid arthritis prevention and treatment: A systematic review of human prospective studies. *Rheumatol. Int.* **2018**, *38*, 737–747. [CrossRef]
72. McKellar, G.; Morrison, E.; McEntegart, A.; Hampson, R.; Tierney, A.; Mackle, G.; Scoular, J.; Scott, J.A.; Capell, H.A. A pilot study of a Mediterranean-type diet intervention in female patients with rheumatoid arthritis living in areas of social deprivation in Glasgow. *Ann. Rheum. Dis.* **2007**, *66*, 1239–1243. [CrossRef]
73. Sköldstam, L.; Hagfors, L.; Johansson, G. An experimental study of a Mediterranean diet intervention for patients with rheumatoid arthritis. *Ann. Rheum. Dis.* **2003**, *62*, 208–214. [CrossRef] [PubMed]
74. Molendijk, I.; Martens, J.E.; van Lingen, E.; van der Marel, S.; van Veen-Lievaart, M.E.; van der Meulen, A.E.; Barnhoorn, M.C.; Ernst-Stegeman, A.M.; Maljaars, J. P592 Towards a Food Pharmacy: increased dietary quality reduces CRP and improves quality of life in IBD patients in remission. *J. Crohn's Colitis* **2019**, *13* (Suppl. 1), S411. [CrossRef]

8

Dietary Composition and Effects in Inflammatory Bowel Disease

Fernando Castro [1] and Heitor S. P. de Souza [1,2,*]

[1] Department of Internal Medicine, School of Medicine, Federal University of Rio de Janeiro, 21941-913 Rio de Janeiro, Brazil; fernandommcastro@gmail.com

[2] Department of Internal Medicine, D'Or Institute for Research and Education (IDOR), 22281-100 Rio de Janeiro, Brazil

[*] Correspondence: heitor.souza@gmail.com or hsouza@hucff.ufrj.br

Abstract: Dramatic changes in the environment and human lifestyle have been associated with the rise of various chronic complex diseases, such as inflammatory bowel disease (IBD). A dysbiotic gut microbiota has been proposed as a crucial pathogenic element, contributing to immune imbalances and fostering a proinflammatory milieu, which may be associated with disease relapses or even the initiation of IBD. In addition to representing important regulators of the mucosal immunity and the composition of the gut microbiota, food components have been shown to be potential environmental triggers of epigenetic modifications. In the context of chronic intestinal inflammation, dietary habits and specific food components have been implicated as important modulators of epigenetic mechanisms, including DNA methylation, which may predispose a person to the increased risk of the initiation and evolution of IBD. This review provides novel insights about how dietary factors may interact with the intestinal mucosa and modulate immune homeostasis by shaping the intestinal ecosystem, as well as the potential influence of diet in the etiopathogenesis and management of IBD.

Keywords: inflammatory bowel disease; dietary habits; food components; gut microbiota; immune homeostasis; epigenetic changes

---

1. Introduction

Inflammatory bowel disease (IBD), including Crohn's disease (CD) and ulcerative colitis (UC), is regarded as a heterogeneous disease of unknown etiology, with an unpredictable clinical course and usually labeled as a chronic disabling disorder [1,2]. Although the mechanisms leading to the development of IBD are rather complex and have not yet been completely elucidated, the current information points to a multifactorial origin. The chronic inflammatory process underlying the pathogenesis of IBD reflects a dysregulated immune response, stemming from a conflicting interaction involving several environmental factors, an altered innate immunity, and a predisposing genetic background [3–6].

Information derived from epidemiological studies has revealed consistent associations between the increase in the occurrence in IBD and other autoimmune and chronic inflammatory disorders, and the decline in infectious diseases, accompanied by the use of antibiotics, immunizations, and overall improvements in sanitary conditions and the quality of water [7]. IBD has progressively become a global disease, affecting newly industrialized nations in Asia, South America, and the Middle East [8–10]. Although the prevalence of IBD in newly industrialized countries is still lower than in developed countries, the incidence rate is increasing rapidly [11]. Among all the environmental changes usually associated with IBD, dietary habits are one element, both from the patients' perspective, including personal observations and common practical concerns, and due to scientific evidence implicating diet as a triggering factor in disease relapses [12]. In this article, we discuss the effects of diet on IBD, especially considering the basic physiological processes that underlie these associations.

2. Diet and Microbiota

Although the influence of dietary habits on the intestinal microbiota has long been speculated, only after the introduction of new technology, including next-generation DNA sequencing and metabolic profiling, was reliable information able to be obtained [13]. For example, the microbiota composition is currently thought of as a dynamic process that changes with age and fluctuates in consonance with environmental exposures, including diet, among other factors [14].

The results of studies analyzing the microbial communities of the gut obtained from mammalian species have endorsed the assumption that diet can influence microbial diversity. Such diversity has been shown to increase from carnivores to omnivores and then to herbivores [15]. Regarding humans, the intestinal microbiota reflects predominant omnivorous habits, but substantial inconsistencies have been reported. For example, opposing patterns of the intestinal microbiota composition were reported when comparing samples from African children living in rural communities with children from a European urban center, a phenomenon that has been attributed to dietary differences [16]. In this case, in terms of health issues, individuals from the European urban center are expected to be at increased risk for the development of several immune-mediated disorders. Such diseases, likely including IBD, are probably associated with the microbiome structure, often resulting from dietary incompatibilities between the current environments and those in which humans evolved.

The Western style of diet, defined by high caloric content due to large amounts of fat and carbohydrates, has been associated with a markedly reduced microbiome diversity [17]. In addition to the plethora of fat, Western diets usually have high concentrations of dietary omega-6 fatty acids, from vegetable oils, resulting in a high omega-6 to omega-3 ratio. Whereas omega-3 fatty acids, such as a-linolenic acid from vegetables and eicosapentaenoic acid and docosahexaenoic acid from fish, have anti-inflammatory properties, omega-6 fatty acids, particularly arachidonic acid, are considered pro-inflammatory. This may explain why the Western diet has been regarded as a key factor for producing intestinal inflammation [18]. Other relevant studies focusing on diet potentially affecting the intestinal microbiota are summarized in Table 1.

Previous studies have analyzed the gut microbiota of infants and children within one population, but few have attempted to compare the microbial composition considering distinct socio-economic, geographic, and cultural aspects [16]. To analyze the potential effect of environmental factors on defining how and from where a gut microbiota may be acquired, investigators characterized bacterial species and gene contents of fecal samples from a cohort of healthy Amerindians from Venezuela, rural Malawian communities, and metropolitan USA inhabitants. The investigators found that bacterial diversity increases with age, and the degree of similarity among members of a family is consistent in all three populations. The fecal microbiota of USA adults was the least diverse compared to the others [19]. Therefore, it appears that differences in social structures and cultural traditions known to impact food and many other environmental factors may also condition the magnitude of the circulation of microbes among members of a family or community.

Table 1. Relationship between gut microbiota alterations and dietary patterns.

Genus	Characteristics	Dietary Component	Gastrointestinal (GI) Effect
Prevotella *Bacteroides*	Gram-negative anaerobic	Diets rich in fat and carbohydrates	Involved in colitis [17,20–23]
Clostridium	Gram-positive anaerobic	Decrease in high-fat but not high-sugar diets	Affects the clinical course of inflammatory bowel disease (IBD) [21–24]
Ruminococcus	Gram-positive anaerobic	Fermentation of dietary fiber and decrease in high-fat but not high-sugar diets	[21,25,26]
Streptococcus *Lactobacillus*	Gram-positive	Constituents of the normal animal microbiota	Induces remission in ulcerative colitis (UC) patients [21]
Escherichia	Gram-negative anaerobic	High-fat and high-sugar diets	Overgrowth of *Escherichia coli* and involved in colitis [16,22,27]
Bifidobacterium	Gram-positive anaerobic	High-fiber diet	Induces remission in UC patients [28,29]
Fusobacterium	Gram-negative anaerobic	-	Involved in colitis and colon cancer [30]
-	-	Alcohol	Decreased butyrate/total short chain fatty acids (SCFA) ratio in stool [31]

Source: adapted from Levine et al. [5] and Rapozo et al. [21].

3. Diet and Immune Response

Western lifestyle factors have been associated with the progressive increase in various metabolic, autoimmune, and chronic inflammatory disorders, including IBD [32–34]. In addition to industrialization, urbanization, the improvement of sanitary conditions, antibiotic usage, and other factors, abundant evidence supports the involvement of dietary habits in shaping the gut microbiota and influencing the interaction with the immune system [35–37].

Dietary fiber has been shown to interfere in host immunity via multiple pathways. Fibers and starches present in fruits and vegetables represent a substrate for the production of butyrate and other short chain fatty acids (SCFAs) by intestinal microbiota. Butyrate, for example, is well-recognized as a critical element in epithelial homeostasis, but also plays an important role in downregulating the immune response by inhibiting the transcription of inflammatory cytokines and promoting the differentiation of lamina propria Tregs [5,38,39]. Low dietary fiber may precipitate the catabolism of the mucous layer, leading to increased permeability and compromising the epithelial barrier against potential pathogenic luminal bacteria [40].

Investigations based on experimental models have provided results regarding the effects of specific diets on the immune response. For instance, a high-fat (HF) and high-sugar diet generated a proinflammatory intestinal environment, associated with an overgrowth of Proteobacteria, reduction in butyrate production, and expression of the butyrate GPR43 receptor, also underexpressed in CD patients [41]. Results from another experimental model showed that HF diets led to the upregulation of tumor necrosis factor-α (TNF-α) and interferon-γ expression, and to the decrease in the densities of colonic Tregs [42]. A high intake of fat has been shown to have several effects on the mucosal immune system, revealing the complex interaction between the lamina propria immune cells and the intestinal microbiota. For example, the ingestion of high-fat meals increases the expression of interlukein-1β (IL-1β), TNF-α, IL-6, and necrosis factor-κB (NF-κB) in the colon [43,44]. Likewise, mice fed with cholesterol-enriched meals displayed acute inflammasome-dependent intestinal inflammation, increasing the production of IL-1β, and driving the accumulation of CD11b+ and CD11c+ cells in the lamina propria [45].

The increasing knowledge about the influence of the gut microbiome on the mucosal and systemic immune response has contributed to the understanding of the mechanisms underlying the pathogenesis of IBD and other chronic inflammatory conditions. Dysbiosis has been confirmed in samples from patients with CD, displaying an increase in Enterobacteriales such as *Escherichia coli*, and a decrease in Clostridiales such as *Faecalibacterium prausnitzii* [46–48]. In a study involving UC, the results supported a role for reduced microbial diversity, although not as prominent as the dysbiosis seen in CD [49]. A large cohort study analyzing fecal samples from four different European countries revealed that CD and UC are distinct in terms of the microbiome [50]. Notably, some specific intestinal microbes can shape the immune response. For example, *Listeria monocytogenes*, *Clostridium difficile*, and *Toxoplasma gondii* have been shown to elicit innate lymphoid cells-1 (ILC1) and Th1 cells, which orchestrate the secretion of cytokines, such as interferon-gamma and TNF-α, critically important in the immunity against those intestinal pathogens [51]. Clostridia strains have been shown to promote the accumulation of Foxp3 Treg cells in the gut [52], which in turn down-regulate inflammatory responses, including those in experimental colitis [53]. Some microorganisms induce the activation of subsets of immune cells responsible for promoting intestinal inflammation, such as Th17 cells [54]. For instance, segmented filamentous bacteria can activate Th17 cells, whereas a decrease in Th17 cell-inducing bacteria can attenuate the severity of colitis in mice [55]. In previous studies, adherent invasive *E. coli* (AIEC) and *Bifidobacteria adolescentis* [56,57], in addition to *E. coli O157* and *Citrobacter rodentium* [54], have been shown to induce populations of Th17 cells.

Dietary habits can affect human health either directly or via changes in the gut microbiota. The gut microbiota is a highly complex and dynamic system that can be shaped by environmental factors, including the diet [58]. Regarding the dietary factors directly or indirectly associated with the immune response and intestinal homeostasis, diets with high concentrations of fat and sugar have been associated with intestinal colonization with potential IBD-related pathobionts. For instance, adherent invasive *E. coli* (AIEC) strains, induced by high-fat high-sugar diets, may become pathogenic when the ligand CEACAM 6 is presented by the intestinal epithelium. Under such circumstances, AIEC may form biofilms, adhere to, and translocate via M cells and the associated epithelium [59]. These findings reinforce the idea that changes in the local environment exert a selective pressure on several species, which in turn shape the microbiota according to the most adaptable microorganisms to the intestinal milieu [60]. A selection of dietary factors that may affect the host immunity is listed in Table 2.

Table 2. Dietary patterns potentially affecting microbiota and immunity.

Dietary Component	GI and Immunological Effect
High-fat, high-sugar diet	• Intestinal mucosa dysbiosis [41] • Higher degree of crypt abscesses • Decreased butyrate production • Overgrowth of *E. coli* [41]
Milk fat (saturated fat)	• Induced pro-inflammatory Th1 immune response [61] • Increased incidence of colitis [61] • Dysbiosis
High-fiber diet	• Protected from acute colitis [62] • Did not increase SCFAs production in patients with UC [62]
Animal versus plant diet	• Animal-based food increased the abundance of bile-tolerant microorganisms and decreased the proportions of *Firmicutes* [27]
Alcohol	• Decreased butyrate/total SCFA ratio in stool [31]
Maltodextrin	• Biofilm formation of adherent invasive *E. coli* [63,64] • Enhanced *E. coli* adhesion independent of cellular receptor CEACAM 6 [63,64]

Source: adapted from Levine et al. [5].

4. Diet and IBD

Advances resulting from clinical and experimental investigations have demonstrated that the microbiome might play a critical role in the pathogenesis of IBD [65,66]. In parallel, results from other studies have supported a link between dietary patterns and the structure of the intestinal microbiome in healthy individuals and in patients with gastrointestinal disorders, including IBD [17,27,67]. Given the potential effects that diet can have on the composition and function of the intestinal microbiome, diet may also be involved in the pathogenesis of IBD, either directly or indirectly. As a consequence, due to the associations with the microbiome and IBD, specific dietary interventions are promising novel therapies.

Data have confirmed that food plays a crucial role in the gut microenvironment, and modifications of dietary habits may have an important impact on the microbial composition and function, but also on the gut barrier and immunity [5]. Previous studies demonstrated that modifications in a single food group might produce various outcomes. For instance, changing the dietary composition from a predominant plant- to animal-based diet results in a change in the intestinal microbial environment and functionality, determining alterations in bile acids and sulfide metabolism, which have been implicated in IBD pathogenesis [27,68]. In an experimental study, investigators demonstrated that a low-fiber diet induces the expansion and activity of colonic mucous-degrading microorganisms, potentially favoring the development of severe colitis by enteric pathogens [40]. In another experimental study, mice fed a Western-style diet (rich in saturated fats and simple carbohydrates, but depleted in dietary fiber), developed an alteration in the colonic microbiota, resulting in increased permeability and a reduced inner mucus layer. Both defects could be prevented by transplanting microbiota from chow-fed mice, whereas the administration of *Bifidobacterium longum* was sufficient to restore the mucus layer [69]. These findings suggest that specific bacteria are crucial for normal mucus and barrier function and, in humans, this information could help us to understand important mechanisms underlying IBD pathogenesis.

Unveiling the association between diet and the development of IBD would ideally require knowledge on dietary details before the onset of the disease. In this regard, large longitudinal studies have been performed that have started to provide information to support specific dietary patterns as risk factors for IBD [17]. For instance, the metabolic activity of the microbiota may present important abnormalities in IBD. A reduced production of SCFAs, which are promoted by the presence of dietary fiber, has been shown in UC and CD. Particularly in patients with UC, a deficient production of SCFAs has been shown, and could not be corrected by increasing the intake of wheat bran-associated fiber and high amylose-associated-resistant starch [5,70].

Among the dietary factors potentially implicated in the development of IBD, dietary fiber has received special attention due to evidence showing associated protective mechanisms, including the conversion to SCFAs [71,72], interference in the structure of the gut microbiota [16], and maintenance of the barrier function [73]. However, a large prospective cohort study evaluating the impact of the intake of dietary fiber from several sources failed to identify any protective effect against the development of IBD [74].

Regarding the presumably harmful Western diet, in addition to its general composition characterized by high animal or dairy fat and animal protein, it is important to draw attention to the ubiquitous presence of emulsifiers, thickeners, and artificial sweeteners, many of which are associated with abnormal intestinal permeability, dysbiosis, and intestinal inflammation in animal models [75,76]. As an integral part of this type of diet, the common use of processed foods, usually rich in phosphate [77], but poor in micronutrients such zinc and other nutrients including omega-3 fatty acids, and vitamins D and E [78–80], may also be involved in the development or the predisposition to chronic intestinal inflammation.

5. Environmental Factors and IBD

The rise of IBD in the developing world has usually been attributed to the industrialization and urbanization of societies [11,81]. The observation of the coincident increase in immune-mediated and inflammatory diseases in the more developed and industrialized nations has long been associated with the hygiene hypothesis [82]. This hypothesis appears to be relatively reductionist, as it does not explain the dynamics of IBD evolution in long-modernized Asian countries, for example. Whereas improvements in sanitation and hygiene practices are usually related to the urban compared to the rural environment, several other concomitant factors affecting the rise of immune-mediated disorders need to be pondered. For example, areas with a higher prevalence of IBD also have fewer infections and are characterized by the widespread use of vaccines and antibiotics, in addition to the availability of clean food and water [83–85]. Other considerations associated with modern urban life in developed and developing nations include, for instance, population density, lifestyle modifications, level of education, and exposure to pollutants [86]. A positive association between ambient air pollution and IBD has been previously suggested [81], and the residential exposures to nitrogen dioxide and sulfur dioxide were shown to increase the risk of early-onset IBD [87].

The increased risk for developing IBD has also been associated with the exposure to different medications. Among them, the use of antibiotics has been shown to increase the risk of IBD, especially CD [88,89]. In a nested case-control analysis of the population-based database of prescription drugs, investigators found that patients diagnosed with IBD in childhood were more likely to have used antibiotics during the first year of life [90]. This positive association was further corroborated, for example, in a prospective study in which the use of antibiotics was strongly associated with the development of CD in childhood [91]. Although causality cannot be firmly established to date, exposure to antibiotics in childhood has been proposed to affect the normal development of tolerance to enteric bacteria, increasing the risk of IBD [92].

Other medications have been linked to IBD. For example, oral contraceptives have been shown to have a positive association with the development of IBD, in particular with CD [93]. In a case-control study, investigators found a positive association between nonsteroidal anti-inflammatory drugs (NSAIDs) and IBD [94]. In a cohort study, investigators found that the regular use of NSAIDs may increase CD activity [95]. However, a systematic review did not find a reliable association between the use of NSAIDs and risk of CD and UC exacerbation [96]. NSAIDs are capable of disrupting the intestinal epithelial barrier, and this may predispose the individual to the invasion of pathogens and may affect the intestinal homeostasis. The conflicting results regarding the association between NSAIDs and IBD may reflect different methodologies but also the participation of other uncontrolled environmental factors generating unanticipated and confounding effects.

Smoking is a well-established modifying factor in IBD, with opposing effects in CD and UC [97], but the mechanism by which it regulates intestinal inflammation is still unclear. The composition of cigarettes is heterogeneous and complex with several chemical elements that may affect different targets in the intestinal cells and modulate the microbiota [98,99]. Other evidence suggests that chemicals released from cigarette smoking can interfere with functions related to the immune response, such as the production of cytokines [100], and significantly impact the microbiota [101].

The functionality of vitamin D, an important regulator of mucosal immunity, is critically related to the exposure to sun with natural UV light [102]. Therefore, low sunlight exposure has been proposed to be a risk factor for the development of IBD, especially CD [103,104]. This is in line with the incidence and prevalence rates of IBD being greater in the Northern Hemisphere, where UV light is markedly lower [105]. However, the proposed association between IBD, particularly CD, and the northern latitudes should be interpreted not only in terms of geography, but in a wider context, where several other variables interact in a complex and dynamic concert, with largely unpredictable outcomes.

6. Epidemiological Associations between Diet and IBD

Although a consistent correlation between environmental factors and the pathogenesis of several disorders is usually difficult to prove due to the intervening effect of potentially confounding variables and the uncertain dynamics of exposures, associations between IBD and diet have been reported. The realization that the increase in the worldwide incidence of IBD and other immune-mediated diseases began in more developed and industrialized countries, particularly in North America and Northern Europe, has led investigators to hypothesize the global spread of a "Westernized" lifestyle [106–108].

The observation that the risk of developing IBD increases when people move from a low-risk to high-risk area appears to further support the role of environmental factors in the detriment of genetic predisposition, and reinforces the utility of studies examining immigration. For example, distinct investigations showed that immigrants to Israel had a higher prevalence of IBD than populations born in Israel [107,109]. Another population-based study demonstrated that in Sweden, a high incidence region, second-generation but not first-generation immigrants developed IBD at rates comparable to the native Swedish population. These results appear to underscore the importance of early-life exposures in determining disease initiation [110].

Epidemiological studies investigating the South Asian population indicate that the incidence and prevalence of adult IBD are significantly lower than in North America or the U.K. [111–114]. However, higher incidences of IBD in patients from South Asia have been reported in adult individuals who subsequently migrated to the U.K. [115], and in children migrating to British Columbia, Canada, at rates higher than in other ethnicities, including children of Western European descent [116]. In another similar study analyzing a migrant group to investigate the role of environmental factors in the development of IBD, Middle Eastern migrants to Australia had a significantly higher risk compared with the Caucasian population. The results, including the analysis of additional exposures such as smoking, antibiotic usage, and hygiene markers, suggested that migrants might be more sensitive to environmental challenges influencing the gut microbiome [117]. This thought is further supported by the results of a population-based study in the Asia-Pacific area in which the investigators suggested that early childhood factors and markers of altered intestinal microbiota may modulate the risk of IBD later in life [118].

Another study analyzing an Asian population combined a series of Chinese patients with IBD with the sequences from RISK and PRISM cohorts of IBD patients from the United States for a meta-analysis comparing gut microbiome profiles across ethnic groups. The investigators found that the gut dysbiosis observed in IBD is similar among Chinese and Western populations [119]. This may lead to the question of whether the gut microbiota provides universal biomarkers in IBD regardless of ethnicity. Results from another study suggest the existence of diverse gut microbial taxa with differential patterns of abundance common to various immune-mediated inflammatory diseases (IMIDs), including IBD [120]. These findings appear to corroborate the possible use of microbial taxa patterns as biomarkers for the detection and diagnosis of IBD, but also support the idea that the gut microbiota may constitute a common component of the etiology of IMIDs.

Several observational studies have attempted to characterize dietary patterns that could contribute to a higher risk of IBD development. These studies pointed to an increased risk of IBD among people consuming larger proportions of meat and fats, and a lower risk among people with diets rich in fiber, fruits, and vegetables [121,122]. However, as in other complex diseases, it may be difficult to interpret the role of individual risk factors, and an analysis of dietary patterns should consider exposures to groups of foods [5], distinct food components, and cultural habits, including specificities in food preparation.

7. Diet and Epigenetic Modifications in IBD

The epigenome, an intersection between the environment and the genome, has been implicated in the regulation of gene expression and cellular functions, and plays an essential role in the delineation of phenotypes and their preservation [21]. Novel information has contributed to an improved understanding of the role of epigenetic modifications in defining the molecular basis of IBD [123,124]. Regarding IBD, the first epigenetic modifications associated with disease pathogenesis were based on DNA methylation studies [125].

Currently, among the environmental factors, dietary factors were found to be powerful stimuli, being associated with peculiar patterns of gene expression and epigenetic signatures [126]. For instance, the diet supplies substrates for DNA methylation and can regulate the enzymatic activity required in the one-carbon cycle. Consequently, elements such as folate, choline, and water-soluble B vitamins have been implicated in methylation patterns [123,127], which are essential elements for the synthesis and repair of DNA that modulate gene expression [128]. Experimental evidence obtained also supports the idea that dietary nutraceuticals possess potential as epigenetic modulators. For example, data from studies involving DNA methylation and chromatin repair indicate that polyphenols can regulate gene expression [129]. Polyphenols are secondary plant metabolites, common components of vegetables, fruits, green tea, and red wine, and have been recognized for their antioxidant properties. In addition, studies have shown beneficial effects of polyphenols through the modulation of NF-κB expression, and chromatin remodeling via the modulation of histone deacetylases and DNA methyltransferase activities, reversing altered gene expression [130]. In experimental IBD, resveratrol, a natural phenolic compound, was shown to decrease inflammatory cytokines and profibrotic factors, supporting a potential therapeutic benefit [131].

Curcumin, another natural product commonly used in cooking, has been investigated in experimental models of IBD, demonstrating beneficial effects mediated by the suppression of proinflammatory mediators [132]. In a randomized, multicenter, double-blind, placebo-controlled trial, curcumin has shown beneficial results in maintenance therapy for patients with UC [133]. Although the exact mechanisms by which curcumin may exert a wide range of biological actions have not been established, effects have been attributed to the regulation of histone acetylation/deacetylation and the expression of various microRNAs [134].

Several nutrients have been shown to modulate immune responses, potentially counteracting inflammatory processes [135], in actions also mediated through epigenetic regulation [123,136]. Processed foods, deficient in micronutrients including selenium and folate, have been implicated in the progression of diseases, such as colorectal cancer and possibly IBD [21,137–139]. In an experimental model, a selenium-deficient diet was shown to result in markedly hypomethylated colon DNA [140]. Selenium supplementation was able to prevent tissue damage by modulating the expression of key genes responsible for inflammation in experimental IBD [141]. Although low levels of selenium have been detected in the serum of patients with IBD [142], studies in human IBD involving potential effects of selenium supplementation are still limited [21].

To investigate the mechanisms underlying the potential beneficial effects of the Mediterranean diet, an intervention with two different diets, one rich in nuts and the other one in extra-virgin olive oil, was conducted. The evaluation of the methylation status of peripheral white blood cells genes showed that both diets influenced methylation, characteristically of genes such as *CPT1B* and *GNAS* involved in intermediate metabolism, inflammation, and the signal transduction process. Therefore, the investigators concluded that the expected beneficial effects of the Mediterranean diet, supplemented with nuts or extra-virgin olive oil, could be mediated, at least in part, through epigenetic modifications [16,143,144].

In addition to the direct effects of dietary constituents on epigenetic modifications in human intestinal tissues, the resident microbiota has been shown to alter host histone acetylation and methylation. In this regard, particularly short-chain fatty acids such as acetate, butyrate, and propionate, mostly produced by the microbial fermentation of fiber, appear to play a critical role in the epigenetic control of the inflammatory response. In a diet poor in fiber, the inhibition of SCFA production was correlated with disturbed chromatin effects, which were restored following supplementation with SCFA [145]. In human IBD, SCFA-producing bacteria (*Roseburia*) and butyrate-producing bacteria (*Faecalibacterium*) are reduced [146]. However, the application of butyrate-producing bacteria as nutraceuticals in humans has been questioned and needs further investigation [123,147]. Figure 1 summarizes the potential interactions between diet and the microbiota and other environmental factors, resulting in epigenetic modifications, exemplifying the effects of different diets with their respective major characteristics.

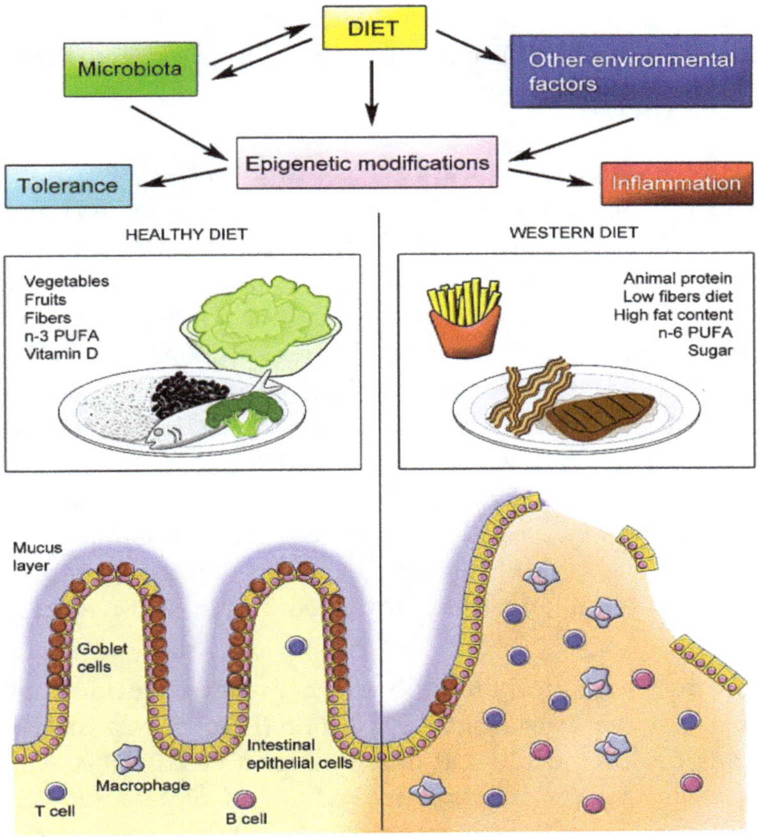

Figure 1. Schematic model of diet–host interactions in the intestine. The interaction between dietary elements and the intestinal mucosa is highly complex and, in normal conditions, results in a tolerogenic response. However, in genetically predisposed individuals, the interplay of specific dietary constituents with the resident microbiota and other environmental factors induces epigenetic modifications that affect the immune response, further compromising the epithelial barrier and defense mechanisms, leading to chronic inflammation, as observed in inflammatory bowel disease (IBD).

8. Clinical Effects of Dietary Factors

Clinical experience shows that patients usually associate their symptoms or disease relapses with the ingestion of certain foods and, as a result, they often change their diet empirically, with variable and, at most, temporary effects. In practice, decisions on dietary modifications usually do not follow professional nutritional advice and may have detrimental consequences [17,148–150]. In a prospective study investigating the dietary influence in the course of UC, researchers observed that a large ingestion of meat, more so of red and processed meat, in addition to ethanol, protein, sulfur, and sulfate, enhanced the chances of triggering a flare [151,152]. In the case of patients with CD, a diet rich in total fat, saturated fat, monounsaturated fatty acids, and a higher ratio of omega-6:omega-3 polyunsaturated fatty acids (PUFAs) was related to disease relapses [153,154]. Of note, the oral administration of iron sulfate or heme in dietary iron, which is present in meat, was shown to increase the severity of chemically-induced colitis in rodents [155,156]. However, although a substantial number of iron-deficient patients tolerate oral iron poorly, only a small percentage of patients with IBD have disease relapses attributed to oral iron [157]. Anemia is a common complication of IBD, mostly multifactorial, but frequently related to iron deficiency due to loss from bleeding and decreased iron absorption or ingestion [158]. Although many physicians have concerns regarding the management of iron deficiency in IBD, current data suggest that oral iron therapy should be preferred in mild cases or during clinical remission, unless patients are intolerant or have an inadequate response [159]. The aggravation of experimental colitis following dietary iron has been associated with a marked reduction in the fecal abundance of

Firmicutes and Bacteroidetes, and an increase in Proteobacteria [160]. Hence, poor outcomes following oral iron replacement in patients with IBD could be related to exacerbation of the intestinal dysbiosis.

9. Dietary Interventions in IBD

Simple dietary interventions usually improve gastrointestinal symptoms in patients with IBD, including a reduction in the ingestion of dairy products and also fermentable oligosaccharides, disaccharides, monosaccharides, and polyols (FODMAPS) [161]. More recent data have demonstrated the possible roles of specific dietary therapy in IBD. For example, dietary therapies, such as exclusive enteral nutrition (EEN), have been successfully used to induce remission in early or new-onset CD [162]. Theoretically, EEN involves the isolated use of medical formulas in a liquid form without exposure to other foods, usually for six to eight weeks [5]. This strategy is apparently more feasible in the pediatric population, in contrast to adults. Investigations have demonstrated that EEN may induce remission in more than 60% of children with CD followed by a significant reduction in inflammatory markers, including the erythrocyte sedimentation rate (ESR), C-reactive protein (CRP), and fecal calprotectin [5,163–165]. Grover et al. conducted a prospective open label study to assess mucosal healing before and after eight weeks of EEN, and concluded that the therapy is effective for inducing early clinical, biochemical, mucosal, and transmural remission, and was associated with improved outcomes at one year [166].

Given practical concerns and clinical limitations, other research groups have employed a different strategy based on the combination of partial enteral nutrition (PEN) with a specific exclusion diet granting access to whole foods. The diet was evaluated in a retrospective cohort of children and young adults with mild-to-moderate CD, and remission was achieved in 70% of patients. Clinical improvement was followed by the reduction in ESR and CRP and was associated with mucosal healing [167]. Afterward, this diet—low in animal fat, rich in complex carbohydrates, and with a moderate exposure to soluble fiber—was evaluated for the induction of remission in children and adults failing biologics. More than 60% of the patients achieved clinical remission, with a marked decrease in inflammatory markers [168].

Other important theoretical dietary elements, fiber, and prebiotics supplements have been evaluated as interventions in CD. However, a systematic review of randomized controlled trials found no evidence for the use of fiber or prebiotics to induce or maintain remission in CD [169]. No evidence for the restriction of fiber in the absence of obstructive symptoms or stricturing disease has been established for CD. In another study, a semi-vegetarian diet with considerable amounts of dietary fiber was shown to induce a high remission rate with no negative effects [170]. The same group investigated the effect of infliximab combined with a plant-based diet as first-line therapy for patients with CD naïve to biologics and found that the combined therapy can induce remission in most cases [171].

Although the most consistent studies regarding dietary interventions in IBD usually refer to CD, previous systematic evaluations performed by independent groups have supported the potential beneficial effects of diet in both CD and UC according to patients' perceptions [149,172]. In an observational prospective cohort study, patients with UC in clinical remission were followed for one year to investigate the effect of diet on disease relapse. The investigators identified an increased risk of UC relapses associated with the consumption of meat (particularly red and processed meat), eggs, and alcoholic beverages, which have been attributed to the high dietary content of sulfur [151]. In addition to red meat and eggs, milk and dairy products contain high concentrations of cysteine, which can be used by sulfate-reducing bacteria (SRB) to produce hydrogen sulfide (H_2S) [173,174]. H_2S, in turn, has been shown to induce proinflammatory effects in the colon and intestinal epithelial cells [175–177]. Some studies have demonstrated the increased presence of SRB and H_2S production in the colon of patients with UC [178–180]. However, despite all evidence suggesting a link between sulfur or sulfate-containing foods and UC, current data do not allow a causal association. While more controlled studies regarding SRB and H_2S in UC are awaited, patients should be aware of the potential detrimental effects of high-sulfur-containing dietary products.

The nutritional theories of IBD pathogenesis involving carbohydrates, for example, have been based on the increasing evidence of the beneficial effects of the Specific Carbohydrate Diet in the treatment of both CD and UC, resulting in improvement in clinical parameters and inflammatory biomarkers [181–183]. The hypothesis that carbohydrate variation increases the predisposition to IBD has been supported by the evidence of resultant immune dysfunction, mucosal barrier defects, and dysbiosis, which are represented by the Westernized dietary features [1,184,185]. Carbohydrate monotony could be beneficial in IBD [186]. This has been corroborated by a successful report using the Paleo diet for a small cohort of patients with IBD [187]. Paleo is also an exclusion diet, supposedly representing habits of the Paleolithic era, consisting of a non-cereal, plant-based diet, including non-domesticated meats, and a low intake of carbohydrates, which are taken from a monotonous source. The rational for the use of carbohydrate monotony derives from the usually lower prevalence of IBD in rural or less developed communities consuming locally-produced seasonal products [16], in contrast to the modern Westernized diet, for which the digestive tract would theoretically not have had time to adapt [188].

In terms of dietary supplements, vitamin D appears to have a role in IBD. Vitamin D3 (animal sources and skin exposure to ultraviolet light) and vitamin D2 (plant sources) are first hydroxylated in the liver, and then in the kidney and extrarenal tissues, including intestinal macrophages, into the active form 1,25-dihydroxyvitamin D. The active vitamin D binds to its specific receptor in different tissues, including immune cells, modulating gene expression. Vitamin D deficiency has been frequently seen in patients with IBD; therefore, it has been regarded as a protective factor against disease development [189,190]. Particularly in patients with CD, vitamin D deficiency has been consistently associated with disease activity [79,191,192]. Vitamin D3 supplementation for patients with CD has been suggested to alleviate clinical manifestations [193]. In another clinical investigation, a randomized double-blind placebo-controlled study, dietary supplementation with 1200 IU vitamin D3 daily for 12 months significantly increased the vitamin D levels, but only modestly reduced the risk of disease relapse [194].

Currently, the exact mechanisms by which vitamin D may reduce the severity of CD are still unclear. In a study using peripheral blood mononuclear cells, investigators found that vitamin D was able to reduce the expression of pro-inflammatory M1 cytokines but did not induce the anti-inflammatory M2 phenotype [195]. In other experimental studies, vitamin D deficiency, or even its impaired signaling, were shown to worsen different models of experimental colitis through multiple effects, including epithelial barrier disruption [196,197], reduced mucosal immunity [198], and an association with gut dysbiosis [199,200].

10. Future Directions

Among the environmental changes associated with the progressive and global expansion of IBD, diet has emerged as an essential regulatory element of the gut microbiome, which in turn has been strongly associated with the pathogenesis of several complex chronic inflammatory and autoimmune disorders. In addition to the involvement in dysbiosis, dietary components have been shown to interfere in intestinal homeostasis, modulating the barrier function and innate immunity mechanisms. Therefore, the accumulated scientific evidence appears to position diet as a central element both in disease pathogenesis as a critical risk factor and also as a potential opportunity for therapeutic interventions. Currently, several clinical trials are being conducted in different institutions and, hopefully, novel approaches to dietary therapy will be available in the near future.

Considering the progressive burden due to IBD anticipated in the next decades, dietary interventions appear particularly interesting, presumably due to the expected irrelevant side effects, lower costs, and potential application in the prevention of disease initiation or relapses. For the moment, however, the simplest approach includes the avoidance of foods that patients self-identify as worsening their symptoms, in addition to high-fat, high-carbohydrate meals and processed foods. Notably, dietary measures should be considered within the wider context of the patient's routine, not only in terms of food quality, but also changes in lifestyle, including dietary habits. For this purpose, while the results of large prospective controlled studies are awaited to provide more specific dietary guidance to patients, it is important to reinforce the role of multidisciplinary teams, including nutritionists, for offering better attention to and individualized support for patients with IBD.

Author Contributions: F.C. participated in the investigation and writing—original draft preparation; H.S.P.d.S. participated in the conceptualization, investigation, data curation, writing—review and editing, supervision, and funding acquisition.

Acknowledgments: This research was funded by Brazilian Research Council (CNPq), grant number 302401/2016-4, and FAPERJ (Fundação Carlos Chagas Filho de Amparo a Pesquisa do Estado do Rio de Janeiro), grant number E26/202.781/2017. The APC was funded by Fundação CAPES/PROEX, grant number 8882.331795/2010-01. We thank Claudio Bernardazzi for his assistance with the figure.

References

1. de Souza, H.S.; Fiocchi, C. Immunopathogenesis of ibd: Current state of the art. *Nat. Rev. Gastroenterol. Hepatol.* **2016**, *13*, 13–27. [CrossRef]
2. Siebert, U.; Wurm, J.; Gothe, R.M.; Arvandi, M.; Vavricka, S.R.; von Kanel, R.; Begre, S.; Sulz, M.C.; Meyenberger, C.; Sagmeister, M. Swiss IBDCSG: Predictors of temporary and permanent work disability in patients with inflammatory bowel disease: Results of the swiss inflammatory bowel disease cohort study. *Inflamm. Bowel Dis.* **2013**, *19*, 847–855. [CrossRef]
3. Knights, D.; Lassen, K.G.; Xavier, R.J. Advances in inflammatory bowel disease pathogenesis: Linking host genetics and the microbiome. *Gut* **2013**, *62*, 1505–1510. [CrossRef]
4. de Souza, H.S.P.; Fiocchi, C.; Iliopoulos, D. The ibd interactome: An integrated view of aetiology, pathogenesis and therapy. *Nat. Rev. Gastroenterol. Hepatol.* **2017**, *14*, 739–749. [CrossRef]
5. Levine, A.; Sigall Boneh, R.; Wine, E. Evolving role of diet in the pathogenesis and treatment of inflammatory bowel diseases. *Gut* **2018**, *67*, 1726–1738. [CrossRef]
6. Uniken Venema, W.T.; Voskuil, M.D.; Dijkstra, G.; Weersma, R.K.; Festen, E.A. The genetic background of inflammatory bowel disease: From correlation to causality. *J. Pathol.* **2017**, *241*, 146–158. [CrossRef]
7. Rook, G.A. Hygiene hypothesis and autoimmune diseases. *Clin. Rev. Allergy Immunol.* **2012**, *42*, 5–15. [CrossRef]
8. Park, S.J.; Kim, W.H.; Cheon, J.H. Clinical characteristics and treatment of inflammatory bowel disease: A comparison of eastern and western perspectives. *World J. Gastroenterol.* **2014**, *20*, 11525–11537. [CrossRef]
9. Ng, S.C.; Tang, W.; Ching, J.Y.; Wong, M.; Chow, C.M.; Hui, A.J.; Wong, T.C.; Leung, V.K.; Tsang, S.W.; Yu, H.H.; et al. Incidence and phenotype of inflammatory bowel disease based on results from the Asia-pacific Crohn's and colitis epidemiology study. *Gastroenterology* **2013**, *145*, 158–165. [CrossRef]
10. Kaplan, G.G. The global burden of ibd: From 2015 to 2025. *Nat. Rev. Gastroenterol. Hepatol.* **2015**, *12*, 720–727. [CrossRef]
11. Bernstein, C.N. Review article: Changes in the epidemiology of inflammatory bowel disease-clues for aetiology. *Aliment. Pharmacol. Ther.* **2017**, *46*, 911–919. [CrossRef]
12. Marion-Letellier, R.; Savoye, G.; Ghosh, S. Ibd: In food we trust. *J. Crohn's Colitis* **2016**, *10*, 1351–1361. [CrossRef]
13. Duffy, L.C.; Raiten, D.J.; Hubbard, V.S.; Starke-Reed, P. Progress and challenges in developing metabolic footprints from diet in human gut microbial cometabolism. *J. Nutr.* **2015**, *145*, 1123S–1130S. [CrossRef]
14. Clemente, J.C.; Ursell, L.K.; Parfrey, L.W.; Knight, R. The impact of the gut microbiota on human health: An integrative view. *Cell* **2012**, *148*, 1258–1270. [CrossRef]
15. Ley, R.E.; Hamady, M.; Lozupone, C.; Turnbaugh, P.J.; Ramey, R.R.; Bircher, J.S.; Schlegel, M.L.; Tucker, T.A.; Schrenzel, M.D.; Knight, R.; et al. Evolution of mammals and their gut microbes. *Science* **2008**, *320*, 1647–1651. [CrossRef]
16. De Filippo, C.; Cavalieri, D.; Di Paola, M.; Ramazzotti, M.; Poullet, J.B.; Massart, S.; Collini, S.; Pieraccini, G.; Lionetti, P. Impact of diet in shaping gut microbiota revealed by a comparative study in children from Europe and rural Africa. *Proc. Natl. Acad. Sci. USA* **2010**, *107*, 14691–14696. [CrossRef]
17. Lewis, J.D.; Abreu, M.T. Diet as a trigger or therapy for inflammatory bowel diseases. *Gastroenterology* **2017**, *152*, 398–414.e6. [CrossRef]
18. Calder, P.C. Polyunsaturated fatty acids and inflammation. *Biochem. Soc. Trans.* **2005**, *33*, 423–427. [CrossRef]

19. Yatsunenko, T.; Rey, F.E.; Manary, M.J.; Trehan, I.; Dominguez-Bello, M.G.; Contreras, M.; Magris, M.; Hidalgo, G.; Baldassano, R.N.; Anokhin, A.P.; et al. Human gut microbiome viewed across age and geography. *Nature* **2012**, *486*, 222–227. [CrossRef]
20. Barcenilla, A.; Pryde, S.E.; Martin, J.C.; Duncan, S.H.; Stewart, C.S.; Henderson, C.; Flint, H.J. Phylogenetic relationships of butyrate-producing bacteria from the human gut. *Appl. Environ. Microbiol.* **2000**, *66*, 1654–1661. [CrossRef]
21. Rapozo, D.C.; Bernardazzi, C.; de Souza, H.S. Diet and microbiota in inflammatory bowel disease: The gut in disharmony. *World J. Gastroenterol.* **2017**, *23*, 2124–2140. [CrossRef]
22. Man, S.M.; Kaakoush, N.O.; Mitchell, H.M. The role of bacteria and pattern-recognition receptors in Crohn's disease. *Nat. Rev. Gastroenterol. Hepatol.* **2011**, *8*, 152–168. [CrossRef]
23. Takahashi, K.; Nishida, A.; Fujimoto, T.; Fujii, M.; Shioya, M.; Imaeda, H.; Inatomi, O.; Bamba, S.; Sugimoto, M.; Andoh, A. Reduced abundance of butyrate-producing bacteria species in the fecal microbial community in Crohn's disease. *Digestion* **2016**, *93*, 59–65. [CrossRef]
24. Zhu, B.; Wang, X.; Li, L. Human gut microbiome: The second genome of human body. *Protein Cell* **2010**, *1*, 718–725. [CrossRef]
25. Harris, R.A.; Shah, R.; Hollister, E.B.; Tronstad, R.R.; Hovdenak, N.; Szigeti, R.; Versalovic, J.; Kellermayer, R. Colonic mucosal epigenome and microbiome development in children and adolescents. *J. Immunol. Res.* **2016**, *2016*, 9170162. [CrossRef]
26. Guslandi, M. Role of probiotics in Crohn's disease and in pouchitis. *J. Clin. Gastroenterol.* **2015**, *49* (Suppl. 1), S46–S49. [CrossRef]
27. David, L.A.; Maurice, C.F.; Carmody, R.N.; Gootenberg, D.B.; Button, J.E.; Wolfe, B.E.; Ling, A.V.; Devlin, A.S.; Varma, Y.; Fischbach, M.A.; et al. Diet rapidly and reproducibly alters the human gut microbiome. *Nature* **2014**, *505*, 559–563. [CrossRef]
28. Sokol, H. Probiotics and antibiotics in ibd. *Dig. Dis.* **2014**, *32* (Suppl. 1), 10–17. [CrossRef]
29. Ishikawa, H.; Akedo, I.; Umesaki, Y.; Tanaka, R.; Imaoka, A.; Otani, T. Randomized controlled trial of the effect of bifidobacteria-fermented milk on ulcerative colitis. *J. Am. Coll. Nutr.* **2003**, *22*, 56–63. [CrossRef]
30. Gevers, D.; Kugathasan, S.; Denson, L.A.; Vazquez-Baeza, Y.; Van Treuren, W.; Ren, B.; Schwager, E.; Knights, D.; Song, S.J.; Yassour, M.; et al. The treatment-naive microbiome in new-onset Crohn's disease. *Cell Host Microbe* **2014**, *15*, 382–392. [CrossRef]
31. Forsyth, C.B.; Shaikh, M.; Bishehsari, F.; Swanson, G.; Voigt, R.M.; Dodiya, H.; Wilkinson, P.; Samelco, B.; Song, S.; Keshavarzian, A. Alcohol feeding in mice promotes colonic hyperpermeability and changes in colonic organoid stem cell fate. *Alcohol. Clin. Exp. Res.* **2017**, *41*, 2100–2113. [CrossRef]
32. Cani, P.D.; Bibiloni, R.; Knauf, C.; Waget, A.; Neyrinck, A.M.; Delzenne, N.M.; Burcelin, R. Changes in gut microbiota control metabolic endotoxemia-induced inflammation in high-fat diet-induced obesity and diabetes in mice. *Diabetes* **2008**, *57*, 1470–1481. [CrossRef]
33. Turnbaugh, P.J.; Ley, R.E.; Mahowald, M.A.; Magrini, V.; Mardis, E.R.; Gordon, J.I. An obesity-associated gut microbiome with increased capacity for energy harvest. *Nature* **2006**, *444*, 1027–1031. [CrossRef]
34. Cox, A.J.; West, N.P.; Cripps, A.W. Obesity, inflammation, and the gut microbiota. *Lancet Diabetes Endocrinol.* **2015**, *3*, 207–215. [CrossRef]
35. Frank, D.N.; Robertson, C.E.; Hamm, C.M.; Kpadeh, Z.; Zhang, T.; Chen, H.; Zhu, W.; Sartor, R.B.; Boedeker, E.C.; Harpaz, N.; et al. Disease phenotype and genotype are associated with shifts in intestinal-associated microbiota in inflammatory bowel diseases. *Inflamm. Bowel Dis.* **2011**, *17*, 179–184. [CrossRef]
36. Maeda, Y.; Kurakawa, T.; Umemoto, E.; Motooka, D.; Ito, Y.; Gotoh, K.; Hirota, K.; Matsushita, M.; Furuta, Y.; Narazaki, M.; et al. Dysbiosis contributes to arthritis development via activation of autoreactive t cells in the intestine. *Arthr. Rheumatol.* **2016**, *68*, 2646–2661. [CrossRef]
37. Ott, S.J.; Musfeldt, M.; Wenderoth, D.F.; Hampe, J.; Brant, O.; Folsch, U.R.; Timmis, K.N.; Schreiber, S. Reduction in diversity of the colonic mucosa associated bacterial microflora in patients with active inflammatory bowel disease. *Gut* **2004**, *53*, 685–693. [CrossRef]
38. Wang, H.; Shi, P.; Zuo, L.; Dong, J.; Zhao, J.; Liu, Q.; Zhu, W. Dietary non-digestible polysaccharides ameliorate intestinal epithelial barrier dysfunction in il-10 knockout mice. *J. Crohn's Colitis* **2016**, *10*, 1076–1086. [CrossRef]

39. Furusawa, Y.; Obata, Y.; Fukuda, S.; Endo, T.A.; Nakato, G.; Takahashi, D.; Nakanishi, Y.; Uetake, C.; Kato, K.; Kato, T.; et al. Commensal microbe-derived butyrate induces the differentiation of colonic regulatory t cells. *Nature* **2013**, *504*, 446–450. [CrossRef]
40. Desai, M.S.; Seekatz, A.M.; Koropatkin, N.M.; Kamada, N.; Hickey, C.A.; Wolter, M.; Pudlo, N.A.; Kitamoto, S.; Terrapon, N.; Muller, A.; et al. A dietary fiber-deprived gut microbiota degrades the colonic mucus barrier and enhances pathogen susceptibility. *Cell* **2016**, *167*, 1339–1353.e21. [CrossRef]
41. Agus, A.; Denizot, J.; Thevenot, J.; Martinez-Medina, M.; Massier, S.; Sauvanet, P.; Bernalier-Donadille, A.; Denis, S.; Hofman, P.; Bonnet, R.; et al. Western diet induces a shift in microbiota composition enhancing susceptibility to adherent-invasive *E. coli* infection and intestinal inflammation. *Sci. Rep.* **2016**, *6*, 19032. [CrossRef]
42. Ma, X.; Torbenson, M.; Hamad, A.R.; Soloski, M.J.; Li, Z. High-fat diet modulates non-cd1d-restricted natural killer t cells and regulatory t cells in mouse colon and exacerbates experimental colitis. *Clin. Exp. Immunol.* **2008**, *151*, 130–138. [CrossRef]
43. Kim, K.A.; Gu, W.; Lee, I.A.; Joh, E.H.; Kim, D.H. High fat diet-induced gut microbiota exacerbates inflammation and obesity in mice via the tlr4 signaling pathway. *PLoS ONE* **2012**, *7*, e47713. [CrossRef]
44. Liu, Z.; Brooks, R.S.; Ciappio, E.D.; Kim, S.J.; Crott, J.W.; Bennett, G.; Greenberg, A.S.; Mason, J.B. Diet-induced obesity elevates colonic tnf-alpha in mice and is accompanied by an activation of wnt signaling: A mechanism for obesity-associated colorectal cancer. *J. Nutr. Biochem.* **2012**, *23*, 1207–1213. [CrossRef]
45. Progatzky, F.; Sangha, N.J.; Yoshida, N.; McBrien, M.; Cheung, J.; Shia, A.; Scott, J.; Marchesi, J.R.; Lamb, J.R.; Bugeon, L.; et al. Dietary cholesterol directly induces acute inflammasome-dependent intestinal inflammation. *Nat. Commun.* **2014**, *5*, 5864. [CrossRef]
46. Joossens, M.; Huys, G.; Cnockaert, M.; De Preter, V.; Verbeke, K.; Rutgeerts, P.; Vandamme, P.; Vermeire, S. Dysbiosis of the faecal microbiota in patients with Crohn's disease and their unaffected relatives. *Gut* **2011**, *60*, 631–637. [CrossRef]
47. Varela, E.; Manichanh, C.; Gallart, M.; Torrejon, A.; Borruel, N.; Casellas, F.; Guarner, F.; Antolin, M. Colonisation by *Faecalibacterium prausnitzii* and maintenance of clinical remission in patients with ulcerative colitis. *Aliment. Pharmacol. Ther.* **2013**, *38*, 151–161. [CrossRef]
48. Wright, E.K.; Kamm, M.A.; Teo, S.M.; Inouye, M.; Wagner, J.; Kirkwood, C.D. Recent advances in characterizing the gastrointestinal microbiome in Crohn's disease: A systematic review. *Inflamm. Bowel Dis.* **2015**, *21*, 1219–1228.
49. Sokol, H.; Leducq, V.; Aschard, H.; Pham, H.P.; Jegou, S.; Landman, C.; Cohen, D.; Liguori, G.; Bourrier, A.; Nion-Larmurier, I.; et al. Fungal microbiota dysbiosis in ibd. *Gut* **2017**, *66*, 1039–1048. [CrossRef]
50. Pascal, V.; Pozuelo, M.; Borruel, N.; Casellas, F.; Campos, D.; Santiago, A.; Martinez, X.; Varela, E.; Sarrabayrouse, G.; Machiels, K.; et al. A microbial signature for Crohn's disease. *Gut* **2017**, *66*, 813–822. [CrossRef]
51. Powell, N.; MacDonald, T.T. Recent advances in gut immunology. *Parasite Immunol.* **2017**, *39*. [CrossRef]
52. Atarashi, K.; Tanoue, T.; Oshima, K.; Suda, W.; Nagano, Y.; Nishikawa, H.; Fukuda, S.; Saito, T.; Narushima, S.; Hase, K.; et al. Treg induction by a rationally selected mixture of clostridia strains from the human microbiota. *Nature* **2013**, *500*, 232–236. [CrossRef]
53. Sefik, E.; Geva-Zatorsky, N.; Oh, S.; Konnikova, L.; Zemmour, D.; McGuire, A.M.; Burzyn, D.; Ortiz-Lopez, A.; Lobera, M.; Yang, J.; et al. Mucosal immunology. Individual intestinal symbionts induce a distinct population of rorgamma(+) regulatory t cells. *Science* **2015**, *349*, 993–997. [CrossRef]
54. Atarashi, K.; Tanoue, T.; Ando, M.; Kamada, N.; Nagano, Y.; Narushima, S.; Suda, W.; Imaoka, A.; Setoyama, H.; Nagamori, T.; et al. Th17 cell induction by adhesion of microbes to intestinal epithelial cells. *Cell* **2015**, *163*, 367–380. [CrossRef]
55. Tan, T.G.; Sefik, E.; Geva-Zatorsky, N.; Kua, L.; Naskar, D.; Teng, F.; Pasman, L.; Ortiz-Lopez, A.; Jupp, R.; Wu, H.J.; et al. Identifying species of symbiont bacteria from the human gut that, alone, can induce intestinal th17 cells in mice. *Proc. Natl. Acad. Sci. USA* **2016**, *113*, E8141–E8150. [CrossRef]
56. Viladomiu, M.; Kivolowitz, C.; Abdulhamid, A.; Dogan, B.; Victorio, D.; Castellanos, J.G.; Woo, V.; Teng, F.; Tran, N.L.; Sczesnak, A.; et al. Iga-coated *E. coli* enriched in Crohn's disease spondyloarthritis promote th17-dependent inflammation. *Sci. Transl. Med.* **2017**, *9*, eaaf9655. [CrossRef]

57. Ivanov, I.I.; Atarashi, K.; Manel, N.; Brodie, E.L.; Shima, T.; Karaoz, U.; Wei, D.; Goldfarb, K.C.; Santee, C.A.; Lynch, S.V.; et al. Induction of intestinal th17 cells by segmented filamentous bacteria. *Cell* **2009**, *139*, 485–498. [CrossRef]
58. Statovci, D.; Aguilera, M.; MacSharry, J.; Melgar, S. The impact of western diet and nutrients on the microbiota and immune response at mucosal interfaces. *Front. Immunol.* **2017**, *8*, 838. [CrossRef]
59. Martinez-Medina, M.; Denizot, J.; Dreux, N.; Robin, F.; Billard, E.; Bonnet, R.; Darfeuille-Michaud, A.; Barnich, N. Western diet induces dysbiosis with increased e coli in ceabac10 mice, alters host barrier function favouring AIEC colonisation. *Gut* **2014**, *63*, 116–124. [CrossRef]
60. Tilg, H.; Moschen, A.R. Food, immunity, and the microbiome. *Gastroenterology* **2015**, *148*, 1107–1119. [CrossRef]
61. Devkota, S.; Wang, Y.; Musch, M.W.; Leone, V.; Fehlner-Peach, H.; Nadimpalli, A.; Antonopoulos, D.A.; Jabri, B.; Chang, E.B. Dietary-fat-induced taurocholic acid promotes pathobiont expansion and colitis in il10-/- mice. *Nature* **2012**, *487*, 104–108. [CrossRef]
62. Silveira, A.L.M.; Ferreira, A.V.M.; de Oliveira, M.C.; Rachid, M.A.; da Cunha Sousa, L.F.; Dos Santos Martins, F.; Gomes-Santos, A.C.; Vieira, A.T.; Teixeira, M.M. Preventive rather than therapeutic treatment with high fiber diet attenuates clinical and inflammatory markers of acute and chronic dss-induced colitis in mice. *Eur. J. Nutr.* **2017**, *56*, 179–191. [CrossRef]
63. Nickerson, K.P.; McDonald, C. Crohn's disease-associated adherent-invasive escherichia coli adhesion is enhanced by exposure to the ubiquitous dietary polysaccharide maltodextrin. *PLoS ONE* **2012**, *7*, e52132. [CrossRef]
64. Nickerson, K.P.; Chanin, R.; McDonald, C. Deregulation of intestinal anti-microbial defense by the dietary additive, maltodextrin. *Gut Microbes* **2015**, *6*, 78–83. [CrossRef]
65. Hold, G.L.; Smith, M.; Grange, C.; Watt, E.R.; El-Omar, E.M.; Mukhopadhya, I. Role of the gut microbiota in inflammatory bowel disease pathogenesis: What have we learnt in the past 10 years? *World J. Gastroenterol.* **2014**, *20*, 1192–1210. [CrossRef]
66. Colombel, J.F. Decade in review-ibd: Ibd-genes, bacteria and new therapeutic strategies. *Nat. Rev. Gastroenterol. Hepatol.* **2014**, *11*, 652–654. [CrossRef]
67. Zhernakova, A.; Kurilshikov, A.; Bonder, M.J.; Tigchelaar, E.F.; Schirmer, M.; Vatanen, T.; Mujagic, Z.; Vila, A.V.; Falony, G.; Vieira-Silva, S.; et al. Population-based metagenomics analysis reveals markers for gut microbiome composition and diversity. *Science* **2016**, *352*, 565–569. [CrossRef]
68. Figliuolo, V.R.; Dos Santos, L.M.; Abalo, A.; Nanini, H.; Santos, A.; Brittes, N.M.; Bernardazzi, C.; de Souza, H.S.P.; Vieira, L.Q.; Coutinho-Silva, R.; et al. Sulfate-reducing bacteria stimulate gut immune responses and contribute to inflammation in experimental colitis. *Life Sci.* **2017**, *189*, 29–38. [CrossRef]
69. Schroeder, B.O.; Birchenough, G.M.H.; Stahlman, M.; Arike, L.; Johansson, M.E.V.; Hansson, G.C.; Backhed, F. Bifidobacteria or fiber protects against diet-induced microbiota-mediated colonic mucus deterioration. *Cell Host Microbe* **2018**, *23*, 27–40.e7. [CrossRef]
70. James, S.L.; Christophersen, C.T.; Bird, A.R.; Conlon, M.A.; Rosella, O.; Gibson, P.R.; Muir, J.G. Abnormal fibre usage in uc in remission. *Gut* **2015**, *64*, 562–570. [CrossRef]
71. Vinolo, M.A.; Rodrigues, H.G.; Nachbar, R.T.; Curi, R. Regulation of inflammation by short chain fatty acids. *Nutrients* **2011**, *3*, 858–876. [CrossRef]
72. Hartog, A.; Belle, F.N.; Bastiaans, J.; de Graaff, P.; Garssen, J.; Harthoorn, L.F.; Vos, A.P. A potential role for regulatory t-cells in the amelioration of dss induced colitis by dietary non-digestible polysaccharides. *J. Nutr. Biochem.* **2015**, *26*, 227–233. [CrossRef]
73. Roberts, C.L.; Keita, A.V.; Duncan, S.H.; O'Kennedy, N.; Soderholm, J.D.; Rhodes, J.M.; Campbell, B.J. Translocation of Crohn's disease escherichia coli across m-cells: Contrasting effects of soluble plant fibres and emulsifiers. *Gut* **2010**, *59*, 1331–1339. [CrossRef]
74. Andersen, V.; Chan, S.; Luben, R.; Khaw, K.T.; Olsen, A.; Tjonneland, A.; Kaaks, R.; Grip, O.; Bergmann, M.M.; Boeing, H.; et al. Fibre intake and the development of inflammatory bowel disease: A european prospective multi-centre cohort study (epic-ibd). *J. Crohn's Colitis* **2018**, *12*, 129–136. [CrossRef]
75. Chassaing, B.; Koren, O.; Goodrich, J.K.; Poole, A.C.; Srinivasan, S.; Ley, R.E.; Gewirtz, A.T. Dietary emulsifiers impact the mouse gut microbiota promoting colitis and metabolic syndrome. *Nature* **2015**, *519*, 92–96. [CrossRef]

76. Chassaing, B.; Van de Wiele, T.; De Bodt, J.; Marzorati, M.; Gewirtz, A.T. Dietary emulsifiers directly alter human microbiota composition and gene expression ex vivo potentiating intestinal inflammation. *Gut* **2017**, *66*, 1414–1427. [CrossRef]
77. Khalili, H.; Malik, S.; Ananthakrishnan, A.N.; Garber, J.J.; Higuchi, L.M.; Joshi, A.; Peloquin, J.; Richter, J.M.; Stewart, K.O.; Curhan, G.C.; et al. Identification and characterization of a novel association between dietary potassium and risk of Crohn's disease and ulcerative colitis. *Front. Immunol.* **2016**, *7*, 554. [CrossRef]
78. Mayneris-Perxachs, J.; Bolick, D.T.; Leng, J.; Medlock, G.L.; Kolling, G.L.; Papin, J.A.; Swann, J.R.; Guerrant, R.L. Protein- and zinc-deficient diets modulate the murine microbiome and metabolic phenotype. *Am. J. Clin. Nutr.* **2016**, *104*, 1253–1262. [CrossRef]
79. Del Pinto, R.; Pietropaoli, D.; Chandar, A.K.; Ferri, C.; Cominelli, F. Association between inflammatory bowel disease and vitamin d deficiency: A systematic review and meta-analysis. *Inflamm. Bowel Dis.* **2015**, *21*, 2708–2717. [CrossRef]
80. de Bruyn, J.R.; van Heeckeren, R.; Ponsioen, C.Y.; van den Brink, G.R.; Lowenberg, M.; Bredenoord, A.J.; Frijstein, G.; D'Haens, G.R. Vitamin d deficiency in Crohn's disease and healthy controls: A prospective case-control study in the netherlands. *J. Crohn's Colitis* **2014**, *8*, 1267–1273. [CrossRef]
81. Maaser, C.; Langholz, E.; Gordon, H.; Burisch, J.; Ellul, P.; Ramirez, V.H.; Karakan, T.; Katsanos, K.H.; Krustins, E.; Levine, A.; et al. European Crohn's and colitis organisation topical review on environmental factors in ibd. *J. Crohn's Colitis* **2017**, *11*, 905–920. [CrossRef]
82. Strachan, D.P. Hay fever, hygiene, and household size. *BMJ* **1989**, *299*, 1259–1260. [CrossRef]
83. Yazdanbakhsh, M.; Matricardi, P.M. Parasites and the hygiene hypothesis: Regulating the immune system? *Clin. Rev. Allergy Immunol.* **2004**, *26*, 15–24. [CrossRef]
84. Feillet, H.; Bach, J.F. Increased incidence of inflammatory bowel disease: The price of the decline of infectious burden? *Curr. Opin. Gastroenterol.* **2004**, *20*, 560–564. [CrossRef]
85. Foster, A.; Jacobson, K. Changing incidence of inflammatory bowel disease: Environmental influences and lessons learnt from the south Asian population. *Front. Pediatr.* **2013**, *1*, 34. [CrossRef]
86. Ponder, A.; Long, M.D. A clinical review of recent findings in the epidemiology of inflammatory bowel disease. *Clin. Epidemiol.* **2013**, *5*, 237–247.
87. Kaplan, G.G.; Hubbard, J.; Korzenik, J.; Sands, B.E.; Panaccione, R.; Ghosh, S.; Wheeler, A.J.; Villeneuve, P.J. The inflammatory bowel diseases and ambient air pollution: A novel association. *Am. J. Gastroenterol.* **2010**, *105*, 2412–2419. [CrossRef]
88. Ungaro, R.; Bernstein, C.N.; Gearry, R.; Hviid, A.; Kolho, K.L.; Kronman, M.P.; Shaw, S.; Van Kruiningen, H.; Colombel, J.F.; Atreja, A. Antibiotics associated with increased risk of new-onset Crohn's disease but not ulcerative colitis: A meta-analysis. *Am. J. Gastroenterol.* **2014**, *109*, 1728–1738. [CrossRef]
89. Aniwan, S.; Tremaine, W.J.; Raffals, L.E.; Kane, S.V.; Loftus, E.V., Jr. Antibiotic use and new-onset inflammatory bowel disease in Olmsted county, Minnesota: A population-based case-control study. *J. Crohn's Colitis* **2018**, *12*, 137–144. [CrossRef]
90. Shaw, S.Y.; Blanchard, J.F.; Bernstein, C.N. Association between the use of antibiotics in the first year of life and pediatric inflammatory bowel disease. *Am. J. Gastroenterol.* **2010**, *105*, 2687–2692. [CrossRef]
91. Hviid, A.; Svanstrom, H.; Frisch, M. Antibiotic use and inflammatory bowel diseases in childhood. *Gut* **2011**, *60*, 49–54. [CrossRef]
92. Hildebrand, H.; Malmborg, P.; Askling, J.; Ekbom, A.; Montgomery, S.M. Early-life exposures associated with antibiotic use and risk of subsequent Crohn's disease. *Scand. J. Gastroenterol.* **2008**, *43*, 961–966. [CrossRef]
93. Cornish, J.A.; Tan, E.; Simillis, C.; Clark, S.K.; Teare, J.; Tekkis, P.P. The risk of oral contraceptives in the etiology of inflammatory bowel disease: A meta-analysis. *Am. J. Gastroenterol.* **2008**, *103*, 2394–2400. [CrossRef]
94. Felder, J.B.; Korelitz, B.I.; Rajapakse, R.; Schwarz, S.; Horatagis, A.P.; Gleim, G. Effects of nonsteroidal antiinflammatory drugs on inflammatory bowel disease: A case-control study. *Am. J. Gastroenterol.* **2000**, *95*, 1949–1954. [CrossRef]
95. Long, M.D.; Kappelman, M.D.; Martin, C.F.; Chen, W.; Anton, K.; Sandler, R.S. Role of nonsteroidal anti-inflammatory drugs in exacerbations of inflammatory bowel disease. *J. Clin. Gastroenterol.* **2016**, *50*, 152–156. [CrossRef]
96. Moninuola, O.O.; Milligan, W.; Lochhead, P.; Khalili, H. Systematic review with meta-analysis: Association

between acetaminophen and nonsteroidal anti-inflammatory drugs (nsaids) and risk of Crohn's disease and ulcerative colitis exacerbation. *Aliment. Pharmacol. Ther.* **2018**, *47*, 1428–1439. [CrossRef]

97. Cosnes, J. Tobacco and ibd: Relevance in the understanding of disease mechanisms and clinical practice. *Best Pract. Res. Clin. Gastroenterol.* **2004**, *18*, 481–496. [CrossRef]
98. Parkes, G.C.; Whelan, K.; Lindsay, J.O. Smoking in inflammatory bowel disease: Impact on disease course and insights into the aetiology of its effect. *J. Crohn's Colitis* **2014**, *8*, 717–725. [CrossRef]
99. Biedermann, L.; Fournier, N.; Misselwitz, B.; Frei, P.; Zeitz, J.; Manser, C.N.; Pittet, V.; Juillerat, P.; von Kanel, R.; Fried, M.; et al. High rates of smoking especially in female Crohn's disease patients and low use of supportive measures to achieve smoking cessation—Data from the swiss ibd cohort study. *J. Crohn's Colitis* **2015**, *9*, 819–829. [CrossRef]
100. Sher, M.E.; Bank, S.; Greenberg, R.; Sardinha, T.C.; Weissman, S.; Bailey, B.; Gilliland, R.; Wexner, S.D. The influence of cigarette smoking on cytokine levels in patients with inflammatory bowel disease. *Inflamm. Bowel Dis.* **1999**, *5*, 73–78. [CrossRef]
101. Biedermann, L.; Brulisauer, K.; Zeitz, J.; Frei, P.; Scharl, M.; Vavricka, S.R.; Fried, M.; Loessner, M.J.; Rogler, G.; Schuppler, M. Smoking cessation alters intestinal microbiota: Insights from quantitative investigations on human fecal samples using fish. *Inflamm. Bowel Dis.* **2014**, *20*, 1496–1501. [CrossRef]
102. Adorini, L.; Penna, G. Dendritic cell tolerogenicity: A key mechanism in immunomodulation by vitamin d receptor agonists. *Hum. Immunol.* **2009**, *70*, 345–352. [CrossRef]
103. Jorgensen, S.P.; Hvas, C.L.; Agnholt, J.; Christensen, L.A.; Heickendorff, L.; Dahlerup, J.F. Active Crohn's disease is associated with low vitamin d levels. *J. Crohn's Colitis* **2013**, *7*, e407–e413. [CrossRef]
104. Limketkai, B.N.; Bayless, T.M.; Brant, S.R.; Hutfless, S.M. Lower regional and temporal ultraviolet exposure is associated with increased rates and severity of inflammatory bowel disease hospitalisation. *Aliment. Pharmacol. Ther.* **2014**, *40*, 508–517. [CrossRef]
105. Holmes, E.A.; Xiang, F.; Lucas, R.M. Variation in incidence of pediatric Crohn's disease in relation to latitude and ambient ultraviolet radiation: A systematic review and analysis. *Inflamm. Bowel Dis.* **2015**, *21*, 809–817. [CrossRef]
106. Magnus, P.; Jaakkola, J.J. Secular trend in the occurrence of asthma among children and young adults: Critical appraisal of repeated cross sectional surveys. *BMJ* **1997**, *314*, 1795–1799. [CrossRef]
107. Lee, D.; Albenberg, L.; Compher, C.; Baldassano, R.; Piccoli, D.; Lewis, J.D.; Wu, G.D. Diet in the pathogenesis and treatment of inflammatory bowel diseases. *Gastroenterology* **2015**, *148*, 1087–1106. [CrossRef]
108. Alcalde-Cabero, E.; Almazan-Isla, J.; Garcia-Merino, A.; de Sa, J.; de Pedro-Cuesta, J. Incidence of multiple sclerosis among european economic area populations, 1985–2009: The framework for monitoring. *BMC Neurol.* **2013**, *13*, 58. [CrossRef]
109. Krawiec, J.; Odes, H.S.; Lasry, Y.; Krugliak, P.; Weitzman, S. Aspects of the epidemiology of Crohn's disease in the Jewish population in Beer Sheva, Israel. *Isr. J. Med. Sci.* **1984**, *20*, 16–21.
110. Li, X.; Sundquist, J.; Hemminki, K.; Sundquist, K. Risk of inflammatory bowel disease in first- and second-generation immigrants in Sweden: A nationwide follow-up study. *Inflamm. Bowel Dis.* **2011**, *17*, 1784–1791. [CrossRef]
111. Sood, A.; Midha, V.; Sood, N.; Bhatia, A.S.; Avasthi, G. Incidence and prevalence of ulcerative colitis in Punjab, north India. *Gut* **2003**, *52*, 1587–1590. [CrossRef]
112. Khosla, S.N.; Girdhar, N.K.; Lal, S.; Mishra, D.S. Epidemiology of ulcerative colitis in hospital and select general population of northern India. *J. Assoc. Phys. India* **1986**, *34*, 405–407.
113. Loftus, C.G.; Loftus, E.V., Jr.; Harmsen, W.S.; Zinsmeister, A.R.; Tremaine, W.J.; Melton, L.J., 3rd; Sandborn, W.J. Update on the incidence and prevalence of Crohn's disease and ulcerative colitis in Olmsted county, Minnesota, 1940–2000. *Inflamm. Bowel Dis.* **2007**, *13*, 254–261. [CrossRef]
114. Bernstein, C.N.; Wajda, A.; Svenson, L.W.; MacKenzie, A.; Koehoorn, M.; Jackson, M.; Fedorak, R.; Israel, D.; Blanchard, J.F. The epidemiology of inflammatory bowel disease in Canada: A population-based study. *Am. J. Gastroenterol.* **2006**, *101*, 1559–1568. [CrossRef]
115. Fellows, I.W.; Freeman, J.G.; Holmes, G.K. Crohn's disease in the city of derby, 1951–1985. *Gut* **1990**, *31*, 1262–1265. [CrossRef]
116. Pinsk, V.; Lemberg, D.A.; Grewal, K.; Barker, C.C.; Schreiber, R.A.; Jacobson, K. Inflammatory bowel disease in the south Asian pediatric population of British Columbia. *Am. J. Gastroenterol.* **2007**, *102*, 1077–1083. [CrossRef]

117. Ko, Y.; Butcher, R.; Leong, R.W. Epidemiological studies of migration and environmental risk factors in the inflammatory bowel diseases. *World J. Gastroenterol.* **2014**, *20*, 1238–1247. [CrossRef]
118. Ng, S.C.; Tang, W.; Leong, R.W.; Chen, M.; Ko, Y.; Studd, C.; Niewiadomski, O.; Bell, S.; Kamm, M.A.; de Silva, H.J.; et al. Environmental risk factors in inflammatory bowel disease: A population-based case-control study in Asia-Pacific. *Gut* **2015**, *64*, 1063–1071. [CrossRef]
119. Zhou, Y.; Xu, Z.Z.; He, Y.; Yang, Y.; Liu, L.; Lin, Q.; Nie, Y.; Li, M.; Zhi, F.; Liu, S.; et al. Gut microbiota offers universal biomarkers across ethnicity in inflammatory bowel disease diagnosis and infliximab response prediction. *MSystems* **2018**, *3*, e00188-17. [CrossRef]
120. Forbes, J.D.; Chen, C.Y.; Knox, N.C.; Marrie, R.A.; El-Gabalawy, H.; de Kievit, T.; Alfa, M.; Bernstein, C.N.; Van Domselaar, G. A comparative study of the gut microbiota in immune-mediated inflammatory diseases-does a common dysbiosis exist? *Microbiome* **2018**, *6*, 221. [CrossRef]
121. Hou, J.K.; Abraham, B.; El-Serag, H. Dietary intake and risk of developing inflammatory bowel disease: A systematic review of the literature. *Am. J. Gastroenterol.* **2011**, *106*, 563–573. [CrossRef]
122. Ananthakrishnan, A.N. Epidemiology and risk factors for ibd. *Nat. Rev. Gastroenterol. Hepatol.* **2015**, *12*, 205–217. [CrossRef]
123. Aleksandrova, K.; Romero-Mosquera, B.; Hernandez, V. Diet, gut microbiome and epigenetics: Emerging links with inflammatory bowel diseases and prospects for management and prevention. *Nutrients* **2017**, *9*, 962. [CrossRef]
124. Dabritz, J.; Menheniott, T.R. Linking immunity, epigenetics, and cancer in inflammatory bowel disease. *Inflamm. Bowel Dis.* **2014**, *20*, 1638–1654. [CrossRef]
125. Barnett, M.; Bermingham, E.; McNabb, W.; Bassett, S.; Armstrong, K.; Rounce, J.; Roy, N. Investigating micronutrients and epigenetic mechanisms in relation to inflammatory bowel disease. *Mutat. Res.* **2010**, *690*, 71–80. [CrossRef]
126. Gallou-Kabani, C.; Vige, A.; Gross, M.S.; Junien, C. Nutri-epigenomics: Lifelong remodelling of our epigenomes by nutritional and metabolic factors and beyond. *Clin. Chem. Lab. Med.* **2007**, *45*, 321–327. [CrossRef]
127. Anderson, O.S.; Sant, K.E.; Dolinoy, D.C. Nutrition and epigenetics: An interplay of dietary methyl donors, one-carbon metabolism and DNA methylation. *J. Nutr. Biochem.* **2012**, *23*, 853–859. [CrossRef]
128. Lu, Q.; Qiu, X.; Hu, N.; Wen, H.; Su, Y.; Richardson, B.C. Epigenetics, disease, and therapeutic interventions. *Ageing Res. Rev.* **2006**, *5*, 449–467. [CrossRef]
129. Remely, M.; Lovrecic, L.; de la Garza, A.L.; Migliore, L.; Peterlin, B.; Milagro, F.I.; Martinez, A.J.; Haslberger, A.G. Therapeutic perspectives of epigenetically active nutrients. *Br. J. Pharmacol.* **2015**, *172*, 2756–2768. [CrossRef]
130. Russell, W.R.; Duncan, S.H.; Scobbie, L.; Duncan, G.; Cantlay, L.; Calder, A.G.; Anderson, S.E.; Flint, H.J. Major phenylpropanoid-derived metabolites in the human gut can arise from microbial fermentation of protein. *Mol. Nutr. Food Res.* **2013**, *57*, 523–535. [CrossRef]
131. Rahal, K.; Schmiedlin-Ren, P.; Adler, J.; Dhanani, M.; Sultani, V.; Rittershaus, A.C.; Reingold, L.; Zhu, J.; McKenna, B.J.; Christman, G.M.; et al. Resveratrol has antiinflammatory and antifibrotic effects in the peptidoglycan-polysaccharide rat model of Crohn's disease. *Inflamm. Bowel Dis.* **2012**, *18*, 613–623. [CrossRef]
132. Hanai, H.; Sugimoto, K. Curcumin has bright prospects for the treatment of inflammatory bowel disease. *Curr. Pharm. Des.* **2009**, *15*, 2087–2094. [CrossRef]
133. Hanai, H.; Iida, T.; Takeuchi, K.; Watanabe, F.; Maruyama, Y.; Andoh, A.; Tsujikawa, T.; Fujiyama, Y.; Mitsuyama, K.; Sata, M.; et al. Curcumin maintenance therapy for ulcerative colitis: Randomized, multicenter, double-blind, placebo-controlled trial. *Clin. Gastroenterol. Hepatol. Off. Clin. Prac. J. Am. Gastroenterol. Assoc.* **2006**, *4*, 1502–1506.
134. Reuter, S.; Gupta, S.C.; Park, B.; Goel, A.; Aggarwal, B.B. Epigenetic changes induced by curcumin and other natural compounds. *Genes Nutr.* **2011**, *6*, 93–108. [CrossRef]
135. Burdge, G.C.; Hoile, S.P.; Lillycrop, K.A. Epigenetics: Are there implications for personalised nutrition? *Curr. Opin. Clin. Nutr. Metab. Care* **2012**, *15*, 442–447. [CrossRef]
136. Beaudet, A.L. Epigenetics and complex human disease: Is there a role in ibd? *J. Pediatr. Gastroenterol. Nutr.* **2008**, *46* (Suppl. 1), E2.
137. Garfinkel, M.D.; Ruden, D.M. Chromatin effects in nutrition, cancer, and obesity. *Nutrition* **2004**, *20*, 56–62. [CrossRef]

138. Wani, N.A.; Hamid, A.; Kaur, J. Folate status in various pathophysiological conditions. *IUBMB life* **2008**, *60*, 834–842. [CrossRef]
139. McKay, J.A.; Williams, E.A.; Mathers, J.C. Gender-specific modulation of tumorigenesis by folic acid supply in the APC mouse during early neonatal life. *Br. J. Nutr.* **2008**, *99*, 550–558. [CrossRef]
140. Davis, C.D.; Uthus, E.O.; Finley, J.W. Dietary selenium and arsenic affect DNA methylation in vitro in caco-2 cells and in vivo in rat liver and colon. *J. Nutr.* **2000**, *130*, 2903–2909. [CrossRef]
141. Tirosh, O.; Levy, E.; Reifen, R. High selenium diet protects against tnbs-induced acute inflammation, mitochondrial dysfunction, and secondary necrosis in rat colon. *Nutrition* **2007**, *23*, 878–886. [CrossRef]
142. Castro Aguilar-Tablada, T.; Navarro-Alarcon, M.; Quesada Granados, J.; Samaniego Sanchez, C.; Rufian-Henares, J.A.; Nogueras-Lopez, F. Ulcerative colitis and Crohn's disease are associated with decreased serum selenium concentrations and increased cardiovascular risk. *Nutrients* **2016**, *8*, 780. [CrossRef]
143. Arpon, A.; Milagro, F.I.; Razquin, C.; Corella, D.; Estruch, R.; Fito, M.; Marti, A.; Martinez-Gonzalez, M.A.; Ros, E.; Salas-Salvado, J.; et al. Impact of consuming extra-virgin olive oil or nuts within a mediterranean diet on DNA methylation in peripheral white blood cells within the predimed-navarra randomized controlled trial: A role for dietary lipids. *Nutrients* **2017**, *10*, 15. [CrossRef]
144. Kau, A.L.; Ahern, P.P.; Griffin, N.W.; Goodman, A.L.; Gordon, J.I. Human nutrition, the gut microbiome and the immune system. *Nature* **2011**, *474*, 327–336. [CrossRef]
145. Krautkramer, K.A.; Kreznar, J.H.; Romano, K.A.; Vivas, E.I.; Barrett-Wilt, G.A.; Rabaglia, M.E.; Keller, M.P.; Attie, A.D.; Rey, F.E.; Denu, J.M. Diet-microbiota interactions mediate global epigenetic programming in multiple host tissues. *Mol. Cell* **2016**, *64*, 982–992. [CrossRef]
146. Kostic, A.D.; Xavier, R.J.; Gevers, D. The microbiome in inflammatory bowel disease: Current status and the future ahead. *Gastroenterology* **2014**, *146*, 1489–1499. [CrossRef]
147. Eeckhaut, V.; Ducatelle, R.; Sas, B.; Vermeire, S.; Van Immerseel, F. Progress towards butyrate-producing pharmabiotics: *Butyricicoccus pullicaecorum* capsule and efficacy in tnbs models in comparison with therapeutics. *Gut* **2014**, *63*, 367. [CrossRef]
148. Limdi, J.K.; Aggarwal, D.; McLaughlin, J.T. Dietary practices and beliefs in patients with inflammatory bowel disease. *Inflamm. Bowel Dis.* **2016**, *22*, 164–170. [CrossRef]
149. Zallot, C.; Quilliot, D.; Chevaux, J.B.; Peyrin-Biroulet, C.; Gueant-Rodriguez, R.M.; Freling, E.; Collet-Fenetrier, B.; Williet, N.; Ziegler, O.; Bigard, M.A.; et al. Dietary beliefs and behavior among inflammatory bowel disease patients. *Inflamm. Bowel Dis.* **2013**, *19*, 66–72. [CrossRef]
150. Tanaka, M.; Kawakami, A.; Iwao, Y.; Fukushima, T.; Yamamoto-Mitani, N. Coping strategies for possible flare-ups and their perceived effectiveness in patients with inflammatory bowel disease. Gastroenterology nursing. *Off. J. Soc. Gastroenterol. Nur. Assoc.* **2016**, *39*, 42–47. [CrossRef]
151. Jowett, S.L.; Seal, C.J.; Pearce, M.S.; Phillips, E.; Gregory, W.; Barton, J.R.; Welfare, M.R. Influence of dietary factors on the clinical course of ulcerative colitis: A prospective cohort study. *Gut* **2004**, *53*, 1479–1484. [CrossRef]
152. Magee, E.A.; Edmond, L.M.; Tasker, S.M.; Kong, S.C.; Curno, R.; Cummings, J.H. Associations between diet and disease activity in ulcerative colitis patients using a novel method of data analysis. *Nutr. J.* **2005**, *4*, 7. [CrossRef]
153. Guerreiro, C.S.; Ferreira, P.; Tavares, L.; Santos, P.M.; Neves, M.; Brito, M.; Cravo, M. Fatty acids, il6, and tnfalpha polymorphisms: An example of nutrigenetics in Crohn's disease. *Am. J. Gastroenterol.* **2009**, *104*, 2241–2249. [CrossRef]
154. Ferreira, P.; Cravo, M.; Guerreiro, C.S.; Tavares, L.; Santos, P.M.; Brito, M. Fat intake interacts with polymorphisms of caspase9, fasligand and ppargamma apoptotic genes in modulating Crohn's disease activity. *Clin. Nutr.* **2010**, *29*, 819–823. [CrossRef]
155. Reifen, R.; Matas, Z.; Zeidel, L.; Berkovitch, Z.; Bujanover, Y. Iron supplementation may aggravate inflammatory status of colitis in a rat model. *Dig. Dis. Sci.* **2000**, *45*, 394–397. [CrossRef]
156. Carrier, J.; Aghdassi, E.; Cullen, J.; Allard, J.P. Iron supplementation increases disease activity and vitamin e ameliorates the effect in rats with dextran sulfate sodium-induced colitis. *J. Nutr.* **2002**, *132*, 3146–3150. [CrossRef]
157. de Silva, A.D.; Tsironi, E.; Feakins, R.M.; Rampton, D.S. Efficacy and tolerability of oral iron therapy in inflammatory bowel disease: A prospective, comparative trial. *Aliment. Pharmacol. Ther.* **2005**, *22*, 1097–1105. [CrossRef]

158. Goldberg, N.D. Iron deficiency anemia in patients with inflammatory bowel disease. *Clin. Exp. Gastroenterol.* **2013**, *6*, 61–70. [CrossRef]
159. Nielsen, O.H.; Ainsworth, M.; Coskun, M.; Weiss, G. Management of iron-deficiency anemia in inflammatory bowel disease: A systematic review. *Medicine* **2015**, *94*, e963. [CrossRef]
160. Mahalhal, A.; Williams, J.M.; Johnson, S.; Ellaby, N.; Duckworth, C.A.; Burkitt, M.D.; Liu, X.; Hold, G.L.; Campbell, B.J.; Pritchard, D.M.; et al. Oral iron exacerbates colitis and influences the intestinal microbiome. *PLoS ONE* **2018**, *13*, e0202460. [CrossRef]
161. Colombel, J.F.; Shin, A.; Gibson, P.R. AGA clinical practice update on functional gastrointestinal symptoms in patients with inflammatory bowel disease: Expert review. *Clin. Gastroenterol. Hepatol. Off. Clin. Prac. J. Am. Gastroenterol. Assoc.* **2019**, *17*, 380–390.e1.
162. Ruemmele, F.M.; Veres, G.; Kolho, K.L.; Griffiths, A.; Levine, A.; Escher, J.C.; Amil Dias, J.; Barabino, A.; Braegger, C.P.; Bronsky, J.; et al. Consensus guidelines of ecco/espghan on the medical management of pediatric Crohn's disease. *J. Crohn's Colitis* **2014**, *8*, 1179–1207. [CrossRef]
163. Lee, D.; Baldassano, R.N.; Otley, A.R.; Albenberg, L.; Griffiths, A.M.; Compher, C.; Chen, E.Z.; Li, H.; Gilroy, E.; Nessel, L.; et al. Comparative effectiveness of nutritional and biological therapy in North American children with active Crohn's disease. *Inflamm. Bowel Dis.* **2015**, *21*, 1786–1793. [CrossRef]
164. Connors, J.; Basseri, S.; Grant, A.; Giffin, N.; Mahdi, G.; Noble, A.; Rashid, M.; Otley, A.; Van Limbergen, J. Exclusive enteral nutrition therapy in paediatric Crohn's disease results in long-term avoidance of corticosteroids: Results of a propensity-score matched cohort analysis. *J. Crohn's Colitis* **2017**, *11*, 1063–1070. [CrossRef]
165. Cohen-Dolev, N.; Sladek, M.; Hussey, S.; Turner, D.; Veres, G.; Koletzko, S.; Martin de Carpi, J.; Staiano, A.; Shaoul, R.; Lionetti, P.; et al. Differences in outcomes over time with exclusive enteral nutrition compared with steroids in children with mild to moderate Crohn's disease: Results from the growth cd study. *J. Crohn's Colitis* **2018**, *12*, 306–312. [CrossRef]
166. Grover, Z.; Burgess, C.; Muir, R.; Reilly, C.; Lewindon, P.J. Early mucosal healing with exclusive enteral nutrition is associated with improved outcomes in newly diagnosed children with luminal Crohn's disease. *J. Crohn's Colitis* **2016**, *10*, 1159–1164. [CrossRef]
167. Sigall-Boneh, R.; Pfeffer-Gik, T.; Segal, I.; Zangen, T.; Boaz, M.; Levine, A. Partial enteral nutrition with a Crohn's disease exclusion diet is effective for induction of remission in children and young adults with Crohn's disease. *Inflamm. Bowel Dis.* **2014**, *20*, 1353–1360. [CrossRef]
168. Sigall Boneh, R.; Sarbagili Shabat, C.; Yanai, H.; Chermesh, I.; Ben Avraham, S.; Boaz, M.; Levine, A. Dietary therapy with the Crohn's disease exclusion diet is a successful strategy for induction of remission in children and adults failing biological therapy. *J. Crohn's Colitis* **2017**, *11*, 1205–1212. [CrossRef]
169. Wedlake, L.; Slack, N.; Andreyev, H.J.; Whelan, K. Fiber in the treatment and maintenance of inflammatory bowel disease: A systematic review of randomized controlled trials. *Inflamm. Bowel Dis.* **2014**, *20*, 576–586. [CrossRef]
170. Chiba, M.; Tsuji, T.; Nakane, K.; Komatsu, M. High amount of dietary fiber not harmful but favorable for Crohn disease. *Perm. J.* **2015**, *19*, 58–61. [CrossRef]
171. Chiba, M.; Tsuji, T.; Nakane, K.; Tsuda, S.; Ishii, H.; Ohno, H.; Watanabe, K.; Ito, M.; Komatsu, M.; Sugawara, T. Induction with infliximab and a plant-based diet as first-line (ipf) therapy for Crohn disease: A single-group trial. *Perm. J.* **2017**, *21*, 17-009. [CrossRef] [PubMed]
172. Cohen, A.B.; Lee, D.; Long, M.D.; Kappelman, M.D.; Martin, C.F.; Sandler, R.S.; Lewis, J.D. Dietary patterns and self-reported associations of diet with symptoms of inflammatory bowel disease. *Dig. Dis. Sci.* **2013**, *58*, 1322–1328. [CrossRef] [PubMed]
173. Levine, J.; Ellis, C.J.; Furne, J.K.; Springfield, J.; Levitt, M.D. Fecal hydrogen sulfide production in ulcerative colitis. *Am. J. Gastroenterol.* **1998**, *93*, 83–87. [CrossRef] [PubMed]
174. Magee, E.A.; Richardson, C.J.; Hughes, R.; Cummings, J.H. Contribution of dietary protein to sulfide production in the large intestine: An in vitro and a controlled feeding study in humans. *Am. J. Clin. Nutr.* **2000**, *72*, 1488–1494. [CrossRef] [PubMed]
175. Medani, M.; Collins, D.; Docherty, N.G.; Baird, A.W.; O'Connell, P.R.; Winter, D.C. Emerging role of hydrogen sulfide in colonic physiology and pathophysiology. *Inflamm. Bowel Dis.* **2011**, *17*, 1620–1625. [CrossRef] [PubMed]

176. Attene-Ramos, M.S.; Nava, G.M.; Muellner, M.G.; Wagner, E.D.; Plewa, M.J.; Gaskins, H.R. DNA damage and toxicogenomic analyses of hydrogen sulfide in human intestinal epithelial FHS 74 int cells. *Environ. Mol. Mutagen.* **2010**, *51*, 304–314. [CrossRef] [PubMed]
177. Babidge, W.; Millard, S.; Roediger, W. Sulfides impair short chain fatty acid beta-oxidation at acyl-coa dehydrogenase level in colonocytes: Implications for ulcerative colitis. *Mol. Cell. Biochem.* **1998**, *181*, 117–124. [CrossRef] [PubMed]
178. Pitcher, M.C.; Beatty, E.R.; Cummings, J.H. The contribution of sulphate reducing bacteria and 5-aminosalicylic acid to faecal sulphide in patients with ulcerative colitis. *Gut* **2000**, *46*, 64–72. [CrossRef] [PubMed]
179. Loubinoux, J.; Bronowicki, J.P.; Pereira, I.A.; Mougenel, J.L.; Faou, A.E. Sulfate-reducing bacteria in human feces and their association with inflammatory bowel diseases. *FEMS Microbiol. Ecol.* **2002**, *40*, 107–112. [CrossRef]
180. Khalil, N.A.; Walton, G.E.; Gibson, G.R.; Tuohy, K.M.; Andrews, S.C. In vitro batch cultures of gut microbiota from healthy and ulcerative colitis (uc) subjects suggest that sulphate-reducing bacteria levels are raised in uc and by a protein-rich diet. *Int. j. Food Sci. Nutr.* **2014**, *65*, 79–88. [CrossRef]
181. Suskind, D.L.; Wahbeh, G.; Cohen, S.A.; Damman, C.J.; Klein, J.; Braly, K.; Shaffer, M.; Lee, D. Patients perceive clinical benefit with the specific carbohydrate diet for inflammatory bowel disease. *Dig. Dis. Sci.* **2016**, *61*, 3255–3260. [CrossRef] [PubMed]
182. Burgis, J.C.; Nguyen, K.; Park, K.T.; Cox, K. Response to strict and liberalized specific carbohydrate diet in pediatric Crohn's disease. *World J. Gastroenterol.* **2016**, *22*, 2111–2117. [CrossRef] [PubMed]
183. Obih, C.; Wahbeh, G.; Lee, D.; Braly, K.; Giefer, M.; Shaffer, M.L.; Nielson, H.; Suskind, D.L. Specific carbohydrate diet for pediatric inflammatory bowel disease in clinical practice within an academic ibd center. *Nutrition* **2016**, *32*, 418–425. [CrossRef] [PubMed]
184. Britto, S.; Kellermayer, R. Carbohydrate monotony as protection and treatment for inflammatory bowel disease. *J. Crohn's Colitis* **2019**. [CrossRef] [PubMed]
185. Fiocchi, C. Tailoring treatment to the individual patient—Will inflammatory bowel disease medicine be personalized? *Dig. Dis.* **2015**, *33* (Suppl. 1), 82–89. [CrossRef]
186. Nagy-Szakal, D.; Mir, S.A.; Ross, M.C.; Tatevian, N.; Petrosino, J.F.; Kellermayer, R. Monotonous diets protect against acute colitis in mice: Epidemiologic and therapeutic implications. *J. Pediatr. Gastroenterol. Nutr.* **2013**, *56*, 544–550. [CrossRef]
187. Konijeti, G.G.; Kim, N.; Lewis, J.D.; Groven, S.; Chandrasekaran, A.; Grandhe, S.; Diamant, C.; Singh, E.; Oliveira, G.; Wang, X.; et al. Efficacy of the autoimmune protocol diet for inflammatory bowel disease. *Inflamm. Bowel Dis.* **2017**, *23*, 2054–2060. [CrossRef]
188. Knight-Sepulveda, K.; Kais, S.; Santaolalla, R.; Abreu, M.T. Diet and inflammatory bowel disease. *Gastroenterol. Hepatol.* **2015**, *11*, 511–520.
189. van der Sloot, K.W.J.; Amini, M.; Peters, V.; Dijkstra, G.; Alizadeh, B.Z. Inflammatory bowel diseases: Review of known environmental protective and risk factors involved. *Inflamm. Bowel Dis.* **2017**, *23*, 1499–1509. [CrossRef]
190. Schaffler, H.; Schmidt, M.; Huth, A.; Reiner, J.; Glass, A.; Lamprecht, G. Clinical factors are associated with vitamin d levels in ibd patients: A retrospective analysis. *J. Dig. Dis.* **2018**, *19*, 24–32. [CrossRef]
191. Suibhne, T.N.; Cox, G.; Healy, M.; O'Morain, C.; O'Sullivan, M. Vitamin d deficiency in Crohn's disease: Prevalence, risk factors and supplement use in an outpatient setting. *J. Crohn's Colitis* **2012**, *6*, 182–188. [CrossRef] [PubMed]
192. Alrefai, D.; Jones, J.; El-Matary, W.; Whiting, S.J.; Aljebreen, A.; Mirhosseini, N.; Vatanparast, H. The association of vitamin d status with disease activity in a cohort of Crohn's disease patients in Canada. *Nutrients* **2017**, *9*, 1112. [CrossRef] [PubMed]
193. Narula, N.; Cooray, M.; Anglin, R.; Muqtadir, Z.; Narula, A.; Marshall, J.K. Impact of high-dose vitamin d3 supplementation in patients with Crohn's disease in remission: A pilot randomized double-blind controlled study. *Dig. Dis. Sci.* **2017**, *62*, 448–455. [CrossRef] [PubMed]
194. Jorgensen, S.P.; Agnholt, J.; Glerup, H.; Lyhne, S.; Villadsen, G.E.; Hvas, C.L.; Bartels, L.E.; Kelsen, J.; Christensen, L.A.; Dahlerup, J.F. Clinical trial: Vitamin d3 treatment in Crohn's disease—A randomized double-blind placebo-controlled study. *Aliment. Pharmacol. Ther.* **2010**, *32*, 377–383. [CrossRef] [PubMed]
195. Dionne, S.; Duchatelier, C.F.; Seidman, E.G. The influence of vitamin d on m1 and m2 macrophages in patients with Crohn's disease. *Innate Immun.* **2017**, *23*, 557–565. [CrossRef] [PubMed]

196. Liu, W.; Chen, Y.; Golan, M.A.; Annunziata, M.L.; Du, J.; Dougherty, U.; Kong, J.; Musch, M.; Huang, Y.; Pekow, J.; et al. Intestinal epithelial vitamin d receptor signaling inhibits experimental colitis. *J. Clin. Investig.* **2013**, *123*, 3983–3996. [CrossRef]
197. Wu, S.; Zhang, Y.G.; Lu, R.; Xia, Y.; Zhou, D.; Petrof, E.O.; Claud, E.C.; Chen, D.; Chang, E.B.; Carmeliet, G.; et al. Intestinal epithelial vitamin d receptor deletion leads to defective autophagy in colitis. *Gut* **2015**, *64*, 1082–1094. [CrossRef]
198. Ryz, N.R.; Lochner, A.; Bhullar, K.; Ma, C.; Huang, T.; Bhinder, G.; Bosman, E.; Wu, X.; Innis, S.M.; Jacobson, K.; et al. Dietary vitamin d3 deficiency alters intestinal mucosal defense and increases susceptibility to *Citrobacter rodentium*-induced colitis. *Am. J. Ophysiol. Gastrointest. Liver physiol.* **2015**, *309*, G730–G742. [CrossRef]
199. Ooi, J.H.; Li, Y.; Rogers, C.J.; Cantorna, M.T. Vitamin d regulates the gut microbiome and protects mice from dextran sodium sulfate-induced colitis. *J. Nutr.* **2013**, *143*, 1679–1686. [CrossRef]
200. Jin, D.; Wu, S.; Zhang, Y.G.; Lu, R.; Xia, Y.; Dong, H.; Sun, J. Lack of vitamin d receptor causes dysbiosis and changes the functions of the murine intestinal microbiome. *Clin. Ther.* **2015**, *37*, 996–1009.e7. [CrossRef]

9

Obesity in Inflammatory Bowel Disease: Gains in Adiposity despite High Prevalence of Myopenia and Osteopenia

Robert Venning Bryant [1,2,*], Christopher G. Schultz [3], Soong Ooi [4], Charlotte Goess [4], Samuel Paul Costello [1,2], Andrew D. Vincent [5], Scott N. Schoeman [1], Amanda Lim [1], Francis Dylan Bartholomeusz [3], Simon P.L. Travis [6] and Jane Mary Andrews [2,4]

1 IBD Service, Department of Gastroenterology and Hepatology, The Queen Elizabeth Hospital, 28 Woodville Road, Woodville 5011, Australia; sam.costello@sa.gov.au (S.P.C.); snschoeman@gmail.com (S.N.S.); Amanda.Lim@sa.gov.au (A.L.)

2 School of Medicine, Faculty of Health Sciences, University of Adelaide, Adelaide 5000, Australia; jane.andrews@sa.gov.au

3 Department of Nuclear Medicine, PET and Bone Densitometry, Royal Adelaide Hospital, Port Road, Adelaide 5000, Australia; chris.schultz@sa.gov.au (C.G.S.); Dylan.Bartholomeusz@sa.gov.au (F.D.B.)

4 IBD Service, Department of Gastroenterology and Hepatology, Royal Adelaide Hospital, Port Road, Adelaide 5000, Australia; soongyuan.ooi@uq.edu.au (S.O.); charlotte.goess@sa.gov.au (C.G.)

5 Freemasons Foundation Centre for Men's Health, School of Medicine, University of Adelaide, North Terrace, Adelaide 5000, Australia; andrew.vincent@adelaide.edu.au

6 Translational Gastroenterology Unit, John Radcliffe Hospital, Headley Way, Headington, Oxford OX3 9DU, UK; simon.travis@ndm.ox.ac.uk

* Correspondence: Robert.Bryant@sa.gov.au

Abstract: Background: Rising rates of obesity have been reported in patients with inflammatory bowel disease (IBD); however, prospective data is lacking. The aim of this study is to prospectively evaluate body composition in adults with IBD over 24 months. Methods: Whole body dual energy X-ray absorptiometry (DXA) data was performed at 0 months, 12 months, and 24 months. Bone mineral density (BMD), fat mass index (FMI (kg)/height (m^2)), appendicular skeletal muscle index (ASMI (kg)/height (m^2)), visceral adipose tissue and the visceral adipose height index (VHI, VAT area (cm^3)/height (m^2)), and clinical and anthropometric assessments were performed at each time point. Multivariable linear mixed effects regression analyses were performed. Results: Initially, 154 participants were assessed at baseline (70% Crohn's disease, 55% male, median age 31 years), of whom 129 underwent repeated DXA at 12 months, and 110 underwent repeated DXA at 24 months. Amongst those undergoing repeated DXA, their body mass index (BMI) significantly increased over time, such that by 24 months, 62% of patients were overweight or obese (annual change BMI $\beta = 0.43$, 95%CI = [0.18, 0.67], $p = 0.0006$). Gains in BMI related to increases in both FMI and VHI ($\beta = 0.33$, 95%CI = [0.14, 0.53], $p = 0.0007$; $\beta = 0.08$, 95%CI = [0.02, 0.13], $p = 0.001$; respectively), whereas ASMI decreased ($\beta = -0.07$, 95%CI = [−0.12, −0.01], $p = 0.01$) with a concordant rise in rates of myopenia (OR = 3.1 95%CI = [1.2, 7.7]; $p = 0.01$). Rates of osteopenia and osteoporosis were high (37%), but remained unchanged over time ($p = 0.23$). Conclusion: Increasing rates of obesity in patients with IBD coincide with decreases in lean muscle mass over time, while high rates of osteopenia remain stable. These previously undocumented issues warrant attention in routine care to prevent avoidable morbidity.

Keywords: body composition; obesity; visceral adipose tissue; fat; osteoporosis; osteopenia; sarcopenia; inflammatory bowel disease

1. Introduction

Body composition refers to proportions of bone, fat, and fat-free (lean) mass in the body and may be abnormal in many patients with inflammatory bowel disease (IBD) [1]. Despite the potential negative effects of disturbances in body composition on IBD-related outcomes, response to therapy, cardiovascular disease, and quality of life (QoL), there is a paucity of prospective data on body composition in patients with IBD [1,2].

Rates of obesity are rising in patients with IBD, as in the general population; 15–40% of adults with IBD are obese, and 20–40% are overweight [3]. IBD may be an independent risk factor for obesity that is driven by dysbiosis and aberrations in intestinal microbial metabolism [4,5]. Treatments used for IBD, in particular corticosteroids and anti-tumor necrosis factor alpha therapies, may also play a role in obesity [3]. On the other hand, adipose tissue is metabolically active, and could plausibly contribute to a pro-inflammatory susceptibility to IBD [4,6]. However, existing data on the impact of obesity on IBD susceptibility and disease course are conflicting. This is partly due to the use of the body mass index (BMI) as a blunt instrument for measuring adiposity, which is unable to distinguish between adiposity compartments with distinct metabolic profiles [3,6–10]. Visceral adipose tissue (VAT) is increased in many patients with Crohn's disease (CD) and has been associated with a complicated CD phenotype [3,4,6,11–14]. There are no longitudinal prospective data on direct measures of adiposity in patients with IBD.

There are emerging reports of high rates of both myopenia, which is defined as low lean mass, and sarcopenia, which is defined as a low lean mass coupled with loss of strength, in patients with IBD [1,15–17]. This matters, because low lean mass has been associated with an increased need for surgery and poor surgical outcomes in IBD, as well as with osteopenia [18–20]. Lean mass deficits may be difficult to detect in clinical practice, where BMI can be falsely reassuring [17,18]. Current data on sarcopenia in IBD are limited by small sample sizes and retrospective study designs, as well as a lack of an appropriate incorporation of a functional assessment [1].

A deficit in bone mineral density (BMD) (osteoporosis/osteopenia) is one of the most common complications of IBD, and has been reported in 20% to 50% of patients [21–23]. Reduced BMD is associated with an increased risk of pathological fractures and associated morbidity [22,24]. The pathogenesis of metabolic bone disease in IBD is likely multifactorial; however, clinical data are lacking, and the influence of IBD-related factors beyond conventional risk factors remains poorly explored [25,26].

Dual-energy X-ray absorptiometry (DXA) is in routine use in patients with IBD for the measurement of BMD. Whole body DXA adds little in terms of time and radiation, yet gleans accurate and regional body composition information and is considered a gold-standard tool for the evaluation of body composition as compared to cross-sectional imaging [1,27].

Therefore, the aims of this study were:

1. To evaluate body composition in patients with IBD, with serial prospective measurements over time;
2. To explore the influence of clinical factors on body composition in patients with IBD;
3. To explore whether standard anthropometric testing can detect aberrations in body composition.

2. Materials and Methods

2.1. Subjects

Consecutive patients with IBD (aged 18–50 years and pre-menopausal if female) managed by a tertiary IBD service were invited to participate in a prospective study between April 2012 and September 2013 (Figure 1). Those with significant medical or surgical comorbidity other than IBD, current pregnancy, or steroid use other than that required for IBD, were excluded.

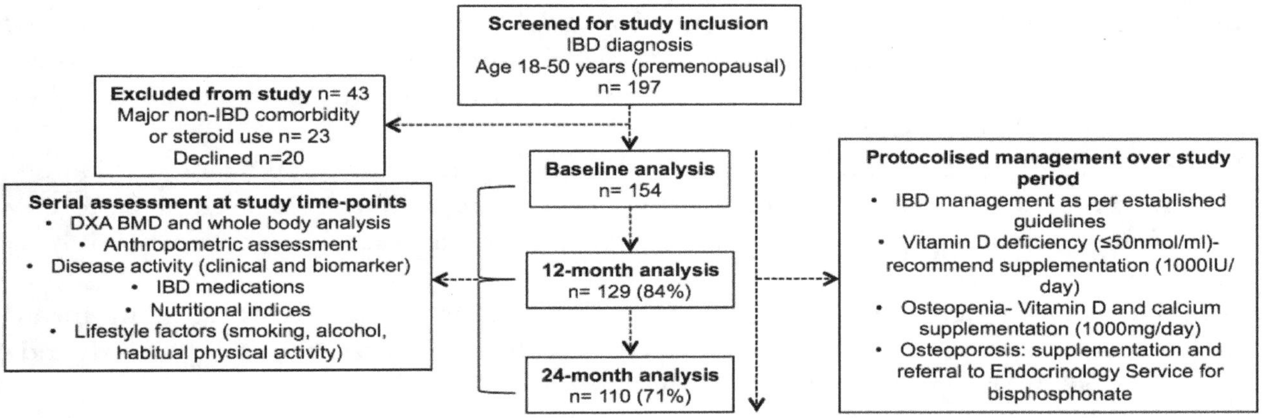

Figure 1. CONSORT diagram—inflammatory bowel disease (IBD) cohort. Legend: DXA, dual energy X-ray absorptiometry, BMD, bone mineral density.

2.2. Subject Data Collection

Prospective data were captured at 0 months, 12 months, and 24 months. At each study time-point case note, an IBD database and medical prescription review was undertaken. Data capture included demographics, Montreal classification at baseline, current IBD therapy, cumulative lifetime corticosteroid use (equivalent to prednisolone $\geq$10 mg/day) and IBD-related surgery [28]. IBD disease activity was assessed at each study time point using clinical indices and biomarkers of inflammation (C-reactive protein (CRP) and faecal calprotectin (FC) using a CALPRO® ELISA test). CRP $\geq$ 5 mg/L and/or FC $\geq$ 100 µg/g were considered consistent with active disease as a composite biomarker assessment.

Lifestyle factors were assessed at 0 months, 12 months, and 24 months. Average alcohol consumption was dichotomised into <20 g/day versus $\geq$20 g/day. Habitual physical activity was assessed using a validated self-administered Short International Physical Activity Questionnaire (IPAQ), which approximates metabolic equivalents MET-minutes per week and allows stratification into low, medium, and high activity groups [29].

2.3. Body Composition, Anthropometric Assessment, and Nutritional Assessment

Dual energy X-ray absorptiometry (DXA, General Electric Lunar Prodigy Vision bone densitometer (system DF + 13727; Encore version 13.60, Madison WI, USA)) of the lumbar spine, total femur, and whole body was used to evaluate BMD and body composition at 0 months, 12 months, and 24 months using standard protocols [30].

Standard calculations of fat and muscle body components were made from DXA data. Appendicular skeletal muscle (ASM) mass, which is considered functionally relevant lean mass, was calculated as the sum of the lean mass of the arms and legs (kg) [31]. The ASM index (ASMI) is the ASM mass in kg divided by the height in metres, squared [32]. Fat mass (FM) is the sum of the body fat mass (kg). The fat mass index (FMI) is calculated as FM in kg divided by height in metres, squared [32]. VAT was measured using CoreScan® analysis software, which correlates well with CT scan measurements [33]. VAT was measured in terms of volume (cm^3), mass (grams), visceral adipose tissue/height index (VHI, VAT volume (cm^3)/height in metres, squared), and VAT: subcutaneous adipose tissue (SAT) ratio. Height (m), weight (kg), waist circumference (cm), and hip circumference (cm) were measured at the time of the DXA and the waist–hip ratio (WHR) was calculated.

World Health Organisation (WHO) standard categories for BMI were used: <18.5 kg/m^2 (underweight), 18.5–24.9 kg/m^2 (normal weight), 25–29.9 kg/m^2 (overweight), $\geq$30 kg/m^2 (obese) [34]. Data from the Australian Bureau of Statistics National Health Survey 2014–2015 provided numerical comparisons with age and sex-matched Australian population for BMI and waist circumference [35]. Population-based, age and gender-matched normative data and standard deviation (SD) values from the National Health and Nutritional Examination Survey (NHANES) were used to calculate the *z*-scores for ASMI and the fat mass index (FMI) [17,32]. WHO population-based, age and sex-matched normative data of the lumbar spine and femur BMD were used to calculate BMD *t*-scores and *z*-scores [36]. The lowest BMD *t*-score at either site was used to stratify patients as normal (>−1), osteopenic (≤−1 >−2.5), or osteoporotic (≤−2.5).

Isometric handgrip strength was measured using a Jamar® Digital Hand Dynamometer, representing a robust surrogate measure of whole body strength [31]. Grip strength *z*-scores were calculated from population-based age and sex-matched normative data derived from healthy adult controls [17].

Myopenia was defined as an ASMI ≥1 SD below the age and gender-matched ASMI mean [31]. Sarcopenia was defined using combined anatomical and functional criteria, as both ASMI and grip strength >1 SD below the age and gender-matched means [31].

Nutritional assessment was performed at each study time point using clinical and laboratory criteria, including albumin, vitamin D (automated chemiluminescent assay), calcium, haemoglobin, iron studies, vitamin B12, and folate. Low vitamin D was defined as serum 25(OH) vitamin D level <50 nmol/L.

2.4. Management during Prospective Study Period

The routine IBD care of enrolled subjects within the tertiary IBD service was consistent with international guidelines (Figure 1) [37,38]. The protocolised management of bone health and nutrition was undertaken during the study period. Oral vitamin D supplementation was recommended to those with low levels (<50 nmol/L). All of the patients were advised to follow a calcium-rich diet and engage in regular exercise. Patients who were found to be osteopenic (or at risk of osteopenia with current corticosteroid use) were advised to take calcium supplementation (1000 mg/day) and oral vitamin D supplementation (≥1000 IU/day). Patients found to be osteoporotic were referred to the Endocrinology service for consideration of bisphosphonate therapy.

2.5. Ethical Considerations

The study was approved by the Royal Adelaide Hospital Research Ethics Committee (#120304). Whole-body DXA does not confer significant additional radiation to standard BMD assessment. Radiation safety reported that the total radiation dose per DXA study visit was 2.56 μSv.

2.6. Statistical Methods

Continuous outcomes are presented using means, standard deviations, medians, and interquartile ranges (IQR), with categorical outcomes as counts and percentages, unless otherwise stated. The lack of existing prospective data on body composition in IBD did not allow a formal power calculation. The enrolment of 150 patients was considered sufficient to provide adequate power for multivariable analysis, allowing for a dropout rate of 30% over the 24 months.

Change over time. Changes in disease activity, treatment, nutrition, and anthropometric and body composition variables in individual patients who underwent repeated measures testing over the 24-month study period were assessed using either linear or logistic mixed effects models, where appropriate. The β coefficient describes the change in the body composition variable per unit of time in the study (12 months). In all of the models, time since baseline assessment (years) was the linear fixed effect, with random intercepts per individual. Compound symmetric and unstructured variance–covariance were assumed for the linear and logistic models respectively. In all of the models, residuals and random effect estimates were examined to ensure that the model distributional assumptions appeared satisfied. As a consequence, VHI was log transformed. Missing data values were not included in the analysis.

Assessment of factors associated with body composition. Linear mixed-effects models were constructed to explore prospective clinical associations with serial assessments of BMI, FMI, VHI, ASMI, and BMD (lumbar spine t-score) at 0 months, 12 months, and 24 months. Univariable models were constructed, followed by full multivariable models. We report β coefficients that describe the change in the dependent variable per unit change in a covariate. Missing data were imputed with cohort means. Significance was set at the 5% alpha level (two-sided). Analyses were performed on R software v3.4.3 (R Studio, Boston, MA 02210, USA) using the nlme and lme4 packages.

3. Results

3.1. Subject Characteristics

Overall, 197 patients with IBD were assessed for eligibility during the study enrolment period (April 2012–September 2013), 43 of whom were excluded (Figure 1). Initially, 154 patients were enrolled in the study at baseline, of whom 129 (84%) completed the 12-month and 110 (71%) completed the 24-month study assessment. Cross-sectional analysis of the cohort at baseline has been previously published (Supplementary Table S1) [17]. Only those patients who underwent repeated measures (n = 129) were included in the primary analysis (Table 1).

In brief, 95 (74%) patients had CD, and 34 (26%) had ulcerative colitis (UC) (Table 1). The median age of the cohort was 31 years (IQR 25–40), with a median IBD disease duration of 7.7 years (IQR 4.5–12.3). The cohort was predominantly Caucasian (n = 121, 94%). Active disease, defined by composite biomarker assessment, was present in 65 patients (50%) at baseline. Prior to enrolment, 38/95 (40%) patients with CD and 1/34 (1%) patient with UC had undergone abdominal surgery. At baseline, 53 (41%) of patients were prescribed biologic therapy, the use of which increased over the study period (59 (54%) patients were prescribed biologic therapy at 24 months, $p = 0.004$). Oral corticosteroid therapy was currently prescribed for 38 (29%) patients, which significantly decreased over time ($p < 0.0001$). Vitamin D levels were low in 52 (40%) of the patients at baseline, 50/52 (96%) of whom were prescribed replacement therapy. Accordingly, there was a significant increase in vitamin D levels over the study period ($p = 0.01$).

3.2. Baseline Body Composition

A detailed cross-sectional analysis of the body composition of this cohort at baseline (n = 137, as enrolled until July 2013) has been previously published [17].

In brief, of those who underwent repeated measures testing (n = 129), the mean BMI at baseline was 26.5 ± 5.1; with 33 (26%) patients classified as overweight and 30 (23%) patients classified as obese (Table 2). Myopenia was evident in 24 (19%) patients, and functional sarcopenia was evident in 12 (9%) patients. Low BMD was prevalent at baseline; with 45 (35%) patients classified as osteopenic and 3 (2%) patients classified as osteoporotic (48 (37%), with either osteopenia or osteoporosis).

3.3. Changes in Body Composition over 24 Months

Anthropometrics. BMI increased over the study period (annual change β = 0.43, 95%CI = [0.18, 0.67], $p = 0.0006$), as did the proportion of patients categorised as overweight and obese (at 24 months 31% overweight and 31% obese) (Table 2, Figure 2). Waist circumference increased over time (β = 1.4, 95%CI = [0.4, 2.3], $p = 0.003$), although no significant change in WHR was observed. Mean BMI, waist circumference, and the proportions of people characterised as overweight or obese, were each numerically higher in the IBD cohort compared to the Australian population stratified by age and gender (Supplementary Table S2).

Table 1. Clinical and Nutritional Characteristics of IBD Cohort over 24 Months.

		Baseline	12 Months	24 Months	Δ *p* Value
Demographics	Patients (*n*, %)	129 (84%)	129 (84%)	110 (71%)	-
	Male (*n*, %)	75 (58%)	75 (58%)	62 (58%)	-
	Age (years) (median, IQR)	31 (25–40)	32 (26–41)	33 (27–42)	-
IBD phenotype	Crohn's disease (*n*, %)	95 (74%)	92 (71%)	79 (72%)	
	Ulcerative colitis (*n*, %)	34 (26%)	37 (29%)	28 (25%)	
	IBD-related abdominal surgery (*n*, %)	39 (30%)	7 (5%)	12 (11%)	-
	IBD-related hospitalisation (*n*, %)	-	22 (17%)	12 (11%)	-
IBD Disease Activity	IBD clinical disease activity score				-
	Crohn's Disease CDAI Mean ± SD	90 ± 99	71 ± 67	65 ± 58	
	Median, IQR	60 (26–126)	62 (26–110)	49 (20–90)	
	Ulcerative colitis partial Mayo mean ± SD	1.5 ± 2.2	1.4 ± 2.2	1.5 ± 1.9	
	Median, IQR	0.5 (0–2)	0 (0–2)	0 (0–4)	
	C-reactive protein (mg/L)				0.40
	Mean ± SD	8.7 ± 21	5.2 ± 11	5.3 ± 8	
	Median, IQR	1.7 (0.5–7.7)	1.9 (0.5–5.8)	1.6 (0.4–6.3)	
	Faecal calprotectin (µg/g)				0.49
	Mean ± SD	247.5 ± 305	155.9 ± 206	179.4 ± 227	
	Median, IQR	84 (20–450)	50 (20–205)	93 (20–245)	
	Composite disease activity assessment § (*n* active disease, %)	65 (50%)	59 (46%)	57 (52%	-
IBD Therapy	Oral corticosteroids ^ Current (*n*, %)	38 (29%)	11 (9%)	7 (6%)	<0.0001 *
	Duration usage (mths) Mean ± SD	28 ± 57			
	Median, IQR	6 (1-24)			
	Biologic therapy overall (*n*, %)	53 (41%)	63 (49%)	59 (54%)	0.0004 *
	Infliximab (*n*, %)	35 (27%)	41 (32%)	35 (32%)	
	Adalimumab (*n*, %)	16 (12%)	19 (15%)	22 (20%)	
	Vedolizumab (*n*, %)	2 (2%)	3 (2%)	2 (2%)	
	5-aminosalicylic acid therapy (*n*, %)	55 (43%)	58 (45%)	53 (48%)	0.18
	Immunomodulator therapy Overall (*n*, %)	73 (57%)	78 (60%)	67 (61%)	0.12
	Azathioprine (*n*, %)	46 (36%)	47 (36%)	41 (37%)	
	Mercaptopurine (*n*, %)	6 (5%)	6 (5%)	5 (5%)	
	Methotrexate (*n*, %)	3 (2%)	5 (3%)	4 (4%)	
	Thiopurine/allopurinol (*n*, %)	18 (14%)	20 (16%)	17 (15%)	

Table 1. *Cont.*

			Baseline	12 Months	24 Months	Δ p Value
Exercise (IPAQ) ¶	Continuous	Mean ± SD	4385 ± 5908	5570 ± 8952	4935 ± 6879	0.36
		Median, IQR	2284 (693–5690)	2106 (862–5745)	2445 (942–5558)	
	Categorical	Inactive	50 (39%)	47 (36%)	37 (34%)	
		Minimally active	30 (23%)	24 (19%)	23 (21%)	
		Active	28 (22%)	41 (32%)	35 (32%)	
Nutritional assessment	Albumin (g/dL)	Mean ± SD	40 ± 4.6	40 ± 3.8	40 ± 3.5	0.64
		Median, IQR	40 (37–43)	40 (37–42)	40 (38–42)	
	Haemoglobin (g/L)	Mean ± SD	141 ± 15	141 ± 14	143 ± 13	0.07
		Median, IQR	141 (132–150)	141 (130–149)	144 (136–152)	
	Ferritin (ng/mL)	Mean ± SD	87 ± 85	93 ± 122	115 ± 186	0.09
		Median, IQR	62 (34–106)	63 (35–104)	71 (42–123)	
		Calcium Mean ± SD	2.35 ± 0.11	2.34 ± 0.1	2.34 ± 0.09	0.16
		Median, IQR	2.35 (2.28–2.42)	2.36 (2.29–2.4)	2.34 (2.30–2.4)	
	Vitamin D (nmol/mL) #	Mean ± SD	64 ± 28	65 ± 25	70 ± 25	0.01 *
		Median, IQR	63 (41–84)	65 (48–80)	67 (53–85)	
		Low Vitamin D level	52 (40%)	40 (31%)	38 (35%)	
		Vitamin D supplementation	50 (39%)	40 (31%)	37 (34%)	
		Bisphosphonate therapy	2 (1%)	4 (3%)	4 (4%)	

Analysis performed using linear and logistic mixed effects regressions. Data presented as mean ± standard deviation (SD), median (interquartile range (IQR)), counts and percentage. CDAI, Crohn's Disease Activity Index; § C-reactive protein (CRP) ≥5 mg/L and/or faecal calprotectin (FC) ≥100 μg/g were considered consistent with active disease as a composite biomarker assessment. ^ Cumulative months equivalent to prednisolone ≥10 mg daily. ¶ International Physical Activity Questionnaire (Short). # Low Vitamin D level classified as <50 nmol/L, Vitamin D supplementation (≥1000 IU/day), * significant p value < 0.05.

Table 2. Body composition in IBD patients over 24 months.

Body Composition			Baseline (n = 129)	Year 1 (n = 129)	Year 2 (n = 110)	p Value
	Body mass index (BMI)	Mean ± SD (kg/m^2)	26.5 ± 5.1	27.4 ± 5.8	27.7 ± 5.6	0.0006 *
	Δ ± SD		-	0.52 ± 2.51	0.84 ± 2.66	
	Median (IQR)		25.1 (22.9–29.7)	26.5 (23.2–30.7)	26.8 (23.8–30.8)	
	BMI categorical ¶	Underweight < 18.5	4 (3%)	3 (2%)	3 (3%)	0.0006 *
	Normal 18.5–25		58 (45%)	47 (36%)	38 (35%)	
	Overweight 25–30		33 (26%)	38 (29%)	34 (31%)	
	Obese ≥ 30		30 (23%)	35 (27%)	34 (31%)	
Anthropometric assessment	Waist circumference (cm)	Mean ± SD	90.8 ± 15.9	92.4 ± 14.5	94.1 ± 14.4	0.003 *
	Δ ± SD		-	0.73 ± 10.32	2.26 ± 9.18	
	Median (IQR)		88 (80–101)	91 (81–102)	93 (83–103)	
	Waist:hip ratio	Mean ± SD	0.88 ± 0.11	0.88 ± 0.10	0.89 ± 0.10	0.31
	Δ ± SD		-	−0.004 ± 0.11	0.01 ± 0.12	
	Median (IQR)		0.86 (0.81–0.95)	0.87 (0.82–0.92)	0.89 (0.83–0.94)	
	Grip strength (PSI)	Mean ± SD	40.2 ± 12.0	39.5 ± 12.2	39.8 ± 12.4	0.68
	Δ ± SD		-	−0.48 ± 5.56	−0.30 ± 5.01	
	Median (IQR)		37.8 (30.0–50.0)	38.0 (29.0–49.3)	37.4 (31.1–49.1)	
	Grip strength z-score	Mean ± SD	−0.63 ± 1.30	−0.9 ± 1.49	−0.67 ± 1.23	0.46
	Δ ± SD		-	−0.27 ± 1.55	−0.01 ± 1.27	
	Median (IQR)		−0.48 (−1.29–0.15)	−0.75 (−1.41–0.12)	−0.6 (−1.32–0.15)	
Fat mass index (FMI) (kg/height m^2)	FMI (kg/m^2)	Mean ± SD	8.83 ± 4.57	9.07 ± 4.50	9.64 ± 4.59	0.0007 *
	Δ ± SD		-	0.26 ± 1.54	0.70 ± 2.05	
	Median (IQR)		7.67 (5.67–10.60)	8.09 (6.07–11.32)	8.61 (5.82–11.81)	
	FMI z-score	Mean ± SD	0.24 ± 1.26	0.30 ± 1.26	0.42 ± 1.24	0.006 *
	Δ ± SD		-	0.06 ± 0.48	0.17 ± 0.61	
	Median (IQR)		−0.13 (−0.59–0.93)	0.08 (−0.57–0.89)	0.25 (−0.47–1.15)	
Visceral adipose tissue (VAT)	VAT volume (cm^3)	Mean ± SD	834.2 ± 821.7	903.9 ± 901.6	949.9 ± 826.7	0.01 *
	Δ ± SD		-	67.8 ± 331.8	102.1 ± 376.6	
	Median (IQR)		493.7 (216.9, 1175.9)	600.5 (248.8, 1291)	702.1 (266.6–1354)	
	VAT (grams) ^	Mean ± SD	786.9 ± 775.2	852.76 ± 850.53	896.09 ± 779.94	0.01 *
	Δ ± SD		-	64.0 ± 313.0	96.3 ± 355.3	
	Median (IQR)		465.74 (204.59–1109.38)	566.51 (241.63–1209.85)	662.35 (256.23–1274.44)	
	VAT:SAT ^	Mean ± SD	0.64 ± 0.68	0.64 ± 0.55	0.63 ± 0.49	0.36
	Δ ± SD		-	−0.005 ± 0.50	0.026 ± 0.585	
	Median (IQR)		0.45 (0.24–0.8)	0.46 (0.31–0.83)	0.49 (0.28–0.89)	

Table 2. *Cont.*

Body Composition			Baseline (n = 129)	Year 1 (n = 129)	Year 2 (n = 110)	p Value
Visceral adipose tissue (VAT)	VHI ^	Mean ± SD	0.26 ± 0.25	0.28 ± 0.28	0.3 ± 0.25	0.01 *
	Δ ± SD		-	0.022 ± 0.10	0.127 ± 0.604	
	Median (IQR)		0.15 (0.07–0.35)	0.2 (0.08–0.41)	0.23 (0.1–0.41)	
Bone mineral density (BMD)	WHO *t*-score femur	Mean ± SD	−0.18 ± 1.02	−0.1 ± 1.03	−0.13 ± 1.03	0.001 *
	Δ ± SD		-	0.075 ± 0.191	0.081 ±0.266	
	Median (IQR)		−0.21 (−0.96–0.52)	−0.20 (−0.99–0.55)	−0.17 (−0.97–0.69)	
	WHO *t*-score spine	Mean ± SD	−0.35 ± 1.1	−0.29 ± 1.11	−0.38 ± 1.17	0.47
	Δ ± SD		-	0.033 ± 0.34	0.027 ± 0.357	
	Median (IQR)		−0.48 (−1.06–0.4)	−0.37 (−1.05–0.39)	−0.36 (−1.21–0.33)	
	WHO *z*-score femur	Mean ± SD	−0.16 ± 1.06	−0.11 ± 1.03	−0.19 ± 0.93	0.86
	Δ ± SD		-	0.049 ± 0.31	0.007 ± 0.52	
	Median (IQR)		−0.24 (−0.93–0.46)	−0.14 (−0.90–0.51)	−0.12 (−0.91–0.48)	
	WHO *z*-score spine	Mean ± SD	−0.46 ± 1.08	−0.47 ± 1.09	−0.62 ± 1.14	0.51
	Δ ± SD		-	0.004 ± 0.385	−0.025 ± 0.41	
	Median (IQR)		−0.52 (−1.19–0.29)	−0.52 (−1.22–0.23)	−0.58 (−1.4–0.18)	
	Bone status #	Osteopenia (n, %)	45 (35%)	41 (32%)	37 (34%)	0.23
	Osteoporosis (n, %)		3 (2%)	2 (2%)	3 (3%)	
	Overall osteopenia/porosis (n, %)		48 (37%)	43 (34%)	40 (37%)	
Appendicular skeletal muscle index (ASMI) (kg/height m^2)	ASMI (kg/m^2)	Mean ± SD	7.76 ± 1.40	7.80 ± 1.45	7.68 ± 1.40	0.01 *
	Δ ± SD		-	0.014 ± 0.49	−0.127 ± 0.55	
	Median (IQR)		7.60 (6.57–8.48)	7.84 (6.74–8.62)	7.64 (6.66–8.45)	
	ASMI *z*-score	Mean ± SD	−0.21 ± 0.96	−0.21 ± 0.98	−0.32 ± 0.99	0.002 *
	Δ ± SD		-	−0.006 ± 0.392	−0.0129 ± 0.444	
	Median (IQR)		−0.31 (−0.95–0.17)	−0.3 (−0.88–0.24)	−0.45 (−0.93–0.29)	
	Myopenia (Low ASMI §)		24 (19%)	25 (19%)	25 (23%)	0.01 *
	Functional sarcopenia (Low ASMI AND low grip strength §)		12 (9%)	21 (16%)	17 (15%)	0.05

Table Legend: Reported are baseline distributions and change from baseline at 12 months and 24 months. Statistical analysis performed using linear and logistic mixed effects regressions. Data presented as mean ± standard deviation, median (interquartile range), counts, and percentage. SD, standard deviation; ^ Data log-transformed prior to analysis: ^ VAT, visceral adipose tissue; ^ VAT:SAT, visceral adipose tissue: subcutaneous adipose tissue ratio; VHI, visceral adipose tissue area (cm^3) divided by height (m^2); § Low appendicular skeletal muscle index (ASMI) and grip strength defined as ≥1 standard deviation below mean. Δ, mean difference from baseline at Year 1 and Year 2 (±standard deviation). # BMI categories and bone status according to World Health Organisation criteria; * significant p value < 0.05.

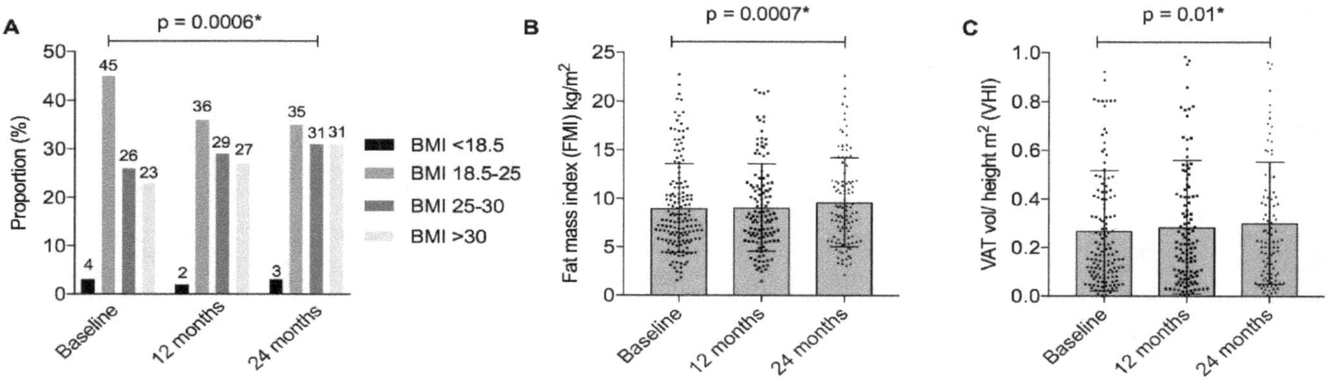

Figure 2. BMI and measures of adiposity in patients with IBD over 24 months. **Figure Legend:** (**A**) Body mass index (BMI) categories according to World Health Organisation criteria; (**B**) Fat mass index (kg/height m^2). Mean and standard deviation presented; (**C**) Visceral adipose tissue (VAT) height index (VAT volume cm^3 /height m^2). Mean and standard deviation presented. * $p < 0.05$, denoting statistical significance.

Adiposity. FMI increased significantly over the study period ($\beta = 0.33$, 95%CI = [0.14, 0.53], $p = 0.0007$), with a concordant increase in FMI *z*-score ($\beta = 0.08$, 95%CI = [0.02, 0.14], $p = 0.006$). (Table 2, Figures 2 and 3) Similarly, VAT volume increased ($\beta = 0.08$, 95%CI = [0.02, 0.14], $p = 0.01$), which resulted in an increase in VHI ($\beta = 0.08$, 95%CI = [0.02, 0.13], $p = 0.01$), but not VAT:SAT ($\beta = 0.027$, 95%CI = [−0.032, 0.087], $p = 0.36$) (Table 2).

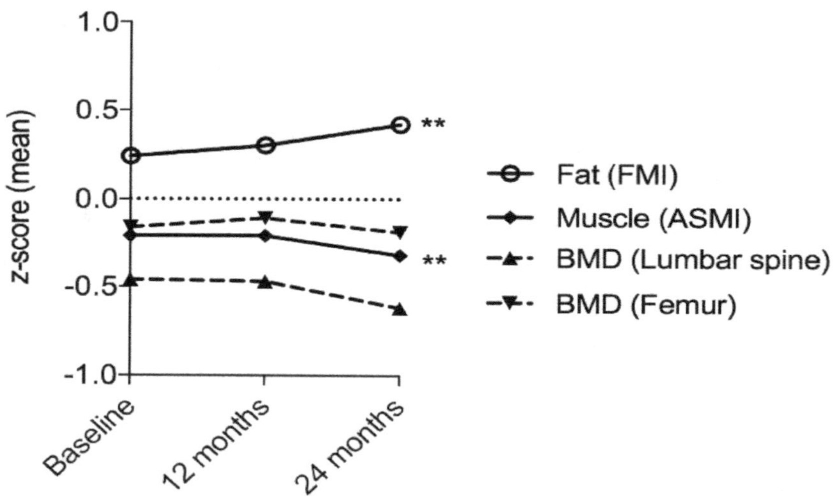

Figure 3. Changes in bone, muscle, and fat in patients with IBD over 24 months. **Figure Legend:** Summary of mean *z*-scores for fat mass index (FMI), appendicular skeletal muscle mass index (ASMI), and bone mineral density (BMD), at the femur and lumbar spine. ** $p < 0.01$, denoting statistical significance.

Muscle. ASMI decreased significantly over the study period (ASMI $\beta = -0.07$, 95%CI = [−0.12, −0.01], $p = 0.01$; ASMI *z*-score $\beta = -0.07$, 95%CI = [−0.11, −0.02], $p = 0.002$) (Table 2). There was a significant increase in myopenia over the study period (19%, 19%, and 24% at 0 months, 12 months, and 24 months, respectively; OR = 3.1 95%CI = [1.2, 7.7]; $p = 0.01$) (Figure 4). There was a trend towards an increase in the proportion of patients classified as sarcopenic; however, this did not reach statistical significance (OR = 2.4, 95%CI = [1.0, 6.0]; $p = 0.05$).

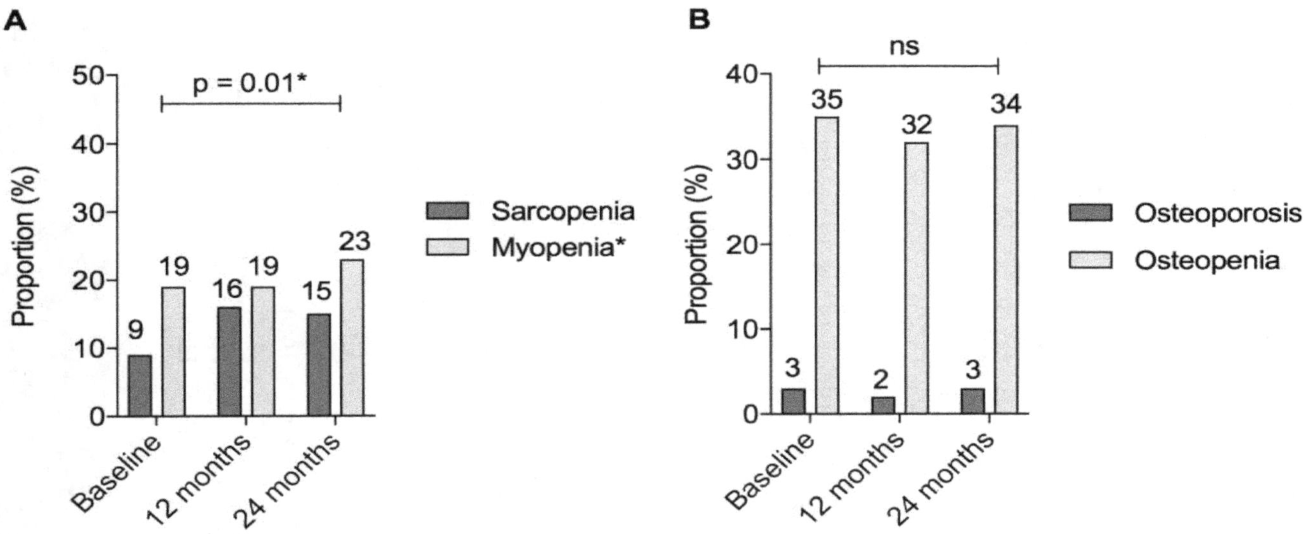

Figure 4. Myopenia, sarcopenia, and metabolic bone disease in patients with IBD over 24 months. **Figure Legend:** (**A**) Sarcopenia defined as BOTH appendicular skeletal muscle index (ASMI) and grip strength <1 standard deviation below gender and age-matched mean. Myopenia defined as appendicular skeletal muscle index (ASMI) <1 standard deviation below gender and age-matched mean; (**B**) osteopenia and osteoporosis according to World Health Organisation criteria. Osteopenia defined as bone mineral density (BMD) 1–2.5 standard deviations and osteoporosis as ≥2.5 standard deviations below the young adult mean. * $p < 0.05$, denoting statistical significance; ns, non-significant p value > 0.05.

Bone. Femur BMD t-score increased significantly over the study period, but there was no change in lumbar spine BMD t-score (β = 0.041, 95%CI = [0.016, 0.066], $p = 0.001$; β = 0.013, 95%CI = [−0.022, 0.048], $p = 0.47$, respectively). No difference in BMD z-scores at either site was detected over time (Table 2). Overall, there was no significant change in the proportion of patients classified with osteopenia 37/110 (34%) or osteoporosis 3/110 (3%) ($p = 0.23$), despite the proactive management of bone health over the study period (Figure 4).

3.4. Clinical Associations with Serial BMI Measurements

BMI was positively associated with vitamin D levels (β = 0.006, 95%CI = [0.00, 0.0.11], $p = 0.03$). FMI, ASMI, and grip strength were also positively associated with BMI over time (β = 1.0, 95%CI = [1.0, 1.1], $p < 0.0001$; β = 1.3, 95%CI = [1.1, 1.5], $p < 0.0001$; β = 0.028, 95%CI = [0.008, 0.049], $p = 0.006$, respectively) (Table 3).

3.5. Clinical Associations with Serial FM and VAT Measurements

Older age was positively associated with VHI (β = 0.040, 95%CI = [0.023, 0.057], $p < 0.0001$) (Supplementary Tables S3 and S4). Male gender was positively associated with VHI, but negatively associated with FMI (β = 0.67, 95%CI = [0.39, 0.95], $p < 0.0001$; β = −2.2, 95%CI = [−2.8, −1.6], $p < 0.0001$, respectively). Serum vitamin D was negatively associated with FMI (β = −0.007, 95%CI = [−0.013, −0.001], $p = 0.02$, $p = 0.02$).

Anthropometric measures (BMI and waist circumference) were associated with a higher FMI (β = 0.52, 95%CI = [0.45, 0.59], $p < 0.0001$; β = 0.07, 95%CI = [0.04, 0.10], $p < 0.0001$, respectively) and VHI (β = 0.08, 95%CI = [0.06, 0.11], $p < 0.0001$; β = 0.015, 95%CI = [0.005, 0.026], $p = 0.003$ respectively). In contrast, grip strength was negatively associated with FMI (β = −0.044, 95%CI = [−0.066, −0.021], $p < 0.0001$).

Table 3. Clinical associations with serial body mass index (BMI) measurements over 24 months.

Variable		Univariable Est. (95%CI)	Univariable *p* Value	Full Multivariable Model Est. (95%CI)	Full Multivariable Model *p* Value
Time	Repeated measures over 24 m	0.43 [0.21, 0.65]	<0.0001	0.08 [−0.08, 0.24]	0.28
Demographics	Age at study entry	0.24 [0.15, 0.33]	<0.0001	0.021 [−0.004, 0.046]	0.08
	Gender (Male vs. female)	0.0 [−2.0, 2.0]	0.99	0.38 [−0.18, 0.95]	0.17
IBD-related factors	IBD phenotype (Ulcerative colitis vs. Crohn's disease)	−0.7 [−2.9, 1.5]	0.52	−0.04 [−0.46, 0.38]	0.86
	IBD disease duration	0.014 [0.005, 0.022]	0.002	0.0003 [−0.0020, 0.0026]	0.78
	Faecal calprotectin (μg/g)	−0.0015 [−0.0025, 0.004]	0.007	0.00021 [−0.00044, 0.00086]	0.48
	C-reactive protein (mg/L)	−0.011 [−0.027, 0.006]	0.19	0.001 [−0.009, 0.011]	0.85
	Current corticosteroid use	−0.4 [−1.0, 0.2]	0.22	−0.10 [−0.49, 0.29]	0.55
	Biologic therapy	0.25 [−0.31, 0.81]	0.38	0.04 [−0.18, 0.25]	0.69
	Immunomodulator therapy	0.42 [−0.03, 0.88]	0.06	0.11 [−0.02, 0.23]	0.08
Lifestyle and nutritional factors	Smoking status				
	Current vs. never	0.8 [−1.9, 3.4]	0.23	−0.24 [−0.75, 0.28]	0.07
	Ex vs. never	2.0 [−0.4, 4.4]		0.34 [−0.11, 0.78]	
	Excess alcohol intake ^	0.2 [−4.9, 5.3]	0.95	0.8 [−0.1, 1.8]	0.06
	Vitamin D level (nmol/mL)	0.006 [−0.005, 0.017]	0.25	0.006 [0.000, 0.011]	0.03
	Habitual exercise (IPAQ score, continuous) §	0.002 [−0.036, 0.041]	0.91	0.009 [−0.011, 0.029]	0.36
	Albumin (g/dL)	0.06 [−0.02, 0.13]	0.16	0.008 [−0.034, 0.049]	0.76
Body composition factors	Fat mass index (FMI)	1.1 [1.0, 1.2]	<0.0001	1.0 [1.0, 1.1]	<0.0001
	Appendicular skeletal muscle index (ASMI)	2.1 [1.8, 2.5]	<0.0001	1.3 [1.1, 1.5]	<0.0001
	Functional sarcopenia ¶	−1.5 [−2.5, −0.4]	0.0006	0.11 [−0.41, 0.62]	0.65
	Grip strength (pounds per square inch, PSI)	0.024 [−0.024, 0.072]	0.32	0.028 [0.008, 0.049]	0.006

^ Data log-transformed prior to analysis: ^ VAT, visceral adipose tissue; ^ VAT:SAT, visceral adipose tissue: subcutaneous adipose tissue ratio; VHI, visceral adipose tissue area (cm^3) divided by height (m^2); ¶ Low ASMI and grip strength ≥1 standard deviation below mean. ^ Excess alcohol use defined according to the Australian Healthy Drinking Guidelines; § IPAQ, International Physical Active Questionnaire; FMI, fat mass index (kg/height m^2); ASMI, appendicular skeletal muscle index (kg/height m^2); Linear mixed effects regression models with missing data imputed with cohort means.

3.6. Clinical Associations with Serial ASMI Measurements

Male gender was associated with a higher ASMI ($\beta = 1.2$, 95%CI = [0.9, 1.4], $p < 0.0001$) (Supplementary Table S5). FC was negatively associated with ASMI ($\beta = -0.00043$, 95%CI = [−0.00067, −0.00018], $p = 0.0004$), whereas anthropometric measures, BMI, and grip strength were positively associated with ASMI ($\beta = 0.13$, 95%CI = [0.11, 0.15], $p < 0.0001$; $\beta = 0.020$, 95%CI = [0.011, 0.028], $p < 0.0001$, respectively).

3.7. Clinical Associations with Serial BMD Measurements

IBD disease duration was negatively associated with lumbar spine *t*-score ($\beta = 0.0031$, 95%CI = [−0.0057, −0.0005], $p = 0.01$), as was grip strength ($\beta = 0.009$, 95%CI = [0.002, 0.017], $p = 0.01$) (Supplementary Table S6). Both biologic therapy and corticosteroids (cumulative use) were associated with increase lumbar spine *t*-scores ($\beta = 0.08$, 95%CI = [0.01, 0.16], $p = 0.02$; $\beta = 0.10$, 95%CI = [0.01, 0.18], $p = 0.02$; respectively). *Neither IBD phenotype nor vitamin D level was associated with changes in the* lumbar spine *t*-score.

4. Discussion

This prospective study has demonstrated persistent and progressive disturbances in body composition in people with IBD over a relatively short time frame. The most striking finding was a significant increase in the proportion of patients classified as overweight and obese, driven by gains in adiposity. Conversely, muscle mass decreased, with a concordant rise in rates of myopenia. Despite the proactive management of bone health, rates of osteopenia remained high and unchanged. Abnormal body composition may go frequently unrecognised in clinical practice using BMI alone, leaving patients with IBD at risk of potentially avoidable morbidity.

After 24 months of follow-up, 62% of patients with IBD were overweight or obese despite a median age of just 33 years, which is numerically higher than age and gender- matched Australian population data [35]. Earlier studies of obesity in IBD have failed to take into account direct measures of adiposity [3,10]. This study demonstrates that gains in BMI were associated with significant increases in both overall FM and VAT. VAT is a strong independent predictor of incident cardiovascular disease after adjustment for clinical risk factors, including BMI [39,40]. Similar to to other chronic inflammatory conditions, there is emerging evidence to suggest that patients with IBD are at increased risk of cardiovascular disease, which is now recognised as a prime cause of morbidity in this young demographic [2,41].

How can a link between IBD and obesity be explained? In contrast to retrospective reports, we found no association between measures of adiposity and IBD phenotype, inflammatory burden, or medications over time [3,6–10]. The lack of correlation between obesity and IBD therapy, in particular cumulative corticosteroid use is surprising, yet may be in part accounted for by the significant decrease in rates of corticosteroid use over the study period. Interestingly, serum vitamin D levels were negatively associated with FMI, which may be related to the sequestration of vitamin D in adipose tissue, coupled with lifestyle factors associated with obesity (less outdoor activity) [42]. The majority of patients were classified as either inactive or minimally active, which is likely reflective of the burden of chronic illness in this cohort, yet this was not shown to be associated with BMI. It is possible that dysbiosis in IBD, which is characterised by reduced microbial diversity and an altered microbial metabolic profile, is a predisposing factor to obesity [43–45], but this is speculation despite gut metabolomic associations with post-prandial glucose [43–46].

While adiposity increased, muscle mass (ASMI) decreased. FC, as a measure of luminal inflammation in IBD, was negatively associated with ASMI, which is consistent with the known catabolic effects of chronic inflammation [18,20,47]. Lean mass is important in patients with IBD, and has been shown to have a bearing on response to therapy, surgical outcomes, and quality of life [15,18,20,48,49]. Grip strength proved to be a simple anthropometric test that was independently and positively associated with ASMI, while also negatively associated with FMI.

IBD disease duration was shown to be negatively associated with BMD; however, inflammation was not associated with BMD over time, which is consistent with existing data showing a minimal impact of IBD-related inflammation on longitudinal bone loss [21,23,25,26,50]. Likewise, vitamin D levels were not associated with BMD, which is similar to other studies showing an uncertain benefit of vitamin D supplementation on BMD in IBD patients [21,23,25,26,50]. Biologic therapy was found to be positively associated with BMD over time, which is in line with current data [50,51]. The positive association between corticosteroid use and BMD is surprising, and may be a spurious result due to multiple comparisons. *Nevertheless, rates of osteopenia remained high in this cohort, despite not only protocolised management of bone health, but also a warm climate and readily accessible dairy products.*

The limitations of this study are the relatively small sample size, which may have limited statistical power. The study was neither structured nor powered to evaluate the influence of body composition on hospitalisation or surgery over time, nor could it evaluate the impact of these factors on body composition. It did not account for dietary intake, nor were other factors associated with cardiometabolic risk measured (cholesterol, family history, blood pressure). Although a control group was not included, the findings were compared to population-based data [35]. The predominantly Caucasian cohort, which was derived from a single tertiary IBD referral centre, may also limit the generalisability of the findings. On the other hand, it is the first prospective study that has incorporated serial measures of body composition in IBD. Furthermore, DXA, in routine use for measuring BMD, is an affordable tool for monitoring body composition, adding little to the time or radiation of the test [21,33].

This study illustrates the rising rates of obesity in patents with IBD over time, driven by gains in fat mass, while lean mass decreases and metabolic bone disease remains unchanged. Apart from raising concerns about the cardiometabolic risk profile of patients with IBD, it is important that clinicians recognise that an increase in BMI may obscure a decrease in muscle mass (myopenia). The study provides a rationale for measuring body composition, as well as a means to do so with DXA, and supports recommendations for the use of grip strength as a discriminatory anthropometric test in clinical practice.

Supplementary Materials: Supplementary Table S1: Baseline clinical and nutritional characteristics of IBD Cohort; Supplementary Table S2: Body mass index and waist circumference by age as compared to data from the Australian Bureau of Statistic National Health Survey First Results 2014, 2015; Supplementary Table S3: Clinical associations with serial visceral adipose tissue (VHI)^ measurements over 24 months; Supplementary Table S4: Clinical associations with serial fat mass index (FMI) measurements over 24 months; Supplementary Table S5: Clinical associations with serial appendicular skeletal muscle index (ASMI) measurements over 24 months; Supplementary Table S6: Clinical associations with serial bone mineral density measurements (lumbar spine *t*-score) over 24 months.

Author Contributions: R.V.B.: C.G.S., F.D.B., S.P.L.T. and J.M.A. were involved in the conception and design of the project. R.V.B., C.G.S., S.O., C.G., S.N.S., A.D.V., A.L., F.D.B., and J.M.A. were involved in data acquisition and management. All authors were involved in analysis and interpretation of research data, and drafting and revision of the article. All authors approved the final version of the manuscript.

Acknowledgments: Thank you to the Royal Adelaide Hospital IBD Nurses, Rachel Grafton and Julie Hughes for their assistance of this project. Thank you to the Royal Adelaide Hospital, Hospital Research Foundation for providing the salary scholarship to R.V.B. (AR Clarkson Award) during 2016.

References

1. Bryant, R.V.; Trott, M.J.; Bartholomeusz, F.D.; Andrews, J.M. Systematic review: Body composition in adults with inflammatory bowel disease. *Aliment. Pharmacol. Ther.* **2013**, *38*, 213–225. [CrossRef] [PubMed]
2. Kirchgesner, J.; Beaugerie, L.; Carrat, F.; Andersen, N.N.; Jess, T.; Schwarzinger, M. Increased risk of acute arterial events in young patients and severely active IBD: A nationwide French cohort study. *Gut* **2017**. [CrossRef] [PubMed]
3. Singh, S.; Dulai, P.S.; Zarrinpar, A.; Ramamoorthy, S.; Sandborn, W.J. Obesity in IBD: Epidemiology, pathogenesis, disease course and treatment outcomes. *Nat. Rev. Gastroenterol. Hepatol.* **2017**, *14*, 110–121. [CrossRef] [PubMed]

4. Winer, D.A.; Luck, H.; Tsai, S.; Winer, S. The intestinal immune system in obesity and insulin resistance. *Cell Metab.* **2016**, *23*, 413–426. [CrossRef] [PubMed]
5. Karmiris, K.; Koutroubakis, I.E.; Xidakis, C.; Polychronaki, M.; Voudouri, T.; Kouroumalis, E.A. Circulating levels of leptin, adiponectin, resistin, and ghrelin in inflammatory bowel disease. *Inflamm. Bowel Dis.* **2006**, *12*, 100–105. [CrossRef] [PubMed]
6. Fink, C.; Karagiannides, I.; Bakirtzi, K.; Pothoulakis, C. Adipose tissue and inflammatory bowel disease pathogenesis. *Inflamm. Bowel Dis.* **2012**, *18*, 1550–1557. [CrossRef] [PubMed]
7. Flores, A.; Burstein, E.; Cipher, D.J.; Feagins, L.A. Obesity in inflammatory bowel disease: A marker of less severe disease. *Dig. Dis. Sci.* **2015**, *60*, 2436–2445. [CrossRef] [PubMed]
8. Seminerio, J.L.; Koutroubakis, I.E.; Ramos-Rivers, C.; Hashash, J.G.; Dudekula, A.; Regueiro, M.; Baidoo, L.; Barrie, A.; Swoger, J.; Schwartz, M.; et al. Impact of obesity on the management and clinical course of patients with inflammatory bowel disease. *Inflamm. Bowel Dis.* **2015**, *21*, 2857–2863. [CrossRef] [PubMed]
9. Hass, D.J.; Brensinger, C.M.; Lewis, J.D.; Lichtenstein, G.R. The impact of increased body mass index on the clinical course of crohn's disease. *Clin. Gastroenterol. Hepatol. Off. Clin. Pract. J. Am. Gastroenterol. Assoc.* **2006**, *4*, 482–488. [CrossRef] [PubMed]
10. Chan, S.S.; Luben, R.; Olsen, A.; Tjonneland, A.; Kaaks, R.; Teucher, B.; Lindgren, S.; Grip, O.; Key, T.; Crowe, F.L.; et al. Body mass index and the risk for crohn's disease and ulcerative colitis: Data from a european prospective cohort study (the IBD in EPIC study). *Am. J. Gastroenterol.* **2013**, *108*, 575–582. [CrossRef] [PubMed]
11. Buning, C.; von Kraft, C.; Hermsdorf, M.; Gentz, E.; Wirth, E.K.; Valentini, L.; Haas, V. Visceral adipose tissue in patients with crohn's disease correlates with disease activity, inflammatory markers, and outcome. *Inflamm. Bowel Dis.* **2015**, *21*, 2590–2597. [CrossRef] [PubMed]
12. Erhayiem, B.; Dhingsa, R.; Hawkey, C.J.; Subramanian, V. Ratio of visceral to subcutaneous fat area is a biomarker of complicated crohn's disease. *Clin. Gastroenterol. Hepatol. Off. Clin. Pract. J. Am. Gastroenterol. Assoc.* **2011**, *9*, 684–687.e681.[CrossRef] [PubMed]
13. Holt, D.Q.; Moore, G.T.; Strauss, B.J.; Hamilton, A.L.; De Cruz, P.; Kamm, M.A. Visceral adiposity predicts post-operative crohn's disease recurrence. *Aliment. Pharmacol. Ther.* **2017**, *45*, 1255–1264. [CrossRef] [PubMed]
14. Liu, G.; Wu, X.; Li, Y.; Rui, Y.; Stocchi, L.; Remzi, F.H.; Shen, B. Postoperative excessive gain in visceral adipose tissue as well as body mass index are associated with adverse outcomes of an ileal pouch. *Gastroenterol. Rep.* **2016**, *5*, 29–35. [CrossRef] [PubMed]
15. Van Langenberg, D.R.; Gatta, P.D.; Hill, B.; Zacharewicz, E.; Gibson, P.R.; Russell, A.P. Delving into disability in crohn's disease: Dysregulation of molecular pathways may explain skeletal muscle loss in crohn's disease. *J. Crohn Colitis* **2013**, *8*, 626–634. [CrossRef] [PubMed]
16. Schneider, S.M.; Al-Jaouni, R.; Filippi, J.; Wiroth, J.B.; Zeanandin, G.; Arab, K.; Hebuterne, X. Sarcopenia is prevalent in patients with crohn's disease in clinical remission. *Inflamm. Bowel Dis.* **2008**, *14*, 1562–1568. [CrossRef] [PubMed]
17. Bryant, R.V.; Ooi, S.; Schultz, C.G.; Goess, C.; Grafton, R.; Hughes, J.; Lim, A.; Bartholomeusz, F.D.; Andrews, J.M. Low muscle mass and sarcopenia: Common and predictive of osteopenia in inflammatory bowel disease. *Aliment. Pharmacol. Ther.* **2015**, *41*, 895–906. [CrossRef] [PubMed]
18. Adams, D.W.; Gurwara, S.; Silver, H.J.; Horst, S.N.; Beaulieu, D.B.; Schwartz, D.A.; Seidner, D.L. Sarcopenia is common in overweight patients with inflammatory bowel disease and may predict need for surgery. *Inflamm. Bowel Dis.* **2017**, *23*, 1182–1186. [CrossRef] [PubMed]
19. Pedersen, M.; Cromwell, J.; Nau, P. Sarcopenia is a predictor of surgical morbidity in inflammatory bowel disease. *Inflamm. Bowel Dis.* **2017**, *23*, 1867–1872. [CrossRef] [PubMed]
20. Bamba, S.; Sasaki, M.; Takaoka, A.; Takahashi, K.; Imaeda, H.; Nishida, A.; Inatomi, O.; Sugimoto, M.; Andoh, A. Sarcopenia is a predictive factor for intestinal resection in admitted patients with crohn's disease. *PLoS ONE* **2017**, *12*, e0180036. [CrossRef] [PubMed]
21. Harbord, M.; Annese, V.; Vavricka, S.R.; Allez, M.; Barreiro-de Acosta, M.; Boberg, K.M.; Burisch, J.; De Vos, M.; De Vries, A.M.; Dick, A.D.; et al. The first european evidence-based consensus on extra-intestinal manifestations in inflammatory bowel disease. *J. Crohn Colitis* **2016**, *10*, 239–254. [CrossRef] [PubMed]
22. Targownik, L.E.; Bernstein, C.N.; Nugent, Z.; Johansson, H.; Oden, A.; McCloskey, E.; Kanis, J.A.; Leslie, W.D. Inflammatory bowel disease and the risk of fracture after controlling for frax. *J. Bone Miner. Res.* **2013**, *28*, 1007–1013. [CrossRef] [PubMed]

23. Targownik, L.E.; Bernstein, C.N.; Nugent, Z.; Leslie, W.D. Inflammatory bowel disease has a small effect on bone mineral density and risk for osteoporosis. *Clin. Gastroenterol. Hepatol. Off. Clin. Pract. J. Am. Gastroenterol. Assoc.* **2013**, *11*, 278–285. [CrossRef] [PubMed]
24. Bernstein, C.N.; Blanchard, J.F.; Leslie, W.; Wajda, A.; Yu, B.N. The incidence of fracture among patients with inflammatory bowel disease. A population-based cohort study. *Ann. Intern. Med.* **2000**, *133*, 795–799. [CrossRef] [PubMed]
25. Casals-Seoane, F.; Chaparro, M.; Mate, J.; Gisbert, J.P. Clinical course of bone metabolism disorders in patients with inflammatory bowel disease: A 5-year prospective study. *Inflamm. Bowel Dis.* **2016**, *22*, 1929–1936. [CrossRef] [PubMed]
26. Targownik, L.E.; Leslie, W.D.; Carr, R.; Clara, I.; Miller, N.; Rogala, L.; Graff, L.A.; Walker, J.R.; Bernstein, C.N. Longitudinal change in bone mineral density in a population-based cohort of patients with inflammatory bowel disease. *Calcif. Tissue Int.* **2012**, *91*, 356–363. [CrossRef] [PubMed]
27. Tosato, M.; Marzetti, E.; Cesari, M.; Savera, G.; Miller, R.R.; Bernabei, R.; Landi, F.; Calvani, R. Measurement of muscle mass in sarcopenia: From imaging to biochemical markers. *Aging Clin. Exp. Res.* **2017**, *29*, 19–27. [CrossRef] [PubMed]
28. Satsangi, J.; Silverberg, M.S.; Vermeire, S.; Colombel, J.F. The montreal classification of inflammatory bowel disease: Controversies, consensus, and implications. *Gut* **2006**, *55*, 749–753. [CrossRef] [PubMed]
29. Ainsworth, B.E.; Macera, C.A.; Jones, D.A.; Reis, J.P.; Addy, C.L.; Bowles, H.R.; Kohl, H.W. Comparison of the 2001 BRFSS and the IPAQ physical activity questionnaires. *Med. Sci. Sports Exerc.* **2006**, *38*, 1584–1592. [CrossRef] [PubMed]
30. Hans, D.B.; Shepherd, J.A.; Schwartz, E.N.; Reid, D.M.; Blake, G.M.; Fordham, J.N.; Fuerst, T.; Hadji, P.; Itabashi, A.; Krieg, M.A.; et al. Peripheral dual-energy X-ray absorptiometry in the management of osteoporosis: The 2007 ISCD official positions. *J. Clin. Densitom. Off. J. Int. Soc. Clin. Densitom.* **2008**, *11*, 188–206. [CrossRef] [PubMed]
31. Cruz-Jentoft, A.J.; Baeyens, J.P.; Bauer, J.M.; Boirie, Y.; Cederholm, T.; Landi, F.; Martin, F.C.; Michel, J.P.; Rolland, Y.; Schneider, S.M.; et al. Sarcopenia: European consensus on definition and diagnosis: Report of the european working group on sarcopenia in older people. *Age Ageing* **2010**, *39*, 412–423. [CrossRef] [PubMed]
32. Kelly, T.L.; Wilson, K.E.; Heymsfield, S.B. Dual energy X-ray absorptiometry body composition reference values from NHANES. *PLoS ONE* **2009**, *4*, e7038. [CrossRef] [PubMed]
33. Kaul, S.; Rothney, M.P.; Peters, D.M.; Wacker, W.K.; Davis, C.E.; Shapiro, M.D.; Ergun, D.L. Dual-energy X-ray absorptiometry for quantification of visceral fat. *Obesity* **2012**, *20*, 1313–1318. [CrossRef] [PubMed]
34. Clinical Guidelines on the Identification; Evaluation; Treatment of Overweight and Obesity in Adults: Executive Summary. Expert panel on the identification, evaluation, and treatment of overweight in adults. *Am. J. Clin. Nutr.* **1998**, *68*, 899–917. [CrossRef] [PubMed]
35. Australian Bureau of Statistics. *National Health Survey: First Results, 2014–2015*, 8 December 2015 ed.; Australian Bureau of Statistics: Canberra, Australia, 2015.
36. World Health Organization. Assessment of fracture risk and its application to screening for postmenopausal osteoporosis. Report of a WHO study group. *World Health Organ. Tech. Rep. Ser.* **1994**, *843*, 1–129.
37. Dignass, A.; Lindsay, J.O.; Sturm, A.; Windsor, A.; Colombel, J.F.; Allez, M.; D'Haens, G.; D'Hoore, A.; Mantzaris, G.; Novacek, G.; et al. Second european evidence-based consensus on the diagnosis and management of ulcerative colitis part 2: Current management. *J. Crohn Colitis* **2012**, *6*, 991–1030. [CrossRef] [PubMed]
38. Dignass, A.; Van Assche, G.; Lindsay, J.O.; Lemann, M.; Soderholm, J.; Colombel, J.F.; Danese, S.; D'Hoore, A.; Gassull, M.; Gomollon, F.; et al. The second european evidence-based consensus on the diagnosis and management of crohn's disease: Current management. *J. Crohn Colitis* **2010**, *4*, 28–62. [CrossRef] [PubMed]
39. Britton, K.A.; Massaro, J.M.; Murabito, J.M.; Kreger, B.E.; Hoffmann, U.; Fox, C.S. Body fat distribution, incident cardiovascular disease, cancer, and all-cause mortality. *J. Am. Coll. Cardiol.* **2013**, *62*, 921–925. [CrossRef] [PubMed]
40. Preis, S.R.; Massaro, J.M.; Robins, S.J.; Hoffmann, U.; Vasan, R.S.; Irlbeck, T.; Meigs, J.B.; Sutherland, P.; D'Agostino, R.B., Sr.; O'Donnell, C.J.; et al. Abdominal subcutaneous and visceral adipose tissue and insulin resistance in the framingham heart study. *Obesity* **2010**, *18*, 2191–2198. [CrossRef] [PubMed]
41. Singh, S.; Singh, H.; Loftus, E.V., Jr.; Pardi, D.S. Risk of cerebrovascular accidents and ischemic heart disease

in patients with inflammatory bowel disease: A systematic review and meta-analysis. *Clin. Gastroenterol. Hepatol. Off. Clin. Pract. J. Am. Gastroenterol. Assoc.* **2014**, *12*, 382–393. [CrossRef] [PubMed]

42. Cheng, S.; Massaro, J.M.; Fox, C.S.; Larson, M.G.; Keyes, M.J.; McCabe, E.L.; Robins, S.J.; O'Donnell, C.J.; Hoffmann, U.; Jacques, P.F.; et al. Adiposity, cardiometabolic risk, and vitamin d status: The framingham heart study. *Diabetes* **2010**, *59*, 242–248. [CrossRef] [PubMed]
43. Pedersen, H.K.; Gudmundsdottir, V.; Nielsen, H.B.; Hyotylainen, T.; Nielsen, T.; Jensen, B.A.; Forslund, K.; Hildebrand, F.; Prifti, E.; Falony, G.; et al. Human gut microbes impact host serum metabolome and insulin sensitivity. *Nature* **2016**, *535*, 376–381. [CrossRef] [PubMed]
44. Qin, J.; Li, Y.; Cai, Z.; Li, S.; Zhu, J.; Zhang, F.; Liang, S.; Zhang, W.; Guan, Y.; Shen, D.; et al. A metagenome-wide association study of gut microbiota in type 2 diabetes. *Nature* **2012**, *490*, 55–60. [CrossRef] [PubMed]
45. Le Chatelier, E.; Nielsen, T.; Qin, J.; Prifti, E.; Hildebrand, F.; Falony, G.; Almeida, M.; Arumugam, M.; Batto, J.M.; Kennedy, S.; et al. Richness of human gut microbiome correlates with metabolic markers. *Nature* **2013**, *500*, 541–546. [CrossRef] [PubMed]
46. Zeevi, D.; Korem, T.; Zmora, N.; Israeli, D.; Rothschild, D.; Weinberger, A.; Ben-Yacov, O.; Lador, D.; Avnit-Sagi, T.; Lotan-Pompan, M.; et al. Personalized nutrition by prediction of glycemic responses. *Cell* **2015**, *163*, 1079–1094. [CrossRef] [PubMed]
47. Subramaniam, K.; Fallon, K.; Ruut, T.; Lane, D.; McKay, R.; Shadbolt, B.; Ang, S.; Cook, M.; Platten, J.; Pavli, P.; et al. Infliximab reverses inflammatory muscle wasting (sarcopenia) in crohn's disease. *Aliment. Pharmacol. Ther.* **2015**, *41*, 419–428. [CrossRef] [PubMed]
48. Ding, N.S.; Malietzis, G.; Lung, P.F.C.; Penez, L.; Yip, W.M.; Gabe, S.; Jenkins, J.T.; Hart, A. The body composition profile is associated with response to anti-TNF therapy in crohn's disease and may offer an alternative dosing paradigm. *Aliment. Pharmacol. Ther.* **2017**, *46*, 883–891. [CrossRef] [PubMed]
49. Holt, D.Q.; Varma, P.; Strauss, B.J.G.; Rajadurai, A.S.; Moore, G.T. Low muscle mass at initiation of anti-TNF therapy for inflammatory bowel disease is associated with early treatment failure: A retrospective analysis. *Eur. J. Clin. Nutr.* **2017**, *71*, 773–777. [CrossRef] [PubMed]
50. Krajcovicova, A.; Hlavaty, T.; Killinger, Z.; Miznerova, E.; Toth, J.; Letkovsky, J.; Nevidanska, M.; Cierny, D.; Koller, T.; Zelinkova, Z.; et al. Combination therapy with an immunomodulator and anti-TNFα agent improves bone mineral density in ibd patients. *J. Crohn Colitis* **2014**, *8*, 1693–1701. [CrossRef] [PubMed]
51. Peyrin-Biroulet, L.; Van Assche, G.; Gomez-Ulloa, D.; Garcia-Alvarez, L.; Lara, N.; Black, C.M.; Kachroo, S. Systematic review of tumor necrosis factor antagonists in extraintestinal manifestations in inflammatory bowel disease. *Clin. Gastroenterol. Hepatol. Off. Clin. Pract. J. Am. Gastroenterol. Assoc.* **2017**, *15*, 25–36. [CrossRef] [PubMed]

10

A Review of Dietary Therapy for IBD and a Vision for the Future

Nicole Green, Talya Miller, David Suskind and Dale Lee *

Department of Pediatric Gastroenterology and Hepatology, Seattle Children's Hospital, Seattle, WA 98105, USA; nicole.green@seattlechildrens.org (N.G.); talya.miller@seattlechildrens.org (T.M.); david.suskind@seattlechildrens.org (D.S.)

* Correspondence: dale.lee@seattlechildrens.org

Abstract: Inflammatory bowel disease (IBD) is a chronic inflammatory condition affecting the gastrointestinal tract. The rising incidence of IBD has been associated with urbanization and shifts toward a Westernized diet. The intestinal microbiome has been a focus of disease pathogenesis and also therapeutic intervention. Dietary therapy for IBD has been well-studied with exclusive enteral nutrition, a formula-based diet with the exclusion of foods. In addition, interest in food-based exclusion diets has been increasing, with patients and families leading the charge. Challenges with dietary therapy for IBD include the lack of understanding of a detailed mechanistic pathway to explain the impact of diet on IBD pathogenesis and the difficult nature of designing and implementing dietary clinical trials. Epidemiological studies have demonstrated associations and intervention studies have demonstrated efficacy, but specific dietary targets remain as hypotheses at present. Current IBD therapy focuses on suppression of the immune system, yet the incomplete efficacy of present drugs suggests that other therapies must be developed and employed. Dietary interventions, with known ability to modulate the intestinal microbiome, are a unique opportunity to improve outcomes in IBD. Dietary intervention trials are challenging, and capturing both broad dietary patterns as well as exposure to individual food compounds is important. With increasing patient interest and preliminary research in dietary therapy indicating efficacy, it is imperative to further advance the science of utilizing diet in IBD, as well as to support patients by proactively addressing diet within their care plan.

Keywords: inflammatory bowel disease; Crohn; ulcerative colitis; diet; nutrition; exclusive enteral nutrition

---

1. Background

Nutritional interventions play a central role in the treatment and management of inflammatory bowel disease (IBD). While malnutrition is a common presentation in IBD, nutritional interventions have not only focused on correcting nutrient deficiencies but also on improving disease activity and symptoms. In addition to other societies, the North American Society for Pediatric Gastroenterology Hepatology and Nutrition has issued clinical guidelines emphasizing the importance of nutritional interventions in pediatric IBD. These guidelines focus on the use of exclusive enteral nutrition (EEN), a formula-based therapy, in pediatric Crohn's disease [1–3]. Since the publication of these guidelines, further research has expanded the concept of food-based nutritional intervention in patients with IBD. Recent research has shown the impact of diet on all three components of the IBD paradigm: the intestinal microbiome, mucosal integrity, and the immune system. With known influence on disease pathogenesis and perpetuation, diet in IBD is developing into a powerful, state-of-the-art treatment for IBD.

The history of nutritional therapy for IBD began with initial observations in hospitalized adults with severe Crohn's disease who improved on EEN [4,5]. Since the initial report of EEN in IBD in the late 1970s, there have been over 200 publications on EEN with multiple meta-analyses showing that the use of EEN in children with Crohn's disease is as effective as corticosteroids at inducing remission of active inflammation [6,7]. In adults with Crohn's disease, EEN has shown conflicting results. A 2018 Cochrane Database Systematic Review comparing EEN versus steroids showed greater efficacy of steroids [8]. It is unclear whether the perceived difference between efficacy in pediatric and adult EEN studies is related to compliance with therapy, greater duration of disease, or prior exposures to immunosuppressive drugs. Two studies in adults with newly diagnosed Crohn's disease showed similar efficacy with EEN involving a nasogastric tube option [9,10].

Immunosuppressive therapies are not effective at treating IBD for all patients and carry risk. The foods we eat have been hypothesized to play a role in pathogenesis as well as exacerbation of inflammation for many years. With basic science research showing the effect of dietary exposures on the intestinal microbiome as well as mucosal integrity, renewed interest has emerged on the ability of diet to treat the inflammatory burden characterizing patients with IBD. Despite the complexities and difficulty in doing clinical nutrition research, epidemiologic research has identified dietary components that are protective and risk factors for the development of IBD [11,12]. In addition, many diets have been reported to be efficacious in small case series, including the specific carbohydrate diet (SCD), IBD anti-inflammatory diet (IBD-AID), Crohn's disease exclusion diet (CDED), and semi-vegetarian diet [13]. The SCD developed by Dr. Sydney Haas, a pediatrician, in the 1930s to treat patients with celiac disease has been one of the better studies of exclusion diets used in IBD [14]. It was popularized in the late 20th century by Elaine Gottschall, whose daughter's ulcerative colitis was successfully treated with the SCD by Dr. Haas [15]. The SCD and other exclusion diets have risen in popularity among patients, and research efforts are underway attempting to keep pace with patient demand.

2. IBD Pathogenesis

The pathogenesis of IBD, while not completely elucidated, is thought to be multifactorial with interplay between genetics, the environment, and the immune system. The major environmental factors associated with IBD include shifts in diet, antibiotics, other medications, air pollution, infections, major life stressors, and smoking [12,16]. Diet is an environmental exposure that has changed over time, is modifiable, and has increasingly become a component of the treatment paradigm for IBD. A look at the epidemiologic patterns of IBD, with highest prevalence in Northern Europe and North America and rapidly increasing incidence in more-industrialized countries, has led to the theory that a Westernized lifestyle, and in particular diet, is linked to the rising incidence of IBD [17].

Understanding the role of dietary therapy in IBD requires an appreciation of the intestinal microbiome and intestinal mucosal integrity or barrier function. The intestinal microbiota consists of thousands of bacterial species with a gene pool 150 times larger than the human genome, with tremendous functional diversity [18]. The intestinal mucosal barrier consists of epithelial cells connected by tight junctions, antimicrobial factors, and overlying inner and outer mucus layers that limit the interaction between the microbiome and immune system [19]. In IBD, the homeostasis between the microbiome, intestinal barrier, and immune system is disrupted resulting in dysbiosis, increased barrier permeability, and inflammation [20].

The intestinal microbiome is highly adaptable and responsive to environmental factors. From the time of birth, environmental factors such as mode of delivery (vaginal versus caesarean section) and feeding method (breast feeding versus formula feeding) influence the microbiome [21,22]. Dietary patterns have a profound effect on the gut microbiome, and Wu et al., demonstrated that a high fat and animal protein diet compared to a high carbohydrate diet was associated with significant differences in the intestinal microbiome [23]. Numerous studies have highlighted differences in the microbiome between individuals with IBD and healthy individuals, with an overall trend towards loss of diversity of the microbiota in IBD [24–27]. A decrease in certain *Clostridium* clusters is a consistent finding among studies [20,25]. These species stimulate regulator T cells, resulting in immune tolerance and reduced gastrointestinal inflammation [20,28]. Conversely, members of the family Enterobacteriaceae are consistently elevated in IBD [20]. These include the well-known intestinal pathogens *Campylobacter* spp., *Salmonella* spp., and *Escherichia coli*. Whether these patterns are a cause or consequence of intestinal inflammation remains debatable. In the healthy state, the microbiota comes into contact with epithelial cells and the immune system in a highly controlled manner [29]. In IBD, the mucosal barrier is compromised, resulting in translocation of the intestinal microbiota and resultant immune system activation and inflammatory response [30].

3. Scientific Basis of Dietary Therapy for IBD

Many studies have evaluated the ability of diet to modulate intestinal microbiota and influence epithelial barrier function. Low fiber diets have been linked to IBD with a posited mechanism of reduction in short-chain fatty acid production by commensal bacteria whose preferred energy source is fiber [31]. Butyrate, a short-chain fatty acid, is essential for colonic health and the major energy source for colonocytes [32]. In addition to supporting intestinal barrier function, short-chain fatty acids also promote immune tolerance by promoting development of T-regulatory cells [33,34]. Food additives are commonly consumed by patients with IBD, and specific dietary emulsifiers (carboxymethylcellulose and polysorbate 80) have been shown to induce low grade inflammation and metabolic syndrome in wild type mice and promote colitis in genetically predisposed IL-10 knockout mice [35,36]. The emulsifiers perturbed the host microbiota, resulting in increased inflammatory potential with a rise in the number of mucolytic bacteria, and erosion of the protective mucous layer. At present, efforts are underway to better evaluate the frequency of exposure to food additives and the effect of these compounds on the intestinal system.

A summary of clinical trials and data reporting on the outcomes of dietary therapies in IBD are well described in greater detail elsewhere [3,37–39]. Importantly, many of these trials are smaller in size, deemed to produce a lower grade of evidence, and limited by the lack of long-term outcome data. In a recently published Cochrane review, Limketkai et al. analyzed 18 randomized controlled trials, comprising 1878 participants, published between 1965 and 2018 [37]. The intervention diets involved complete exclusion or significant limitation of one or more food groups. Diets included low refined carbohydrates; low microparticles; low calcium; low red and processed meat; low disaccharides, grain, saturated fats, red, and processed meat; symptoms-guided diets; highly-restricted organic diet; milk-free; Alberta-based anti-inflammatory diet; and Carrageenan-free diet. The different studies looked at various outcomes, including induction of remission, clinical relapse, surrogate biomarkers of inflammation, endoscopic improvement, health-related quality of life, and the need for surgery. This review concluded that no firm conclusions could be reached about the effect of these dietary interventions on IBD.

Though these included studies may be superior in that they are randomized controlled studies, additional studies on EEN and broader restrictions diets have shown clearer impact on IBD [40–42]. A key distinction from the randomized trials is the more profound nature of dietary intervention with EEN and many restrictions diets. Though not all controlled studies, the findings in these numerous, heterogeneous studies suggest the impact of dietary interventions on inflammation and clinical outcomes. Together with strong patient desire for dietary guidance and the opportunity for greater efficacy with conventional immunosuppression, larger more definitive studies are needed.

The most rigorously studied dietary interventions in IBD is exclusive enteral nutrition (EEN), a formula-based therapy for Crohn's disease. Numerous studies in children and adolescents have demonstrated the ability of EEN to induce remission of active Crohn's disease in 80–85% of patients [43,44]. EEN is equivalent to corticosteroid therapy in inducing clinical remission and superior at achieving endoscopic mucosal healing [43,45]. EEN is a first-line therapy for pediatric Crohn's disease in many parts of the world, and the treatment protocol typically involves administration of formula to provide 100% of caloric needs and exclusion of food for 6–8 weeks [1].

The exact mechanism by which EEN exerts its effect is unknown. Hypothesized mechanisms (Table 1) include limiting antigen exposure, antigenic monotony, enhancing nutritional status and nutrient delivery, altering the microbiome and immune response, and avoidance of deleterious compounds [3,5,20,46]. As EEN and exclusion diets are extremely different interventions, it is likely that the mechanism by which they impact disease is likewise different. Despite disease activity improvement, studies looking at fecal metagenomics in children with Crohn's disease have found that EEN seems to decrease gut microbiota diversity and promote a more "dysbiotic" state when compared to healthy controls [47]. Microbial functional capacity also decreased with EEN as did genes encoding proteins involved in B-complex vitamin biosynthesis [47]. In studies evaluating changes to the intestinal microbiome in patients with IBD treated with conventional medical therapies, dysbiosis improved with therapy [48]. Clearly therefore, the relationship between the beneficial effects of EEN and alterations in the gut microbiota needs further characterization and may result from alterations in beneficial or harmful metabolites produced by the bacteria.

Table 1. Hypothesized Mechanisms of Action for Diet Therapy in Inflammatory Bowel Disease (IBD).

Category of Mechanism	Hypothesized Mechanism	EEN	Exclusion Diets
Mechanical/physical	Liquid nutrition	x	
	Alteration of gut motility	x	x
	Gut rest	x	
Nutritional status	Improved nutrient delivery	x	
	Improved caloric delivery	x	
Epithelial barrier	Decreased permeability	x	x
	Restitution of intestinal barrier	x	x
	Improved delivery of fiber (SCFA * production)		x
Immune system	Limited antigen exposure	x	
	Antigenic monotony	x	
	Direct anti-inflammatory effect	x	x
	Alteration in bile acids	x	x
Microbiome	Shift of gut microbiome	x	x
	Stabilize gut microbiome	x	x
Specific avoidances	Avoidance of food additives		x
	Avoidance of deleterious food substances	x	x
Anti-inflammatory effect	Provide beneficial substance	x	x
	Increased antioxidant consumption		x

* SCFA: short-chain fatty acid.

EEN established the ability of diet to drive Crohn's disease into remission, but EEN is difficult to sustain as long-term maintenance therapy and is not effective for ulcerative colitis. Exclusion diets, though, are practical as long-term therapy and have been found to be useful in both Crohn's disease and ulcerative colitis. One of the most studied exclusion diets is the specific carbohydrate diet (SCD). This diet removes all grains, sweeteners (except for honey), processed food, and all milk products except for hard cheeses and yogurt fermented longer than 24 h. Both clinical and laboratory improvement have been reported in pediatric and adult patients with IBD [49–52]. One study over 12 weeks in children and adolescents used capsule endoscopy and demonstrated mucosal healing [53]. Therapy with the SCD has been shown to result in significant changes in microbial composition [49]. The SCD has been the best-studied food-based diet for IBD, and one survey with 417 respondents found patients reported significant improvement in symptoms, but that only 17% of patients partnered with a healthcare professional in the implementation of the SCD [50].

The Crohn's disease exclusion diet (CDED) is based on the hypothesis that components of the Western diet promote a pro-inflammatory microbiome and may disrupt the mucosal barrier. The diet focuses on excluding gluten, dairy, gluten-free baked goods, animal fat, emulsifiers, and all canned or processed foods. A prospective cohort of pediatric and adult participants with mild to moderate Crohn's disease treated with partial enteral nutrition (formula providing approximately 50% of daily calories) and the CDED showed success in achieving induction of clinical remission [41]. The IBD anti-inflammatory diet (IBD-AID) is derived from the SCD. It is a whole foods-based diet that restricts the intake of complex carbohydrates such as refined sugar, gluten-based grains, and certain starches from the diet, but also incorporates ingestion of prebiotics and probiotics. The diet also incorporates phases of food textures. In a small retrospective case series of patients with IBD on the IBD-AID for at least 4 weeks, all demonstrated improvement in clinical symptoms [54].

In a study of a semi-vegetarian diet in patients with remission of Crohn's disease induced by either medical therapy or surgery, patients maintained a greater rate of clinical remission over 2 years [55]. The CD-TREAT diet hypothesizes that a whole-food diet based on the composition of Modulen^{TM}, a commonly utilized formula for EEN in Europe, can emulate the efficacy of EEN [56]. In the component of the study evaluating healthy adults, similar microbiome and metabolome changes were seen with both the CD-TREAT diet and EEN. In the part of the study evaluating five children with active Crohn's disease, the CD-TREAT diet resulted in a significant decline in fecal calprotectin, though this surrogate marker of intestinal inflammation remained elevated at both 4 and 8 weeks.

The worsening of dysbiosis and decrease in butyrate production demonstrated with EEN therapy is seemingly counterintuitive, as is the lack of any fiber content in the formulas commonly utilized for EEN [57,58]. It may be the case that EEN acts via a unique mechanism of action to impact inflammation in IBD in comparison to the action of restrictions diets. As the gut microbiome can both drive inflammation and respond to underlying inflammation, further elucidation of the complex interaction between diet, microbiome, and host will help guide future therapy. With the paradoxical findings seen in EEN versus whole food restriction diets, changes occurring while transitioning from one diet to another may provide unique insights into mechanisms.

Epidemiologic studies have demonstrated greater risk of developing IBD with increased intake of total fat, polyunsaturated fatty acids, omega-6 fatty acids, and meat, while fruits, vegetables, and fiber intake have been shown to have protective effects [11]. Greater meat intake has been associated with both increased risk of ulcerative colitis relapse in adults and decreased rate of achieving remission of Crohn's disease in children on partial enteral nutrition therapy [59,60]. Conversely the only existing randomized study on red meat showed no association between red meat or processed meat consumption and risk of Crohn's disease relapse, as measured by self-reported symptoms [61]. A limitation of these studies evaluating individual dietary components is the potential for confounding factors due to numerous associations between individual foods consumed [62].

While some dietary interventions have demonstrated impacts on inflammation, other interventions, such as the low FODMAP diet, have been demonstrated to impact functional gastrointestinal symptoms in patients with IBD [63–65]. A variety of exclusion diets have shown efficacy at treating inflammation in small case series reports, but additional studies are needed to better substantiate these findings. While these studies suggest that specific food components may be deleterious, it may be the complex interactions of food components within the food matrix with the intestinal microbiome that trigger and perpetuate the cycle of inflammation in IBD. At present, the mechanism by which dietary interventions impact inflammation in IBD remains unknown. Studies involving the microbiome, metabolome, and proteome are beginning to shed insight, and will help guide the movement to more targeted dietary therapeutic approaches in the future. The mechanism of action for dietary therapies requires further study in both clinical and preclinical models.

4. Contrasting Pharmacological and Dietary Therapy

The goals of IBD therapy include resolution of symptoms, mucosal healing, improved quality of life, nutritional restitution, and minimizing adverse effects associated with therapy. For both nutritional therapy and conventional medical therapy, disease remission is often a singular focus, but the broader goals of the patient are important in the discussions about therapy. Primary outcomes in dietary and drug trials for IBD, though, should be the same, with a focus on evaluation of objective markers of inflammation, including labs, imaging, endoscopic findings, and surrogate markers of intestinal inflammation. An ongoing challenge for dietary trials is the ability to fund trials that are not sponsored by corporations with a financial incentive to drive development of a new therapeutic.

EEN in pediatric Crohn's disease has been demonstrated to lead to high rates of remission (85%) and superior mucosal healing when compared to treatment with corticosteroids [40,43,66]. Immunosuppressive therapy for IBD with monoclonal antibody anti-TNF-alpha drugs (e.g., infliximab or adalimumab), with or without concomitant immunomodulatory drugs are widely viewed as one of the most efficacious approaches to inducing clinical remission. A randomized-controlled trial in adults with newly diagnosed Crohn's disease demonstrated steroid-free remission at week 26 for 56.8% of patients on infliximab plus azathioprine, and 44.4% for those on infliximab alone [67]. A trial of infliximab in children demonstrated clinical remission at week 10 in 58.9% of participants, and 55.8% at week 54 [68]. In the ACT1 and ACT2 trials of infliximab in adult ulcerative colitis, clinical remission at week 8, 30, and 54 was never above 40% [69]. Similarly, a pediatric trial of infliximab in ulcerative colitis showed week 54 remission in less than 40% of study participants [70]. These data suggest that medications, though effective, do not induce remission in all patients with IBD, and room exists to further optimize therapy with newer medical therapies, and dietary interventions.

Like drugs, dietary therapy is not effective for all patients, and future personalization of dietary therapy is an opportunity. Dietary therapy can be utilized as stand-alone monotherapy, or diet can also be utilized concomitant with immunosuppressive drugs. A study in Japan evaluating the utility of partial enteral nutrition therapy (greater than 900 kcal/day from enteral nutrition with formula) with infliximab demonstrated a significant decrease in disease recurrence over the course of nearly 2 years [71]. Patients commonly employ dietary modifications to address symptoms but also attempt to control inflammation with diet [72]. Implementation of dietary changes is often guided by individual research and anecdotal experience, and the majority of patients are not guided by their medical team to involve diet as part of their IBD therapy plan [13]. At present the push to study and employ dietary measures is strongly driven by patients, while many medical practitioners remain skeptical and poorly informed about dietary interventions. As an example, despite overwhelming evidence for the use of EEN in pediatric CD, U.S. physicians still use EEN to a much lesser extent than their European and Canadian colleagues [73].

That patients and families will employ dietary therapy despite the rigor this involves suggests that tangible benefits exist. Given that therapies may be intensive for weeks to months (e.g., EEN), or require changes to dietary patterns long-term, the presence of family and community support can be key in the success of the patient's ability to adhere to the treatment. There has been limited data published on the patient experience while on EEN; however, a study of 29 families of patients with CD who chose EEN as induction therapy showed 59% of patients would repeat EEN if needed. However, 72% of parents would be more interested in a solid food based exclusion diet option [74].

There is generally a lesser degree of concern regarding the safety of nutritional therapy when compared to immunosuppressive drug therapies (Table 2). However, potential side effects can include nutritional inadequacy, psychosocial impact, and a potential for loss to medical follow-up. Psychosocial impact in the setting of nutritional therapy was evaluated by the measure of quality of life (QOL) in children and adolescents in a trial over 8 weeks with anti-TNF therapy, partial enteral nutrition, and exclusive enteral nutrition therapy [60]. This study demonstrated that children with Crohn's disease who achieved clinical remission on any of the three intervention arms had a significant increase in the quality of life measured by the IMPACT-III questionnaire, a validated disease-specific measure of QOL in pediatric IBD. This study evaluated sub-domains of QOL and found that body image-associated QOL was superior in the EEN group compared to the anti-TNF therapy group. Exclusion diets can be isolating and difficult to maintain, and certain patients may not be a good fit for dietary therapy. For those who demonstrate interest in dietary therapy, close monitoring, support of their family and friends, and partnership with the broader medical team (including physician, dietitian, and psychologist) helps with maintaining compliance and ensuring appropriateness of an ongoing dietary approach to IBD.

Table 2. Comparison of Dietary Therapy and Drug Therapy.

	Dietary Therapy	Drug Therapy
Driven by patient/family interest	++	
Ability to personalize	++	+
Directly impacts quality of life *	++	
Importance of family support	++	+
Challenges with compliance	++	+
Challenges with study design	++	
Risk of nutrient deficiency	++	
Works in combination with other therapies	++	++
Physician-driven		++
Targets known pathway		++
Greater risk of infection		++
Greater risk of cancers		++
Insurance coverage		++
Partnership with large industry to study **		++

* Independent of disease activity. ** Formula companies have supported the design and implementation of some studies on EEN, but the majority of dietary trials do not have corporate backing.

Since dietary therapies can be employed without physician prescription, there is potential for loss of medical follow-up. Without partnership with the medical team, dietary therapy may result in inadequate nutritional intake and a lack of appropriate objective evaluation of clinical, laboratory, and mucosal remission. When considering potential side effects of nutritional therapy, medical professionals must acknowledge that many patients are on dietary therapy as treatment for their IBD without formal medical guidance [50]. At a minimum, the medical team should engage patients in discussion about their dietary patterns, understand the basics of commonly utilized IBD exclusion diets, and partner with patients to closely monitor nutritional status and disease activity. Medical therapies require formal prescription from a healthcare professional and insurance provides coverage, or at least provides coverage of alternative medications. At present, dietary therapy for IBD is not broadly reimbursed by insurance. Further data on efficacy of exclusion diets is needed, but even for established therapy like EEN for Crohn's disease, insurance companies do not provide reimbursement in the United States.

Despite the many challenges around utilizing dietary therapy for IBD, dietary interventions are eagerly sought and employed by patients. The desire to avoid or lessen the degree of immunosuppression or supplement existing medical therapies are common drivers. Given the burden associated with dietary modification when considering cost, time for food preparation, and dietary restriction, it is important to recognize that nutritional therapy may not be an appealing option for many patients. For these reasons, not all patients and families will have equitable access to or interest in nutritional therapies. No studies have yet shown the variation in average costs between the different dietary interventions.

5. Vision for the Future of Diet and IBD

Dietary trials present challenges, but the ability to use nutrition to treat disease is a unique opportunity. It has long been accepted that dietary exposures are associated with risk of developing IBD, but diet as therapy has not been fully integrated into the broader paradigm of IBD therapy (Table 3). Diet represents a fundamental aspect of daily living and has infinite variability; diet is a potential target for profound intervention. Dietary intervention with EEN or even a shift in fat and fiber consumption results in a tangible shift in the intestinal microbiome [23,47,75]. Efforts have been placed into the development of therapeutic approaches to selectively modulate the intestinal microbiome, including prebiotics, probiotics, antibiotics, and fecal transplantation, but persistent shaping of the microbiome requires ongoing maintenance of these therapies [76]. Dietary therapies that reshape patterns of food consumption may alter exposures to deleterious substances such as select food additives, directly influence the intestinal microbiome, and also have a direct impact on the functioning of the host immune system [3].

Table 3. Dietary Therapy for IBD: Now and the Future.

Current Accepted Place of Dietary Therapy
EEN in pediatric Crohn's disease
Dietary therapies for symptom control
Nutritional therapy to support malnutrition
Major Areas Requiring Research
Impact of dietary therapies with/without concomitant immunosuppression
Impact of dietary therapies long-term
Mechanism of action for dietary therapies
Exclusion diets—dietary components of importance
Cost-benefit analysis of dietary interventions
Targeted dietary approaches to selectively modulate microbiome

Many individuals institute dietary changes based on varied sources of information and also as a reaction to the onset of IBD symptoms [13,77]. Recommendations are of variable validity, and better data on the role of diet in the setting of active IBD is needed. The data on EEN therapy has led to the utilization of this as standard therapy for induction of remission in pediatric Crohn's disease. The limitation of EEN is the difficulty in sustaining the intervention. Food-based IBD trials can involve exclusion, supplementation, or dramatic changes in dietary pattern [62]. Thus far, it appears unlikely that focused exclusion or supplementation have a role in IBD therapy, but more profound changes in dietary pattern have shown promise. Though individual dietary components may be deleterious (such as refined sugars, high fat, and specific food additives), it may be the case that the effect of these components are balanced or attenuated by other components (e.g., fiber, antioxidants, bioactive molecules). As such, we suggest that future dietary trials in IBD should consider the global dietary pattern, while also considering the role of individual dietary components. At present, published trials for exclusion diets in IBD often include a description of the general principles of the diet, but do not further characterize the variability within the proposed intervention and the impact this has on clinical outcomes. Challenges to consider in food-based dietary trials in IBD include issues with participant compliance, the measurement of compliance, and variability within a particular dietary intervention.

Though randomized controlled trials are the gold standard for the generation of evidence to drive clinical practice, innovative study design such as n-of-1 studies, and data from larger cohort studies, together with preclinical data, will also help to better substantiate the existing literature supporting dietary therapies in IBD. The paradigm of relying only on data from controlled trials is challenging in the setting of dietary interventions requiring profound changes to habitual diet, the need to maintain compliance, and the cost of implementing such trials.

As diet can be a primary or adjunctive therapy, the magnitude of effect considered as significant may be different for dietary trials as compared to drug trials. For example, if a dietary intervention results in lack of endoscopic mucosal healing but significantly decreases inflammatory burden as measured by biochemical markers, this may suggest that the intervention has a promising role as an adjunct to conventional immunosuppressive therapy. As the mechanism by which dietary therapy impacts IBD involves gut luminal exposures, the microbiome, and triggering of the mucosal immune system, diet has the potential to be utilized alongside medications to improve outcomes and durability, and minimize risks associated with immunosuppression. Drugs are not commonly brought to market with known partial efficacy, and they are not tested as frequently as adjuncts to existing therapies, but this is different for dietary therapy. Dietary trials demonstrating complete remission or even some response to therapy may have utility, as the cost and side-effect profile of dietary therapy is generally favorable for dietary therapy.

For novel pharmacologic therapeutics, often the initial identification and targeting of a specific molecular pathway guides drug development. The mechanism by which diet impacts IBD has yet to be fully elucidated [38,78]. Though the microbiome and specific deleterious substances have been identified, as of yet no definitive molecular pathway target exists for dietary therapy. At present, basic scientific research is ongoing to better elucidate mechanisms of action for both EEN and exclusion diets on treatment of active IBD, but empiric clinical trials are being pushed forward as well. Unlike drugs, with guidance, diet can be modulated within the bounds of safety, balance, and nutritionally-adequacy. Empiric dietary changes guided by experience may have value, but systematic evaluation of dietary interventions with trials is needed to produce the data to demonstrate efficacy beyond anecdote. Publication bias in favor of positive studies and poorly designed clinical studies are a limitation to the existing data for dietary therapy in IBD and need to be better addressed moving forward. A variety of exclusion diets have been proposed as therapy for IBD, and with systematic evaluation these trials will inform pre-clinical research, which in turn will help guide future trials.

Close partnership between the patient, gastroenterologist, and dietitian is necessary when utilizing dietary therapy to treat IBD. The discussion about the concept of integrating dietary therapy, goals of therapy, concerns, and a close monitoring plan should begin early. In some situations, diet will be used as monotherapy and it is of particular importance that close follow-up and monitoring of objective markers of inflammation occur, so as to prevent disease progression, select nutrient deficiencies, or global malnutrition. For physicians, the most common IBD treatment paradigms have dismissed the role of diet. A partnership with acknowledgement of the need for further clinical trial data, inherent uncertainty of efficacy for all IBD therapies, and the potential for benefit with dietary interventions will help guide progress towards better understanding of the utility of dietary therapy for individuals with IBD.

Author Contributions: N.G. contributed in design, authorship, and editing of the manuscript. She has approved of the final draft submitted. T.M. contributed in design, authorship, and editing of the manuscript. She has approved of the final draft submitted. D.S. contributed in design, authorship, and editing of the manuscript. He has approved of the final draft submitted. D.L. contributed in design, authorship, and editing of the manuscript. He has approved of the final draft submitted.

References

1. Critch, J.; Day, A.S.; Otley, A.; King-Moore, C.; Teitelbaum, J.E.; Shashidhar, H.; NASPGHAN IBD Committee. Use of enteral nutrition for the control of intestinal inflammation in pediatric Crohn disease. *J. Pediatr. Gastroenterol. Nutr.* **2012**, *54*, 298–305. [CrossRef] [PubMed]
2. Kleinman, R.E.; Baldassano, R.N.; Caplan, A.; Griffiths, A.M.; Heyman, M.B.; Issenman, R.M.; Lake, A.M. Nutrition support for pediatric patients with inflammatory bowel disease: A clinical report of the North American society for pediatric gastroenterology, hepatology and nutrition. *J. Pediatr. Gastroenterol. Nutr.* **2004**, *39*, 15–27. [CrossRef]
3. Lee, D.; Albenberg, L.; Compher, C.; Baldassano, R.; Piccoli, D.; Lewis, J.D.; Wu, G.D. Diet in the pathogenesis and treatment of inflammatory bowel diseases. *Gastroenterology* **2015**, *148*, 1087–1106. [CrossRef]
4. Voitk, A.J.; Brown, R.A.; McArdle, A.H.; Hinchey, E.J.; Gurd, F.N. Clinical uses of an elemental diet: Preliminary studies. *Can. Med. Assoc. J.* **1972**, *107*, 123–129. [PubMed]
5. Voitk, A.J.; Echave, V.; Feller, J.H.; Brown, R.A.; Gurd, F.N. Experience with elemental diet in the treatment of inflammatory bowel disease. Is this primary therapy? *Arch. Surg.* **1973**, *107*, 329–333. [CrossRef] [PubMed]
6. Ricour, C.; Duhamel, J.F.; Nihoul-Fekete, C. Use of parenteral and elementary enteral nutrition in the treatment of Crohn's disease and ulcerative colitis in children. *Arch. Fr. Pediatr.* **1977**, *34*, 505–513. [PubMed]
7. Navarro, J.; Vargas, J.; Cezard, J.P.; Charritat, J.L.; Polonovski, C. Prolonged constant rate elemental enteral nutrition in Crohn's disease. *J. Pediatr. Gastroenterol. Nutr.* **1982**, *1*, 541–546. [CrossRef] [PubMed]
8. Narula, N.; Dhillon, A.; Zhang, D.; Sherlock, M.E.; Tondeur, M.; Zachos, M. Enteral nutritional therapy for induction of remission in Crohn's disease. *Cochrane Database Syst. Rev.* **2018**, *4*, CD000542. [CrossRef] [PubMed]

9. Okada, M.; Yao, T.; Yamamoto, T.; Takenaka, K.; Imamura, K.; Maeda, K.; Fujita, K. Controlled trial comparing an elemental diet with prednisolone in the treatment of active Crohn's disease. *Hepatogastroenterology* **1990**, *37*, 72–80.
10. O'Morain, C.; Segal, A.W.; Levi, A.J. Elemental diet as primary treatment of acute Crohn's disease: A controlled trial. *Br. Med. J. (Clin. Res. Ed.)* **1984**, *288*, 1859–1862. [CrossRef]
11. Hou, J.K.; Abraham, B.; El-Serag, H. Dietary intake and risk of developing inflammatory bowel disease: A systematic review of the literature. *Am. J. Gastroenterol.* **2011**, *106*, 563–573. [CrossRef]
12. Ananthakrishnan, A.N. Epidemiology and risk factors for IBD. *Nat. Rev. Gastroenterol. Hepatol.* **2015**, *12*, 205–217. [PubMed]
13. Hou, J.K.; Lee, D.; Lewis, J. Diet and inflammatory bowel disease: Review of patient-targeted recommendations. *Clin. Gastroenterol. Hepatol.* **2014**, *12*, 1592–1600. [CrossRef] [PubMed]
14. Haas, S.V.; Haas, M.P. The treatment of celiac disease with the specific carbohydrate diet; report on 191 additional cases. *Am. J. Gastroenterol.* **1955**, *23*, 344–360. [PubMed]
15. Gottschall, E. *Breaking the Viscious Cycle*, 2nd ed.; Kirkton Press Limited: Baltimore, ON, Canada, 1994.
16. Ananthakrishnan, A.N.; Bernstein, C.N.; Iliopoulos, D.; Macpherson, A.; Neurath, M.F.; Ali, R.A.R.; Vavricka, S.R.; Fiocchi, C. Environmental triggers in IBD: A review of progress and evidence. *Nat. Rev. Gastroenterol. Hepatol.* **2018**, *15*, 39–49. [CrossRef] [PubMed]
17. Ng, S.C.; Shi, H.Y.; Hamidi, N.; Underwood, F.E.; Tang, W.; Benchimol, E.I.; Panaccione, R.; Ghosh, S.; Wu, J.C.Y.; Chan, F.K.L.; et al. Worldwide incidence and prevalence of inflammatory bowel disease in the 21st century: A systematic review of population-based studies. *Lancet* **2018**, *390*, 2769–2778. [CrossRef]
18. Qin, J.; Li, R.; Raes, J.; Arumugam, M.; Burgdorf, K.S.; Manichanh, C.; Nielsen, T.; Pons, N.; Levenez, F.; Yamada, T.; et al. A human gut microbial gene catalogue established by metagenomic sequencing. *Nature* **2010**, *464*, 59–65. [CrossRef] [PubMed]
19. Turner, J.R. Intestinal mucosal barrier function in health and disease. *Nat. Rev. Immunol.* **2009**, *9*, 799–809. [PubMed]
20. Vindigni, S.M.; Zisman, T.L.; Suskind, D.L.; Damman, C.J. The intestinal microbiome, barrier function, and immune system in inflammatory bowel disease: A tripartite pathophysiological circuit with implications for new therapeutic directions. *Ther. Adv. Gastroenterol.* **2016**, *9*, 606–625. [CrossRef]
21. Fallani, M.; Young, D.; Scott, J.; Norin, E.; Amarri, S.; Adam, R.; Aguilera, M.; Khanna, S.; Gil, A.; Edwards, C.A.; et al. Intestinal microbiota of 6-week-old infants across Europe: Geographic influence beyond delivery mode, breast-feeding, and antibiotics. *J. Pediatr. Gastroenterol. Nutr.* **2010**, *51*, 77–84. [CrossRef]
22. Penders, J.; Thijs, C.; Vink, C.; Stelma, F.F.; Snijders, B.; Kummeling, I.; Van den Brandt, P.A.; Stobberingh, E.E. Factors influencing the composition of the intestinal microbiota in early infancy. *Pediatrics* **2006**, *118*, 511–521. [CrossRef] [PubMed]
23. Wu, G.D.; Chen, J.; Hoffmann, C.; Bittinger, K.; Chen, Y.Y.; Keilbaugh, S.A.; Meenakshi, B.; Dan, K.; William, A.W.; Rob, K.; et al. Linking long-term dietary patterns with gut microbial enterotypes. *Science* **2011**, *334*, 105–108. [CrossRef]
24. Michail, S.; Durbin, M.; Turner, D.; Griffiths, A.M.; Mack, D.R.; Hyams, J.; Leleiko, N.; Kenche, H.; Stolfi, A.; Wine, E. Alterations in the gut microbiome of children with severe ulcerative colitis. *Inflamm. Bowel Dis.* **2012**, *18*, 1799–1808. [CrossRef] [PubMed]
25. Manichanh, C.; Rigottier-Gois, L.; Bonnaud, E.; Gloux, K.; Pelletier, E.; Frangeul, L.; Nalin, R.; Jarrin, C.; Marteau, P.; Roca, J. Reduced diversity of faecal microbiota in Crohn's disease revealed by a metagenomic approach. *Gut* **2006**, *55*, 205–211. [CrossRef]
26. Ott, S.J.; Musfeldt, M.; Wenderoth, D.F.; Hampe, J.; Brant, O.; Fölsch, U.R.; Timmis, K.N.; Schreiber, S. Reduction in diversity of the colonic mucosa associated bacterial microflora in patients with active inflammatory bowel disease. *Gut* **2004**, *53*, 685–693. [CrossRef] [PubMed]
27. Sheehan, D.; Moran, C.; Shanahan, F. The microbiota in inflammatory bowel disease. *J. Gastroenterol.* **2015**, *50*, 495–507. [CrossRef] [PubMed]
28. Atarashi, K.; Tanoue, T.; Shima, T.; Imaoka, A.; Kuwahara, T.; Momose, Y.; Cheng, G.; Yamasaki, S.; Saito, T.; Ohba, Y. Induction of colonic regulatory T cells by indigenous Clostridium species. *Science* **2011**, *331*, 337–341. [CrossRef]
29. de Souza, H.S.; Fiocchi, C. Immunopathogenesis of IBD: Current state of the art. *Nat. Rev. Gastroenterol. Hepatol.* **2016**, *13*, 13–27. [CrossRef]

30. Merga, Y.; Campbell, B.J.; Rhodes, J.M. Mucosal barrier, bacteria and inflammatory bowel disease: Possibilities for therapy. *Dig. Dis.* **2014**, *32*, 475–483. [CrossRef]
31. Canani, R.B.; Costanzo, M.D.; Leone, L.; Pedata, M.; Meli, R.; Calignano, A. Potential beneficial effects of butyrate in intestinal and extraintestinal diseases. *World J. Gastroenterol.* **2011**, *17*, 1519–1528. [CrossRef]
32. Van Immerseel, F.; Ducatelle, R.; De Vos, M.; Boon, N.; Van De Wiele, T.; Verbeke, K.; Rutgeerts, P.; Sas, B.; Louis, P.; Flint, H.J. Butyric acid-producing anaerobic bacteria as a novel probiotic treatment approach for inflammatory bowel disease. *J. Med. Microbiol.* **2010**, *59*, 141–143. [CrossRef]
33. Smith, P.M.; Howitt, M.R.; Panikov, N.; Michaud, M.; Gallini, C.A.; Bohlooly-y, M.; Glickman, J.N.; Garrett, W.S. The microbial metabolites, short-chain fatty acids, regulate colonic Treg cell homeostasis. *Science* **2013**, *341*, 569–573. [CrossRef] [PubMed]
34. Thorburn, A.N.; Macia, L.; Mackay, C.R. Diet, metabolites, and "western-lifestyle" inflammatory diseases. *Immunity* **2014**, *40*, 833–842. [CrossRef] [PubMed]
35. Chassaing, B.; Koren, O.; Goodrich, J.K.; Poole, A.C.; Srinivasan, S.; Ley, R.E.; Gewirtz, A.T. Dietary emulsifiers impact the mouse gut microbiota promoting colitis and metabolic syndrome. *Nature* **2015**, *519*, 92–96. [CrossRef] [PubMed]
36. Lee, D.; Swan, C.K.; Suskind, D.; Wahbeh, G.; Vanamala, J.; Baldassano, R.N.; Leonard, M.B.; Lampe, J.W. Children with Crohn's disease frequently consume select food additives. *Dig. Dis. Sci.* **2018**, *63*, 2722–2728. [CrossRef] [PubMed]
37. Limketkai, B.N.; Iheozor-Ejiofor, Z.; Gjuladin-Hellon, T.; Parian, A.; Matarese, L.E.; Bracewell, K.; MacDonald, J.K.; Gordon, M.; Mullin, G.E. Dietary interventions for induction and maintenance of remission in inflammatory bowel disease. *Cochrane Database Syst. Rev.* **2019**, *2*, CD012839. [CrossRef]
38. Knight-Sepulveda, K.; Kais, S.; Santaolalla, R.; Abreu, M.T. Diet and inflammatory bowel disease. *Gastroenterol. Hepatol.* **2015**, *11*, 511–520.
39. Halmos, E.P.; Gibson, P.R. Dietary management of IBD–insights and advice. *Nat. Rev. Gastroenterol. Hepatol.* **2015**, *12*, 133–146. [CrossRef]
40. Day, A.S.; Lopez, R.N. Exclusive enteral nutrition in children with Crohn's disease. *World J. Gastroenterol.* **2015**, *2*, 6809–6816. [CrossRef]
41. Sigall-Boneh, R.; Pfeffer-Gik, T.; Segal, I.; Zangen, T.; Boaz, M.; Levine, A. Partial enteral nutrition with a Crohn's disease exclusion diet is effective for induction of remission in children and young adults with Crohn's disease. *Inflamm. Bowel Dis.* **2014**, *20*, 1353–1360. [CrossRef]
42. Suskind, D.L.; Cohen, S.A.; Brittnacher, M.J.; Wahbeh, G.; Lee, D.; Shaffer, M.L.; Braly, K.; Hayden, H.S.; Klein, J.; Gold, B.; et al. Clinical and fecal microbial changes with diet therapy in active inflammatory bowel disease. *J. Clin. Gastroenterol.* **2018**, *52*, 155. [CrossRef] [PubMed]
43. Borrelli, O.; Cordischi, L.; Cirulli, M.; Paganelli, M.; Labalestra, V.; Uccini, S.; Russo, P.M.; Cucchiara, S. Polymeric diet alone versus corticosteroids in the treatment of active pediatric Crohn's disease: A randomized controlled open-label trial. *Clin. Gastroenterol. Hepatol.* **2006**, *4*, 744–753. [CrossRef] [PubMed]
44. Day, A.S.; Whitten, K.E.; Sidler, M.; Lemberg, D.A. Systematic review: Nutritional therapy in paediatric Crohn's disease. *Aliment. Pharmacol. Ther.* **2008**, *27*, 293–307. [CrossRef]
45. Gorard, D.A.; Hunt, J.B.; Payne-James, J.J.; Palmer, K.R.; Rees, R.G.; Clark, M.L.; Farthing, M.J.; Misiewicz, J.J.; Silk, D.B. Initial response and subsequent course of Crohn's disease treated with elemental diet or prednisolone. *Gut* **1993**, *34*, 1198–1202. [CrossRef]
46. Rajendran, N.; Kumar, D. Role of diet in the management of inflammatory bowel disease. *World J. Gastroenterol.* **2010**, *16*, 1442–1448. [CrossRef]
47. Quince, C.; Ijaz, U.Z.; Loman, N.; Eren, A.M.; Saulnier, D.; Russell, J.; Haig, S.; Calus, S.; Quick, J.; Barclay, A.; et al. Extensive modulation of the fecal metagenome in children with crohn's disease during exclusive enteral nutrition. *Am. J. Gastroenterol.* **2015**, *110*, 1718–1729. [CrossRef]
48. Ni, J.; Wu, G.D.; Albenberg, L.; Tomov, V.T. Gut microbiota and IBD: Causation or correlation? *Nat. Rev. Gastroenterol. Hepatol.* **2017**, *14*, 573–584. [CrossRef]
49. Lane, E.R.; Lee, D.; Suskind, D.L. Dietary therapies in pediatric inflammatory bowel disease: An evolving inflammatory bowel disease paradigm. *Gastroenterol. Clin.* **2017**, *46*, 731–744. [CrossRef]
50. Suskind, D.L.; Wahbeh, G.; Cohen, S.A.; Damman, C.J.; Klein, J.; Braly, K.; Shaffer, M.; Lee, D. Patients perceive clinical benefit with the specific carbohydrate diet for inflammatory bowel disease. *Dig. Dis. Sci.* **2016**, *61*, 3255–3260. [CrossRef]

51. Suskind, D.L.; Wahbeh, G.; Gregory, N.; Vendettuoli, H.; Christie, D. Nutritional therapy in pediatric Crohn disease: The specific carbohydrate diet. *J. Pediatr. Gastroenterol. Nutr.* **2014**, *58*, 87–91. [CrossRef]
52. Kakodkar, S.; Farooqui, A.J.; Mikolaitis, S.L.; Mutlu, E.A. The specific carbohydrate diet for inflammatory bowel disease: A case series. *J. Acad. Nutr. Diet.* **2015**, *115*, 1226–1232. [CrossRef]
53. Cohen, S.A.; Gold, B.D.; Oliva, S.; Lewis, J.; Stallworth, A.; Koch, B.; Laura, E.; Mason, D. Clinical and mucosal improvement with specific carbohydrate diet in pediatric Crohn disease. *J. Pediatr. Gastroenterol. Nutr.* **2014**, *59*, 516–521. [CrossRef]
54. Olendzki, B.C.; Silverstein, T.D.; Persuitte, G.M.; Ma, Y.; Baldwin, K.R.; Cave, D. An anti-inflammatory diet as treatment for inflammatory bowel disease: A case series report. *Nutr. J.* **2014**, *13*, 5. [CrossRef]
55. Chiba, M.; Abe, T.; Tsuda, H.; Sugawara, T.; Tsuda, S.; Tozawa, H.; Fujiwara, K.; Imai, H. Lifestyle-related disease in Crohn's disease: Relapse prevention by a semi-vegetarian diet. *World J. Gastroenterol.* **2010**, *16*, 2484–2495. [CrossRef]
56. Svolos, V.; Hansen, R.; Nichols, B.; Quince, C.; Ijaz, U.Z.; Papadopoulou, R.T.; Ewards, C.A.; Watson, D.; Alghamdi, A.; Brejnrod, A.; et al. Treatment of active crohn's disease with an ordinary food-based diet that replicates exclusive enteral nutrition. *Gastroenterology* **2019**, *56*, 1354–1367. [CrossRef]
57. MacLellan, A.; Moore-Connors, J.; Grant, S.; Cahill, L.; Langille, M.G.I.; Van Limbergen, J. The impact of Exclusive Enteral Nutrition (EEN) on the gut microbiome in crohn's disease: A review. *Nutrients* **2017**, *9*, 447. [CrossRef]
58. Gerasimidis, K.; Bertz, M.; Hanske, L.; Junick, J.; Biskou, O.; Aguilera, M.; Garrick, V.; Russell, R.K.; Blaut, M.; McGrogan, P.; Edwards, C.A. Decline in presumptively protective gut bacterial species and metabolites are paradoxically associated with disease improvement in pediatric Crohn's disease during enteral nutrition. *Inflamm. Bowel Dis.* **2014**, *20*, 861–871. [CrossRef]
59. Jowett, S.L.; Seal, C.J.; Pearce, M.S.; Phillips, E.; Gregory, W.; Barton, J.R.; Welfare, M.R. Influence of dietary factors on the clinical course of ulcerative colitis: A prospective cohort study. *Gut* **2004**, *53*, 1479–1484. [CrossRef]
60. Lee, D.; Baldassano, R.N.; Otley, A.R.; Albenberg, L.; Griffiths, A.M.; Compher, C.; Chen, E.Z.; Li, H.; Gilroy, E.; Nessel, L.; et al. Comparative effectiveness of nutritional and biological therapy in North American children with active crohn's disease. *Inflamm. Bowel Dis.* **2015**, *21*, 1786–1793. [CrossRef]
61. Albenberg, L.; Brensinger, C.M.; Wu, Q.; Gilroy, E.; Kappelman, M.D.; Sandler, R.S.; Lewis, J.D. A diet low in red and processed meat does not reduce rate of crohn's disease flares. *Gastroenterology* **2019**. [CrossRef]
62. Lewis, J.D.; Albenberg, L.; Lee, D.; Kratz, M.; Gottlieb, K.; Reinisch, W. The Importance and challenges of dietary intervention trials for inflammatory bowel disease. *Inflamm. Bowel Dis.* **2017**, *23*, 181–191. [CrossRef]
63. Pedersen, N.; Ankersen, D.V.; Felding, M.; Wachmann, H.; Végh, Z.; Molzen, L.; Burisch, J.; Andersen, J.R.; Munkholm, P. Low-FODMAP diet reduces irritable bowel symptoms in patients with inflammatory bowel disease. *World J. Gastroenterol.* **2017**, *23*, 3356–3366. [CrossRef] [PubMed]
64. Cox, S.R.; Prince, A.C.; Myers, C.E.; Irving, P.M.; Lindsay, J.O.; Lomer, M.C.; Whelan, K. Fermentable carbohydrates [FODMAPs] exacerbate functional gastrointestinal symptoms in patients with inflammatory bowel disease: A randomised, double-blind, placebo-controlled, cross-over, re-challenge trial. *J. Crohn's Colitis* **2017**, *11*, 1420–1429. [CrossRef] [PubMed]
65. Prince, A.C.; Myers, C.E.; Joyce, T.; Irving, P.; Lomer, M.; Whelan, K. Fermentable carbohydrate restriction (Low FODMAP Diet) in clinical practice improves functional gastrointestinal symptoms in patients with inflammatory bowel disease. *Inflamm. Bowel. Dis.* **2016**, *22*, 1129–1136. [CrossRef] [PubMed]
66. Heuschkel, R.B. Enteral nutrition in children with Crohn's disease. *J. Pediatr. Gastroenterol. Nutr.* **2000**, *31*, 575. [CrossRef]
67. Colombel, J.F.; Sandborn, W.J.; Reinisch, W.; Mantzaris, G.J.; Kornbluth, A.; Rachmilewitz, D.; Lichtiger, S.; D'Haens, G.; Diamond, R.H.; Broussard, D.L.; et al. Infliximab, azathioprine, or combination therapy for Crohn's disease. *N. Engl. J. Med.* **2010**, *362*, 1383–1395. [CrossRef]
68. Hyams, J.; Crandall, W.; Kugathasan, S.; Griffiths, A.; Olson, A.; Johanns, J.; Liu, G.; Travers, S.; Heuschkel, R.; Markowitz, J.; et al. Induction and maintenance infliximab therapy for the treatment of moderate-to-severe Crohn's disease in children. *Gastroenterology* **2007**, *132*, 863–873. [CrossRef]
69. Rutgeerts, P.; Sandborn, W.J.; Feagan, B.G.; Reinisch, W.; Olson, A.; Johanns, J.; Travers, S.; Rachmilewitz, D.; Hanauer, S.B.; Lichtenstein, G.R.; et al. Infliximab for induction and maintenance therapy for ulcerative colitis. *N. Engl. J. Med.* **2005**, *353*, 2462–2476. [CrossRef]

70. Hyams, J.; Damaraju, L.; Blank, M.; Johanns, J.; Guzzo, C.; Winter, H.S.; Kugathasan, S.; Cohen, S.; Markowitz, J.; Escher, J.C.; et al. Induction and maintenance therapy with infliximab for children with moderate to severe ulcerative colitis. *Clin. Gastroenterol. Hepatol.* **2012**, *10*, 391–399. [CrossRef]
71. Hirai, F.; Ishihara, H.; Yada, S.; Esaki, M.; Ohwan, T.; Nozaki, R.; Ashizuka, S.; Inatsu, H.; Ohi, H.; Aoyagi, K.; et al. Effectiveness of concomitant enteral nutrition therapy and infliximab for maintenance treatment of Crohn's disease in adults. *Dig. Dis. Sci.* **2013**, *58*, 1329–1334. [CrossRef]
72. Zallot, C.; Quilliot, D.; Chevaux, J.B.; Peyrin-Biroulet, C.; Guéant-Rodriguez, R.M.; Freling, E.; Collet-Fenetrier, B.; Williet, N.; Ziegler, O.; et al. Dietary beliefs and behavior among inflammatory bowel disease patients. *Inflamm. Bowel Dis.* **2013**, *19*, 66–72. [CrossRef]
73. Stewart, M.; Day, A.S.; Otley, A. Physician attitudes and practices of enteral nutrition as primary treatment of paediatric Crohn disease in North America. *J. Pediatr. Gastroenterol. Nutr.* **2011**, *52*, 38–42. [CrossRef] [PubMed]
74. Svolos, V.; Gerasimidis, K.; Buchanan, E.; Curtis, L.; Garrick, V.; Hay, J.; Laird, S.; Munro, J.; Gaya, D.R.; Russell, R.K.; Hansen, R. Dietary treatment of Crohn's disease: Perceptions of families with children treated by exclusive enteral nutrition, a questionnaire survey. *BMC Gastroenterol.* **2017**, *17*, 14. [CrossRef] [PubMed]
75. Lewis, J.D.; Chen, E.Z.; Baldassano, R.N.; Otley, A.R.; Griffiths, A.M.; Lee, D.; Bittinger, K.; Bailey, A.; Friedman, E.S.; Hoffmann, C.; et al. Inflammation, antibiotics, and diet as environmental stressors of the gut microbiome in pediatric crohn's disease. *Cell Host Microbe* **2017**, *22*, 247. [CrossRef] [PubMed]
76. Hansen, J.J.; Sartor, R.B. Therapeutic manipulation of the microbiome in IBD: Current results and future approaches. *Curr. Treat. Options Gastroenterol.* **2015**, *13*, 105–120. [CrossRef] [PubMed]
77. Cohen, A.B.; Lee, D.; Long, M.D.; Kappelman, M.D.; Martin, C.F.; Sandler, R.S.; Lewis, J.D. Dietary patterns and self-reported associations of diet with symptoms of inflammatory bowel disease. *Dig. Dis. Sci.* **2013**, *58*, 1322–1328. [CrossRef]
78. Sigall-Boneh, R.; Levine, A.; Lomer, M.; Wierdsma, N.; Allan, P.; Fiorino, G.; Gatti, S.; Jonkers, D.; Kierkus, J.; Melgar, S. Research gaps in diet and nutrition in inflammatory bowel disease. A topical review by D-ECCO working group [Dietitians of ECCO]. *J. Crohns Colitis* **2017**, *11*, 1407–1419. [PubMed]

11

Bases for the Adequate Development of Nutritional Recommendations for Patients with Inflammatory Bowel Disease

Esteban Sáez-González [1,2,†], Beatriz Mateos [1,2,†], Pedro López-Muñoz [1], Marisa Iborra [1,2,3], Inés Moret [1,2,3], Pilar Nos [1,2,3] and Belén Beltrán [1,2,3,*]

1 Inflammatory Bowel Disease Unit, Gastroenterology Department, La Fe University and Polytechnic Hospital, 46026 Valencia, Spain; esteban.digestivo@gmail.com (E.S.-G.); bmateosa@gmail.com (B.M.); pedro.lopez8928@gmail.com (P.L.-M.); marisaiborra@hotmail.com (M.I.); Ines.Moret@uv.es (I.M.); pilarnos@gmail.com (P.N.)

2 Inflammatory Bowel Disease Research Group, Medical Research Institute Hospital La Fe (IIS La Fe), 46026 Valencia, Spain

3 Biomedical Research Network Center for Liver and Digestive Diseases (CIBEREHD), 28029 Madrid, Spain

* Correspondence: belenbeltranniclos@gmail.com

† These authors contribute equally to this manuscript.

Abstract: Inflammatory bowel disease (IBD) is a chronic and relapsing inflammatory condition of the gastrointestinal tract; it is a heterogeneous and multifactorial disorder resulting from a complex interplay between genetic variation, intestinal microbiota, the host immune system and environmental factors such as diet, drugs, breastfeeding and smoking. The interactions between dietary nutrients and intestinal immunity are complex. There is a compelling argument for environmental factors such as diet playing a role in the cause and course of IBD, given that three important factors in the pathogenesis of IBD can be modulated and controlled by diet: intestinal microbiota, the immune system and epithelial barrier function. The aim of this review is to summarize the epidemiological findings regarding diet and to focus on the effects that nutrients exert on the intestinal mucosa–microbiota–permeability interaction. The nature of these interactions in IBD is influenced by alterations in the nutritional metabolism of the gut microbiota and host cells that can influence the outcome of nutritional intervention. A better understanding of diet–host–microbiota interactions is essential for unravelling the complex molecular basis of epigenetic, genetic and environmental interactions underlying IBD pathogenesis as well as for offering new therapeutic approaches for the treatment of IBD.

Keywords: diet; inflammatory bowel disease; microbiota; intestinal barrier; nutrients; immunity

---

1. Introduction

Inflammatory bowel disease (IBD) is a chronic and relapsing inflammatory condition of the gastrointestinal tract. Crohn's disease (CD) and ulcerative colitis (UC) are the two principal types of IBD. Its prevalence has been increasing worldwide, with the highest incidence found in Western countries [1]. The precise etiology of IBD remains unclear; however, interactions between genetic, microbiotic and environmental factors are associated with its pathogenesis [2]. There is a compelling argument for environmental factors such as diet playing a role in the cause and course of IBD [3], given that three important factors in the pathogenesis of IBD can be modulated and controlled by diet: intestinal microbiota, the immune system and epithelial barrier function.

Patients with IBD tend to present with malnutrition, especially when they are having a flare or have chronic, only partially controlled, intestinal inflammation. Currently, to deal appropriately with malnutrition is considered a clinical quality criterion, especially for preventing the complications that can arise under a malnutrition situation (e.g., infections, postsurgical complications, immunity alterations). Thus, there is a tendency to at least consider the patient's nutritional status before surgery [4], and a guide has recently been published with dietary recommendations [5]. However, the gastroenterologist typically gives little advice to patients with IBD regarding daily diet or nutrient considerations. Patients are often told, "eat what you can tolerate," and discussion on diet is typically very limited. Despite the scarce attention gastroenterologists give to nutrients, approximately 40% of patients with CD believe that diet can control symptoms, and approximately 80% believe diet is important in the overall management of the disease [6]. Some 40% of patients with IBD have attempted various diet therapies, often without the assistance of a physician or dietician [7].

Perturbations related to dietary intake are thought to relate to the consumption of a dietary pattern that negatively alters gut microbiota composition and intestinal permeability [8]. Recent experimental evidence has suggested a crucial factor of barrier dysfunction in the onset of IBD [9]. The aim of this review is to summarize the epidemiological findings regarding diet and to focus on the effects that nutrients exert on intestinal mucosa–microbiota–permeability interaction.

2. Diet Influences Inflammatory Bowel Disease: Epidemiological Clues

Epidemiological studies have shown associations between the intake of specific dietary components and the risk of developing IBD [10–17]; however, association does not necessarily imply causality. These studies must be considered with caution, given that methodological inconsistencies and a recall bias could be affecting the results observed. Furthermore, in a complex disease with dietary triggers, it can be difficult to unravel the role of individual dietary risk factors because dietary patterns often involve exposure to clusters of nutrients. These clusters are favored by the industrial processing of food.

Classically, no environmental factor has been claimed to impact directly on the pathogenesis of IBD, apart from tobacco [18]. However, a recent systematic review and meta-analysis have shown that breastfeeding provides a protective factor against the development of CD and UC, both in pediatric and adult-onset disease. This inverse association is consistent in studies worldwide and supports the recommendation of breastfeeding in infancy to reduce the risk of IBD development [19]. Further research on the effects of breast milk on the microbiome and modulation of the innate immune system are needed.

A systematic review of the literature, initially including 2085 publications, was published in 2011 [20]. Nineteen studies fulfilled the inclusion criteria, containing a total of 2609 patients with IBD (1340 UC and 1269 CD). The authors concluded that a high intake of total fats, polyunsaturated fatty acids (PUFAs), omega-6 fatty acids and meat were consistently associated with increased risk of developing UC as well as CD. High vegetable intake was consistently associated with decreased risk of UC, whereas fiber and fruit intake were consistently associated with reduced risk of CD.

Dietary fats are associated with an increased or decreased risk for IBD, depending on the type of fat. Among 170,805 women followed over 26 years, a high intake of dietary long-chain omega-3 PUFAs was associated with a reduced risk of UC. In contrast, high intake of trans-unsaturated fats was associated with an increased risk of UC [15]. Various data have been extracted from an analysis of 366,351 individuals with IBD from the European Prospective Investigation into Cancer and Nutrition study cohort. Globally, a dietary imbalance with a high consumption of sugar and soft drinks and a low consumption of vegetables has been associated with UC risk [12]. Regarding fats, a sub-study analyzing 126 incident cases of UC showed that the patients ranking in the superior quartile of linoleic acid intake had a higher risk of developing UC [21]. Similarly, another analysis considering 70 incident cases of CD has shown that higher intake of the omega-3 PUFA docosahexaenoic acid prevents CD development [22]. A recent population-based study of environmental risk factors shows an increased risk of CD with frequent fast-food consumption (Western diet) before the diagnosis [23]. A Western diet typically contains high levels of omega-6 PUFAs and low levels of omega-3 PUFAs. The ratio between the intake of omega-6 and omega-3 PUFAs is considered a risk factor for IBD.

Data from the Nurses' Health Study including 170,776 participants showed that higher long-term fruit intake was associated with a lower risk of CD but not UC [15]. Multiple studies have reported a negative association between dietary fiber intake from fruits or fruits and vegetables and subsequent risk of CD. Fiber is the dietary component with the greatest agreement in epidemiological studies. In a recent prospective study [24], fiber from fruit has also been implicated in preventing the establishment of pouchitis in patients with UC. It is important to remember that the fiber implicated in these effects is soluble fiber, which is fermentable by bacteria. Soluble fiber is usually less present in food; however, the proportion of insoluble to soluble fiber could be the factor limiting tolerance to various foods.

Animal proteins have also been claimed to increase the risk of IBD [10]. A prospective study (E3N) that included 67,581 French women showed that high animal protein intake was associated with a significantly increased the risk of IBD, particularly with UC. However, other smaller studies have not confirmed this risk [20]. In a separate study evaluating dietary intake and relapse of UC, red meat was found to have the strongest association (odds ratio 5.19; 95% confidence interval 2.09–12.9) with relapse [14].

Food additives have been progressively increasing in processed food. Both sweeteners and emulsifiers, used to enhance the texture and stability of foods, have been shown to disrupt host–microbiota interaction and to facilitate intestinal inflammation [25]. However, it is difficult to ascertain whether the additives are risk factors because most of the questionnaires used to assess dietary intake do not evaluate food additives.

Currently, it seems clear that dietary patterns are more important than individual foods for considering the risk of IBD. The consumption of vegetables, fruits, olive oil, fish, grains and nuts (prudent diet) was associated with a decreased risk of developing CD in both boys and girls in a Canadian pediatric study. A Mediterranean dietary pattern is high in extra-virgin olive oil, vegetables, fruit, legumes, nuts and seeds, with a moderate consumption of fish, poultry and milk products, and is low in processed foods, baked goods and red and processed meat. This dietary pattern is high in monounsaturated fats, omega-3 PUFAs, fermentable fiber and polyphenols, and adherence to a Mediterranean dietary pattern is associated with lower levels of inflammation biomarkers [26].

3. Impact of Nutrients on Intestinal Permeability, Microbiome and Immunity

Dietary fiber is not digested or absorbed by host cells, given that mammalian cells largely lack the necessary enzymes to degrade them. Instead, dietary fiber is subjected to bacterial fermentation in the gastrointestinal tract. Although a wide range of bacteria ferment dietary fiber, each bacterium has a substrate preference based on its enzymatic activity. Thus, dietary intervention can remodel the gut microbial composition by customizing the content of dietary fiber [27]. Short-chain fatty acids (SCFAs), such as acetate, propionate and butyrate, are the major end products of microbial fermentation of dietary fiber. They are key energy substrates used by colonocytes [28]. Butyrate enhances intestinal epithelial barrier function via hypoxia-inducible factor-1, which regulates the integrity of epithelial tight junctions [28–30]. It also increases the synthesis of the MUC2 protein, the main component of intestinal mucus [31,32]. Thus, a lack of dietary fiber might compromise epithelial integrity and mucus production due to insufficient SCFA generation, resulting in impaired intestinal barrier function [33]. Recently, it has been observed that consumption of a low-fiber diet leads to the disruption of intestinal barrier function through a mechanism that is independent of SCFAs. In the absence of dietary fiber, some commensal bacteria use host mucus glycans to meet their energy needs [34]. As a result, these mucolytic bacteria become the predominant species within the gut microbiota. Importantly, a bloom of mucolytic bacteria results in the degradation of the colonic mucus layer that renders the host susceptible to enteric pathogens [34] (Figure 1). These changes facilitate bacterial adherence and translocation into the epithelium, which introduce immunomodulatory effects. In summary, a diet poor in soluble fiber can condition both dysbiosis and a subsequent decrease in the mucus layer, which increases the permeability already affected by the fiber-poor diet.

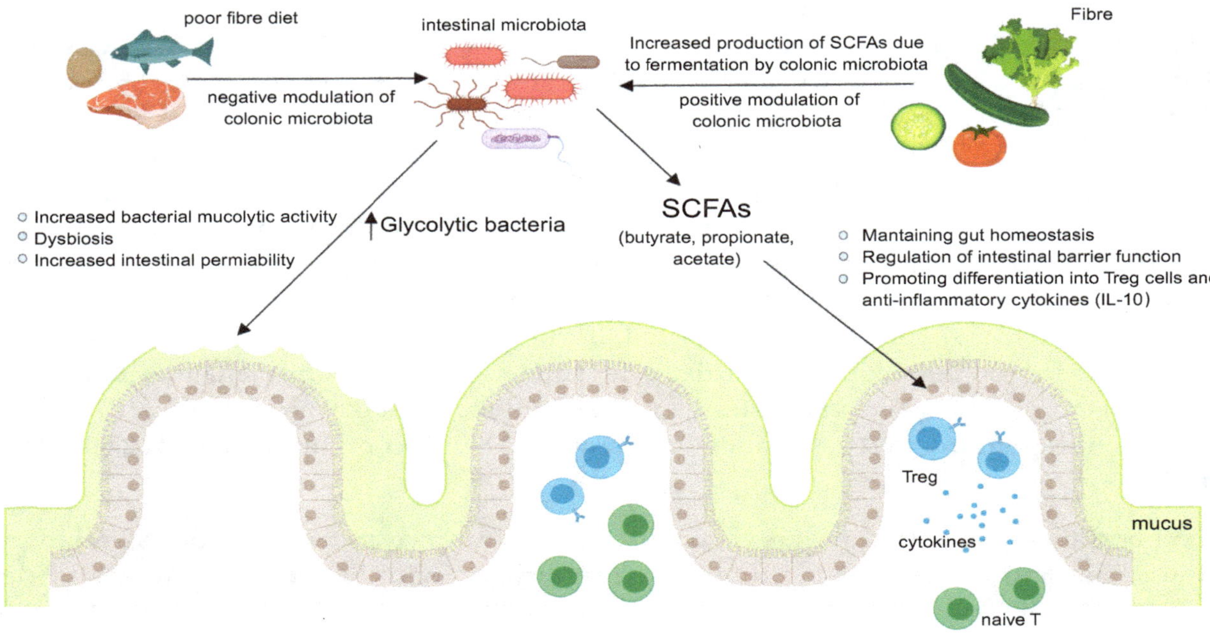

Figure 1. Interaction of dietary fiber with the gut microbiota.

The gut microbiota is thought to play a crucial role in human health and prevention of disease through a variety of mechanisms, including the production of short-chain fatty acids (SCFAs), which are important for maintaining gut homeostasis and optimal immune function. Ingested fiber can influence fecal microbiota profiles, cause changes in the complex gastrointestinal environment and promote the growth of bacteria in general and potentially beneficial bacteria in particular.

Fat- and refined sugar-rich diets can condition a low production of butyrate, which has been described in patients with CD, together with a diminution in the butyrate receptor [35] Butyrate plays an important role in downregulating inflammation by suppressing transcription of cytokines and increasing differentiation and the population of lamina propria Tregs [33,35,36]. Butyrate can also enhance innate immunity by upregulating defensins and cathelicidins in animal models [36]. Defensins have been reported to be permanently decreased in patients with IBD, and whether a dietary intervention could reverse this condition deserves further investigation. High-fat diets (without high sugars) have been shown to increase tumor necrosis factor (TNF)-α and interferon-γ expression, and to decrease levels of colonic Tregs [37].

Dietary amino acids play important roles in gut homeostasis. Amino acid metabolic profiles in the blood, urine, feces and intestinal tissues are also altered in patients with IBD and correlate with the severity of the disease. Additionally, metagenomic studies have revealed that amino acid biosynthesis genes are downregulated and amino acid transporter genes are upregulated in the gut microbiome of patients with IBD, indicating that the gut microbiota lessens the production of amino acids and increases the rate of their use [38,39]. Certain amino acids are critical for immune T-cell function as well as for the proliferation of macrophages [40,41]. Thus, the demand for certain amino acids by host cells and the gut microbiota can increase as a consequence of inflammation.

Tryptophan is an essential amino acid that can be found in fish, meat and cheese. Its metabolites, such as kynurenine, indole-3-aldehyde and indole-3-acetic acid, can act as ligands for the aryl hydrocarbon receptor, a critical regulator of immunity and inflammation involved in adaptive immunity and intestinal barrier function [42–44]. Indoleamine 2,3 dioxygenase-1 (IDO1) is ubiquitously expressed in epithelial cells, dendritic cells and macrophages. IDO1 is the first step in the kynurenine pathway, a major route for tryptophan catabolism. IDO1 regulates the differentiation and maturation of adaptive immune cells [45]. Kynurenine is an initial metabolite of IDO1-mediated tryptophan catabolism and the kynurenine/tryptophan ratio is a surrogate marker of IDO1 activity. A recent clinical study has shown that serum tryptophan levels are lower and the kynurenine/tryptophan ratio is elevated in patients with IBD compared with healthy controls [15]. Additionally, indoleamine 2,3-dioxygenase 1 (IDO1) mRNA expression in colonic tissues is significantly higher in IBD and correlates with disease severity, suggesting the kynurenine pathway is upregulated in IBD.

Arginine and glutamine are two semi-essential amino acids that can impact gut homeostasis and innate immunity. Both are diminished in prospective cohorts of patients with IBD, and both are implicated in wound repair mechanisms [46]. Furthermore, arginine regulates macrophage differentiation into the M1 or M2 phenotype following environmental cytokine guidance, whereas glutamine reduces oxidative stress and cytokine production via downregulation of the NF-kB and signal transducer and activator of transcription proteins (STAT) signaling pathways.

The upregulation of amino acid metabolic pathways is one of the major inflammation-related metabolic shifts in the host and the microbiota. In other words, host cells and resident microbes have an increased demand for certain amino acids in the context of IBD. Thus, dietary supplementation of these amino acids is a key strategy for the treatment of IBD. However, it is noteworthy to mention that other amino acids can fuel pro-inflammatory responses in IBD, and restriction of certain amino acids can attenuate intestinal inflammation. A more thorough understanding of the specific roles various amino acids play in IBD and supplying the optimal amount of anti-inflammatory amino acids while limiting the consumption of proinflammatory amino acids can lead to the development of effective amino acid-based dietary interventions.

4. Mesenteric Fat and Epigenetic Considerations

Today, patients with IBD sometimes have malnutrition with obesity, associated with metabolic syndrome. Obesity has also been associated with the development of more active IBD, with a higher demand for therapeutic resources. Patients with IBD, especially CD, present fat-wrapping or "creeping fat," which corresponds to ectopic adipose tissue extending from the mesenteric attachment and covering the majority of the small and large intestinal surface. Mesenteric adipose tissue in patients with IBD presents several morphological and functional alterations; e.g., it is more infiltrated with immune cells such as macrophages and T-cells. This fat tissue is not an "innocent bystander," but actively contributes to intestinal and systemic inflammatory responses [47]. It overexpresses peroxisome proliferator-activated receptor gamma (PPAR-γ), which is a "master" regulator of the adipogenesis program and the major orchestrator of visceral adipose tissue Treg accumulation, phenotypes and function. Mesenteric adipose tissue is colonized by luminal bacteria, and PPAR-γ expression is modulated by several bacterial stimuli. Thus, the presence of metabolically active adipose tissue should be taken into consideration when attempting to change the alterations facilitating bacterial adherence and/or clearance and permeability regulation of innate/adaptive immunity.

Similarly, epigenetic modulation of gene expression should be contemplated when considering how other environmental factors can affect the mucosa–microbiome–immunity interplay. A Westernized high-fat diet, full of refined carbohydrates, is strongly associated with the development of IBD, contrary to a diet high in fruit, vegetables and omega-3 PUFAs, which is protective against it [26]. Epigenetic mechanisms could explain the connection between genes and environmental factors in triggering the development of IBD. The definition of epigenetics refers to heritable alterations of gene expression events that are caused independently of genetic information carried by the primary DNA sequence. The main epigenetic mechanisms controlling gene expression include DNA methylation, histone modifications and small and long noncoding RNAs [48]. The main objective of epigenetics is to modulate gene expression without modifying the basic DNA sequence. All the mechanisms involved in epigenetics are involved in correct cell development, differentiation, function and homeostasis. Moreover, these mechanisms are influenced by exposure to environmental factors, persist through mitosis and meiosis and, more importantly, can be reversed. Recent advances have indicated that epigenetic variation has an important influence on interactions between nutrients and the genome, which modifies disease risk [49,50]. Diet is known to influence epigenetic changes associated with disease and to modify gene expression patterns in a state of disturbed immunity. A number of nutrients have been shown to modulate immune responses and can potentially counteract inflammatory processes [51]. Some studies have suggested that secondary plant metabolites, such as polyphenols, might modulate gene expression, chromatin remodeling and DNA methylation [52]. Epigenetic effects have also been shown for other dietary components, such as curcumin [53]. Moreover, specific components of the Mediterranean diet, particularly nuts and extra-virgin olive oil, have recently been found to be able to induce methylation changes in several peripheral white blood cells, showing a role for specific fatty acids in epigenetic modulation [54]. Thus, considering the status of epigenetic mechanisms in particular patients, it is important to understand whether a dietary intervention could help or not.

5. Diet as Possible Therapy

Despite the fact that a growing body of knowledge related to diet is emerging in terms of IBD pathogenesis, there is no strong evidence for dietary interventions helping to induce remission or to maintain response. Dietary therapies, such as enteral exclusive nutrition (EEN), have traditionally and primarily been used to induce remission in early or new-onset CD. EEN has been shown to be effective for inducing clinical remission, improving nutritional status, improving body composition, inducing mucosal healing and decreasing proinflammatory cytokines in pediatric and adult patients with CD. EEN has been extensively used for induction of remission in pediatric CD, in which avoidance of steroids is critical for childhood growth. However, EEN has been less often used for adult patients. Although some studies have assessed EEN in adults, most were less conclusive and had multiple confounding factors; thus, this practice is uncommon in adults with CD [55]. EEN involves the exclusive use of liquid nutrition in the form of medical formulas, without exposure to other foods, usually for 6–8 weeks. This effect does not depend on the protein source (a type of formula), but it does depend on the exclusion of ordinary table food [56]. Several recent pediatric studies have demonstrated and confirmed that EEN can induce remission in 60%–86% of children, accompanied by a significant decrease in inflammatory markers, such as the erythrocyte sedimentation rate, C-reactive protein and fecal calprotectin [57–59]. This recent body of literature has evaluated the long-term benefits associated with the use of EEN in mild-to-moderate pediatric CD. In comparison with the use of steroids, and corrected for disease severity, EEN has been associated with higher remission rates, better growth and longer steroid-free periods, but it did not differ in regard to other outcomes such as relapse. The benefit of EEN was lost when partial enteral nutrition (PEN) was used instead, with access to a free diet granted to patients [60]; thus, reaffirming the principle of exclusivity, suggesting that the mechanism depends on the exclusion of a free diet. However, a recent study has shown that PEN can be effective in combination with a "*prudent pattern diet*" [61]. In this study, PEN, with an exclusion diet based on components hypothesized to affect the microbiome or intestinal permeability, was effective for induction of remission in children and young adults with CD. Several randomized controlled trials are being developed in order to confirm this observation (NCT01728870, NCT 02843100, NCT02231814).

The idea of maintaining remission with diet is compelling and challenging at the same time. On the one hand, once remission is established, it is certainly possible that diet will be sufficient to maintain homeostasis and to prevent the cascade of proinflammatory events leading to flare-ups; however, long-term studies are challenging to perform, and adherence becomes a serious concern. Long-term studies on the maintenance of remission have largely focused on the use of semi-elemental EEN [62,63]. These data show promise for the use of semi-elemental EEN in the maintenance of CD. On the other hand, an interesting idea has been revealed by a recent study showing that, in patients with moderate to severe CD undergoing infliximab treatment (anti-TNFα therapy), combined EEN therapy of $\geq$600 kcal/day led to an increase in the remission maintenance rate, preventing loss of response to infliximab therapy [64]. These studies illustrate the potential benefit of elemental nutrition in the maintenance of remission in patients with CD; however, there are as yet no data to support this hypothesis.

Regarding fatty acids, PUFAs comprise two main groups of fats: omega-3 and omega-6 fatty acids. Omega-6 is considered an inflammatory fat, whereas omega-3 is anti-inflammatory. In human IBD, a systematic review has not supported the notion that supplementation of omega-3 fatty acids can induce and maintain remission of IBD [65]. The latest Cochrane review has reached a similar conclusion [66]. Interestingly, several studies have demonstrated that different genotypes can be associated with the variable response to nutritional intervention with omega-3 PUFAs. For example, genetic polymorphisms of TNFα and PPARγ have been associated with an altered response to nutritional intervention with omega-3 PUFAs [67]. In IBD, genetic polymorphisms, such as CYP4F3 and caspase 9+93C/T, modify the association between dietary fatty acid intake and risk of IBD [68]. Thus, specific mutations should also be considered before considering dietary therapeutic interventions.

6. Conclusions

Apart from EEN in specific situations, no strong evidence has been found to provide solid dietary intervention recommendations for patients with IBD. However, evidence and knowledge are accumulating and have suggested that pertinent studies should be prospectively developed in order to characterize potential dietary therapeutic possibilities. This body of knowledge leads us to recommend that a "prudent" diet or a "Mediterranean diet" should be advised to patients. Given that diet has been shown to be important for intestinal homeostasis and to avoid disruption of intestinal permeability, the consumption of vegetables, fruits, olive oil, fish, grains and nuts should be recommended, together with avoidance of the use of excessive additives and industrialized food processing.

Dietary recommendations for patients with IBD should emerge in a personalized manner, taking into consideration nutrient knowledge, the individual mucosa–microbiome–immunity interplay, the status of epigenetic changes and creeping fat metabolism. Dietary recommendations cannot be generalized for all patients, however. Given that the above elements differ per patient, no single dietary intervention can offer the same improvement for all patients. Thus, future studies should take this factor into account and be designed accordingly.

Author Contributions: Conceptualization, B.B., P.N. and I.M.; Writing-Original Draft Preparation, E.S.-G. and B.M.; Writing-Review & Editing, E.S.-G., I.M. and P.L.-M.; Supervision, P.N. and M.I.

References

1. Cosnes, J.; Gowerroisseau-Rousseau, C.; Seksik, P.; Cortot, A. Epidemiology and natural history of inflammatory bowel diseases. *Gastroenterology* **2011**, *140*, 1785–1794. [CrossRef] [PubMed]
2. Ananthakrishnan, A.N. Epidemiology and risk factors for IBD. *Nat. Rev. Gastroenterol. Hepatol.* **2015**, *12*, 205–217. [CrossRef]
3. Dutta, A.K.; Chacko, A. Influence of environmental factors on the onset and course of inflammatory bowel disease. *World J. Gastroenterol.* **2016**, *22*, 1088–1100. [CrossRef] [PubMed]
4. Zangenberg, M.S.; Horesh, N.; Kopylov, U.; El-Hussuna, A. Preoperative optimization of patients with inflammatory bowel disease undergoing gastrointestinal surgery: A systematic review. *Int. J. Colorectal. Dis.* **2017**, *32*, 1663–1676. [CrossRef] [PubMed]
5. Forbes, A.; Escher, J.; Hébuterne, X.; Kłęk, S.; Krznaric, Z.; Schneider, S.; Shamir, R.; Stardelova, K.; Wierdsma, N.; Wiskin, A.E.; et al. ESPEN guideline: Clinical nutrition in inflammatory bowel disease. *Clin. Nutr.* **2017**, *36*, 321–347. [CrossRef] [PubMed]
6. McDonald, P.J.; Fazio, V.W. What can Crohn's patients eat? *Eur. J. Clin. Nutr.* **1988**, *42*, 703–708. [PubMed]
7. Moser, G.; Tillinger, W.; Sachs, G.; Maier-Dobersberger, T.; Wyatt, J.; Vogelsang, H.; Lochs, H.; Gangl, A. Relationship between the use of unconventional therapies and disease-related concerns: A study of patients with inflammatory bowel disease. *J. Psychosom. Res.* **1996**, *40*, 503–509. [CrossRef]
8. Maynard, C.L.; Elson, C.O.; Hatton, R.D.; Weaver, C.T. Reciprocal interactions of the intestinal microbiota and immune system. *Nature* **2012**, *489*, 231–241. [CrossRef] [PubMed]
9. Martini, E.; Krug, S.M.; Siegmund, B.; Neurath, M.F.; Becker, C. Mend Your Fences: The epithelial Barrier and its Relationship With Mucosal Immunity in Inflammatory Bowel Disease. *Cell Mol. Gastroenterol. Hepatol.* **2017**, *23*, 33–46. [CrossRef]

10. Jantchou, P.; Morois, S.; Clavel-Chapelon, F.; Boutron-Ruault, M.C.; Carbonnel, F. Animal protein intake and risk of inflammatory bowel disease: The E3N prospective study. *Am. J. Gastroenterol.* **2010**, *105*, 2195–2201. [CrossRef]
11. D'Souza, S.; Levy, E.; Mack, D.; Israel, D.; Lambrette, P.; Ghadirian, P.; Deslandres, C.; Morgan, K.; Seidman, E.G.; Amre, D.K. Dietary patterns and risk for Crohn's disease in children. *Inflamm. Bowel Dis.* **2008**, *14*, 367–373. [CrossRef]
12. Racine, A.; Carbonnel, F.; Chan, S.S.; Hart, A.R.; Bueno-de-Mesquita, H.B.; Oldenburg, B.; van Schalk, F.D.; Tjønneland, A.; Dahm, C.C.; Key, T.; et al. Dietary patterns and risk of inflammatory bowel disease in Europe: Results from the EPIC study. *Inflamm. Bowel Dis.* **2016**, *22*, 345–354. [CrossRef]
13. Shoda, R.; Matsueda, K.; Yamato, S.; Umeda, N. Epidemiologic analysis of Crohn disease in Japan: Increased dietary intake of n-6 polyunsaturated fatty acids and animal protein relates to the increased incidence of Crohn disease in Japan. *Am. J. Clin. Nutr.* **1996**, *63*, 741–745. [CrossRef] [PubMed]
14. Jowett, S.L.; Seal, C.J.; Pearce, M.S.; Phillips, E.; Gregory, W.; Barton, J.R.; Welfare, M.R. Influence of dietary factors on the clinical course of ulcerative colitis: A prospective cohort study. *Gut* **2004**, *53*, 1479–1484. [CrossRef]
15. Ananthakrishnan, A.N.; Khalili, H.; Konijeti, G.G.; Higuchi, L.M.; de Silva, P.; Korzenik, J.R.; Fuchs, C.S.; Willett, W.C.; Richter, J.M.; Chan, A.T. A prospective study of long-term intake of dietary fiber and risk of crohn's disease and ulcerative colitis. *Gastroenterology* **2013**, *145*, 970–977. [CrossRef]
16. Costea, I.; Mack, D.R.; Lemaitre, R.N.; Israel, D.; Marcil, V.; Ahmad, A.; Amre, D.K. Interactions between the dietary polyunsaturated fatty acid ratio and genetic factors determine susceptibility to pediatric Crohn's disease. *Gastroenterology* **2014**, *146*, 929–931. [CrossRef]
17. Chan, S.S.; Luben, R.; van Schaik, F.; Oldenburg, B.; Bueno-de-Mesquita, H.B.; Hallmans, G.; Karling, P.; Lindgren, S.; Grip, O.; Key, T.; et al. Carbohydrate intake in the etiology of Crohn's disease and ulcerative colitis. *Inflamm. Bowel Dis.* **2014**, *20*, 2013–2021. [CrossRef] [PubMed]
18. Torres, J.; Caprioli, F.; Katsanos, K.H.; Lobatón, T.; Micic, D.; Zerôncio, M.; Van Assche, G.; Lee, J.C.; Lindsay, J.O.; Rubin, D.T.; et al. Predicting outcomes to optimize disease management in inflammatory bowel diseases. *J. Crohns. Colitis.* **2016**, *10*, 1385–1394. [CrossRef] [PubMed]
19. Xu, L.; Lochhead, P.; Ko, Y.; Claggett, B.; Leong, R.W.; Ananthakrishnan, A.N. Systematic review with meta-analysis: Breastfeeding and the risk of Crohn's disease and ulcerative colitis. *Aliment. Pharmacol. Ther.* **2017**, *46*, 780–789. [CrossRef] [PubMed]
20. Hou, J.K.; Abraham, B.; El-Serag, H. Dietary intake and risk of developing inflammatory bowel disease: A systematic review of the literature. *Am. J. Gastroenterol.* **2011**, *106*, 563–573. [CrossRef] [PubMed]
21. Tjonneland, A.; Overvad, K.; Bergmann, M.M.; Nagel, G.; Linseisen, J.; Hallmans, G.; Palmqvist, R.; Sjodin, H.; Hagglund, G.; Berglund, G.; et al. Linoleic acid, a dietary n-6 polyunsaturated fatty acid, and the aetiology of ulcerative colitis: A nested case-control study within a European prospective cohort study. *Gut* **2009**, *58*, 1606–1611, Epub 23 Jul 2009. [CrossRef]
22. Chan, S.S.; Luben, R.; Olsen, A.; Tjonneland, A.; Kaaks, R.; Lindgren, S.; Grip, O.; Bergmann, M.M.; Boeing, H.; Hallmans, G.; et al. Association between high dietary intake of the n-3 polyunsaturated fatty acid docosahexaenoic acid and reduced risk of Crohn's disease. *Aliment. Pharmacol. Ther.* **2014**, *39*, 834–842. [CrossRef]
23. Niewiadomski, O.; Studd, C.; Wilson, J.; Williams, J.; Hair, C.; Knight, R.; Prewett, E.; Dabkowski, P.; Alexander, S.; Allen, B.; et al. Influence of food and lifestyle on the risk of developing inflammatory bowel disease. *Intern. Med. J.* **2016**, *46*, 669–676. [CrossRef] [PubMed]
24. Godny, L.; Maharshak, N.; Reshef, L.; Goren, I.; Yahav, L.; Fliss-Isakov, N.; Gophna, U.; Tulchinsky, H.; Dotan, I. Fruit consumption is associated with alterations in microbial composition and lower rates of pouchitis. *J. Crohns. Colitis.* **2019**, *4*. [CrossRef] [PubMed]
25. Chassaing, B.; Koren, O.; Goodrich, J.K.; Poole, A.C.; Srinivasan, S.; Ley, R.E.; Gewirtz, A.T. Dietary emulsifiers impact the mouse gut microbiota promoting colitis and metabolic syndrome. *Nature* **2015**, *519*, 92–96. [CrossRef] [PubMed]
26. Taylor, L.; Almutairdi, A.; Shommu, N.; Fedorak, R.; Ghosh, S.; Reimer, R.A.; Panaccione, R.; Raman, M. Cross-sectional analysis of overall dietary intake and mediterranean dietary pattern in patients with crohn's disease. *Nutrients* **2018**, *10*, 1761. [CrossRef] [PubMed]

27. Salyers, A.A.; West, S.E.; Vercellotti, J.R.; Wilkins, T.D. Fermentation of mucins and plant polysaccharides by anaerobic bacteria from the human colon. *Appl. Environ. Microbiol.* **1977**, *34*, 529–533. [PubMed]
28. Marsman, K.E.; McBurney, M.I. Dietary fiber increases oxidative metabolism in colonocytes but not in distal small intestinal enterocytes isolated from rats. *J. Nutr.* **1995**, *125*, 273–282. [CrossRef]
29. Kelly, C.J.; Zheng, L.; Campbell, E.L.; Saeedi, B.; Scholz, C.C.; Bayless, A.J.; Wilson, K.E.; Glover, L.E.; Kominsky, D.J.; Magnuson, A.; et al. Crosstalk between Microbiota-Derived Short-Chain Fatty Acids and Intestinal Epithelial HIF Augments Tissue Barrier Function. *Cell Host. Microbe.* **2015**, *17*, 662–671. [CrossRef] [PubMed]
30. Saeedi, B.J.; Kao, D.J.; Kitzenberg, D.A.; Dobrinskikh, E.; Schwisow, K.D.; Masterson, J.C.; Kendrick, A.A.; Kelly, C.J.; Bayless, A.J.; Kominsky, D.J.; et al. HIF-dependent regulation of claudin-1 is central to intestinal epithelial tight junction integrity. *Mol. Biol. Cell.* **2015**, *26*, 2252–2262. [CrossRef] [PubMed]
31. Peng, L.; Li, Z.R.; Green, R.S.; Holzman, I.R.; Lin, J. Butyrate enhances the intestinal barrier by facilitating tight junction assembly via activation of AMP-activated protein kinase in Caco-2 cell monolayers. *J. Nutr.* **2009**, *139*, 1619–1625. [CrossRef] [PubMed]
32. Burger-van Paassen, N.; Vincent, A.; Puiman, P.J.; van der Sluis, M.; Bouma, J.; Boehm, G.; van Goudoever, J.B.; van Seuningen, I.; Renes, I.B. The regulation of intestinal mucin MUC2 expression by short-chain fatty acids: Implications for epithelial protection. *Biochem. J.* **2009**, *420*, 211219. [CrossRef] [PubMed]
33. Furusawa, Y.; Obata, Y.; Fukuda, S.; Endo, T.A.; Nakato, G.; Takahashi, D.; Nakanishi, Y.; Uetake, C.; Kato, K.; Kato, T.; et al. Commensal microbe-derived butyrate induces the differentiation of colonic regulatory T cells. *Nature* **2013**, *504*, 446–450. [CrossRef] [PubMed]
34. Desai, M.S.; Seekatz, A.M.; Koropatkin, N.M.; Kamada, N.; Hickey, C.A.; Wolter, M.; Pudlo, N.A.; Kitamoto, S.; Terrapon, N.; Muller, A.; et al. A dietary fiber-deprived gut microbiota degrades the colonic mucus barrier and enhances pathogen susceptibility. *Cell* **2016**, *167*, 1339–1353.e21. [CrossRef]
35. Bach Knudsen, K.E.; Lærke, H.N.; Hedemann, M.S.; Nielsen, T.S.; Ingerslev, A.K.; Gundelund Nielsen, D.S.; Theil, P.K.; Purup, S.; Hald, S.; Schioldan, A.G.; et al. Impact of Diet-Modulated Butyrate Production on Intestinal Barrier Function and Inflammation. *Nutrients* **2018**, *10*, 1499. [CrossRef]
36. Wang, H.; Shi, P.; Zuo, L.; Dong, J.; Zhao, J.; Liu, Q.; Zhu, W. Dietary Non-digestible polysaccharides ameliorate intestinal epithelial barrier dysfunction in il-10 knockout mice. *J. Crohns. Colitis.* **2016**, *10*, 1076–1086. [CrossRef] [PubMed]
37. Ma, X.; Torbenson, M.; Hamad, A.R.; Soloski, M.J.; Li, Z. High-fat diet modulates non-CD1d-restricted natural killer T cells and regulatory T cells in mouse colon and exacerbates experimental colitis. *Clin. Exp. Immunol.* **2008**, *151*, 130–138. [CrossRef] [PubMed]
38. Morgan, X.; Tickle, T.; Sokol, H.; Gevers, D.; Devaney, K.; Ward, D.; Reyes, J.A.; Shah, S.A.; LeLeiko, N.; Snapper, S.B.; et al. Dysfunction of the intestinal microbiome in inflammatory bowel disease and treatment. *Genome. Biol.* **2012**, *13*, R79. [CrossRef]
39. Davenport, M.; Poles, J.; Leung, J.M.; Wolff, M.J.; Abidi, W.M.; Ullman, T.; Mayer, L.; Cho, I.; Loke, P. Metabolic alterations to the mucosal microbiota inflammatory bowel disease. *Inflamm. Bowel. Dis.* **2014**, *20*, 723–731. [CrossRef]
40. Ren, W.; Liu, G.; Yin, J.; Tan, B.; Wu, G.; Bazer, F.W.; Peng, Y.; Yin, Y. Amino-acid transporters in T-cell activation and differentiation. *Cell Death Dis.* **2017**, *8*, 1–9. [CrossRef]
41. Langston, P.K.; Shibata, M.; Horng, T. Metabolism Supports Macrophage Activation. *Front. Immunol.* **2017**, *8*, 61. [CrossRef] [PubMed]
42. Palego, L.; Betti, L.; Rossi, A.; Giannaccini, G. Tryptophan biochemistry: Structural, nutritional, metabolic, and medical aspects in humans. *J. Amino Acids* **2016**, *2016*, 1–13. [CrossRef]
43. Lee, J.S.; Cella, M.; McDonald, K.G.; Garlanda, C.; Kennedy, G.D.; Nukaya, M.; Mantovani, A.; Kopan, R.; Bradfield, C.A.; Newberry, R.D.; et al. AHR drives the development of gut ILC22 cells and postnatal lymphoid tissues via pathways dependent on and independent of Notch. *Nat. Immunol.* **2012**, *13*, 144–152. [CrossRef] [PubMed]
44. Mezrich, J.D.; Fechner, J.H.; Zhang, X.; Johnson, B.P.; Burlingham, W.J.; Bradfield, C.A. An interaction between kynurenine and the aryl hydrocarbon receptor can generate regulatory T cells. *J. Immunol.* **2010**, *185*, 3190–3198. [CrossRef] [PubMed]

45. El-Zaatari, M.; Bass, A.J.; Bowlby, R.; Zhang, M.; Syu, L.J.; Yang, Y.; Grasberger, H.; Shreiner, A.; Tan, B.; Bishu, S.; et al. Indoleamine 2,3-Dioxygenase 1, increased in human gastric pre-neoplasia, promotes inflammation and metaplasia in mice and is associated with type II hypersensitivity/autoimmunity. *Gastroenterology* **2018**, *154*, 140–153.e17. [CrossRef] [PubMed]
46. Wagner, S.J.; Schmidt, A.; Effenberger, M.J.P.; Gruber, L.; Danier, J.; Haller, D. Semisynthetic diet ameliorates Crohn's disease–like ileitis in TNFΔARE/WT mice through antigen-independent mechanisms of gluten. *Inflamm. Bowel Dis.* **2013**, *19*, 1285–1294. [CrossRef]
47. Gonçalves, P.; Magro, F.; Martel, F. Metabolic inflammation in inflammatory bowel disease: Crosstalk between adipose tissue and bowel. *Inflamm. Bowel Dis.* **2015**, *21*, 453–467. [CrossRef]
48. Ventham, N.T.; Kennedy, N.A.; Nimmo, E.R.; Satsangi, J. Beyond gene discovery in inflammatory bowel disease: The emerging role of epigenetics. *Gastroenterology* **2013**, *145*, 293–308. [CrossRef]
49. Legaki, E.; Gazouli, M. Influence of environmental factors in the development of inflammatory bowel diseases. *World J. Gastrointest. Pharmacol. Ther.* **2016**, *7*, 112–125. [CrossRef]
50. Aleksandrova, K.; Romero-Mosquera, B.; Hernandez, V. Diet, gut microbiome and epigenetics: Emerging links with inflammatory bowel diseases and prospects for management and prevention. *Nutrients* **2017**, *30*, 962. [CrossRef]
51. Burdge, G.C.; Hoile, S.P.; Lillycrop, K.A. Epigenetics: Are there implications for personalised nutrition? *Curr. Opin. Clin. Nutr. Metab. Care* **2012**, *15*, 442–447. [CrossRef]
52. Remely, M.; Lovrecic, L.; de la Garza, A.L.; Migliore, L.; Peterlin, B.; Milagro, F.I.; Martinez, A.J.; Haslberger, A.G. Therapeutic perspectives of epigenetically active nutrients. *Br. J. Pharm.* **2015**, *172*, 2756–2768. [CrossRef]
53. Reuter, S.; Gupta, S.C.; Park, B.; Goel, A.; Aggarwal, B.B. Epigenetic changes induced by curcumin and other natural compounds. *Genes Nutr.* **2011**, *6*, 93–108. [CrossRef] [PubMed]
54. Arpón, A.; Milagro, F.I.; Razquin, C.; Corella, D.; Estruch, R.; Fitó, M.; Marti, A.; Martínez-González, M.A.; Ros, E.; Salas-Salvadó, J.; et al. Impact of consuming extra-virgin olive oil or nuts within a mediterranean diet on dna methylation in peripheral white blood cells within the predimed-navarra randomized controlled trial: A role for dietary lipids. *Nutrients* **2017**, *10*, 15. [CrossRef]
55. Ruemmele, F.M.; Veres, G.; Kolho, K.L.; Griffiths, A.; Levine, A.; Escher, J.C.; Amil-Dias, J.; Barabino, A.; Braegger, C.P.; Bronsky, J.; et al. Consensus guidelines of ECCO/ESPGHAN on the medical management of pediatric Crohn's disease. *J. Crohns Colitis.* **2014**, *8*, 1179–1207. [CrossRef] [PubMed]
56. Lee, D.; Baldassano, R.N.; Otley, A.R.; Albenberg, L.; Griffiths, A.M.; Compher, C.; Chen, E.Z.; Li, H.; Gilroy, E.; Nessel, L.; et al. Comparative effectiveness of nutritional and biological therapy in north american children with active crohn's disease. *Inflamm. Bowel Dis.* **2015**, *21*, 1786–1793. [CrossRef] [PubMed]
57. Levine, A.; Turner, D.; Pfeffer-Gik, T.; Amil-Dias, J.; Veres, G.; Shaoul, R.; Staiano, A.; Escher, J.; Kolho, K.L.; Paerregaard, A.; et al. Comparison of outcomes parameters for induction of remission in new onset pediatric Crohn's disease: Evaluation of the porto IBD group "growth relapse and outcomes with therapy" (GROWTH CD) study. *Inflamm. Bowel Dis.* **2014**, *20*, 278–285. [CrossRef] [PubMed]
58. Connors, J.; Basseri, S.; Grant, A.; Giffin, N.; Mahdi, G.; Noble, A.; Rashid, M.; Otley, A.; Van-Limbergen, J. Exclusive enteral nutrition therapy in paediatric crohn's disease results in long-term avoidance of corticosteroids: Results of a propensity-score matched cohort analysis. *J. Crohns Colitis.* **2017**, *11*, 1063–1070. [CrossRef]
59. Cohen-Dolev, N.; Sladek, M.; Hussey, S.; Turner, D.; Veres, G.; Koletzko, S.; Martin de Carpi, J.; Staiano, A.; Shaoul, R.; Lionetti, P.; et al. Differences in outcomes over time with exclusive enteral nutrition compared with steroids in children with mild to moderate crohn's disease: Results from the growth cd study. *J. Crohns Colitis.* **2018**, *12*, 306–312. [CrossRef]
60. Levine, A.; Wine, E. Effects of enteral nutrition on Crohn's disease: Clues to the impact of diet on disease pathogenesis. *Inflamm. Bowel Dis.* **2013**, *19*, 1322–1329. [CrossRef]
61. Sigall-Boneth, R.; Pfeffer-Gik, T.; Segal, I.; Zangen, T.; Boaz, M.; Levine, A. Partial enteral nutrion with a Crohn's disease exclusion diet is effective for induction of remission in children and young adults with Crohn's disease. *Inflamm. Bowel Dis.* **2014**, *20*, 1353–1360. [CrossRef] [PubMed]
62. Takagi, S.; Utsunomiya, K.; Kuriyama, S.; Yokoyama, H.; Takahashi, S.; Iwabuchi, M.; Takahashi, S.; Kinouchi, Y.; Hiwatashi, N.; Funayama, Y.; et al. Effectiveness of an "half elemental diet" as maintenance

therapy for Crohn's disease: A randomized controlled trial. *Aliment. Pharmacol. Ther.* **2006**, *24*, 1333–1340. [CrossRef]
63. Yamamoto, T.; Nakahigashi, M.; Umegae, S.; Kitagawa, T.; Matsumoto, K. Impact of long-term enteral nutrition on clinical and endoscopic recurrence after resection for Crohn's disease: A prospective, non-randomized, parallel, controlled study. *Aliment. Pharmacol. Ther.* **2007**, *25*, 67–72. [CrossRef]
64. Hisamatsu, T.; Kunisaki, R.; Nakamura, S.; Tsujikawa, T.; Hirai, F.; Nakase, H.; Watanabe, K.; Yokoyama, K.; Nagahori, M.; Kanai, T.; et al. Effect of elemental diet combined with infliximab dose escalation in patients with Crohn's disease with loss of response to infliximab: CERISIER trial. *Intest. Res.* **2018**, *16*, 494–498. [CrossRef]
65. Turner, D.; Shah, P.S.; Steinhart, A.H.; Zlotkin, S.; Griffiths, A.M. Maintenance of remission in inflammatory bowel disease using omega-3 fatty acids (fish oil): A systematic review and meta-analyses. *Inflamm. Bowel. Dis.* **2011**, *17*, 336–345. [CrossRef] [PubMed]
66. Turner, D.; Zlotkin, S.H.; Shah, P.S.; Griffiths, A.M. Omega 3 fatty acids (fish oil) for maintenance of remission in Crohn's disease. *Cochrane Database Syst. Rev.* **2009**, *21*, CD006320. [CrossRef]
67. Paradis, A.M.; Fontaine-Bisson, B.; Bossé, Y.; Robitaille, J.; Lemieux, S.; Jacques, H.; Lamarche, B.; Tchernof, A.; Couture, P.; Vohl, M.C. The peroxisome proliferator-activated receptor alpha Leu162Val polymorphism influences the metabolic response to a dietary intervention altering fatty acid proportions in healthy men. *Am. J. Clin. Nutr.* **2005**, *81*, 523–530. [CrossRef]
68. Ananthakrishnan, A.N.; Khalili, H.; Song, M.; Higuchi, L.M.; Lochhead, P.; Richter, J.M.; Chan, A.T. Genetic polymorphisms in fatty acid metabolism modify the association between dietary n3: n6 intake and risk of ulcerative colitis: A prospective cohort study. *Inflamm. Bowel Dis.* **2017**, *23*, 1898–1904. [CrossRef]

12

Diet in the Pathogenesis and Management of Ulcerative Colitis: A Review of Randomized Controlled Dietary Interventions

Ammar Hassanzadeh Keshteli [1,2], Karen L. Madsen [1,2] and Levinus A. Dieleman [1,2,*]

1 Department of Medicine, University of Alberta, Edmonton, AB T6G 2P5, Canada
2 Centre of Excellence for Gastrointestinal Inflammation and Immunity Research (CEGIIR), Edmonton, AB T6G 2X8, Canada
* Correspondence: l.dieleman@ualberta.ca

Abstract: Epidemiological and experimental studies have suggested that diet is one of the environmental factors that contributes to the onset and pathophysiology of ulcerative colitis. Although many patients suffering from ulcerative colitis attribute their symptoms or disease relapse to dietary factors, only a few well-designed randomized controlled trials have been done to investigate the role of diet in the management of ulcerative colitis. Here, we review the potential mechanisms of the relationship between diet and pathogenesis of ulcerative colitis and summarize randomized controlled dietary interventions that have been conducted in ulcerative colitis patients.

Keywords: diet; inflammatory bowel disease; ulcerative colitis

---

1. Introduction

Ulcerative colitis (UC)—a subtype of inflammatory bowel disease (IBD)—is a chronic, idiopathic inflammatory disease that affects the colon and is characterized by relapsing and remitting mucosal inflammation [1]. UC patients mostly present blood in the stool and diarrhea [1]. UC is associated with major morbidity in Western countries, and its incidence is increasing in developing countries [2]. The multifactorial pathophysiology of UC includes genetic predisposition, epithelial barrier defects, dysregulated immune responses, microbial dysbiosis, and environmental factors [1,2].

It has been suggested that environmental factors play a major role in the pathogenesis of IBD. Early-life events such as mode of birth, breastfeeding, and exposure to antibiotics and other factors such as air pollution, smoking, psychological state, exercise, and diet are among the potential environmental contributors of IBD development or disease activity [3].

Significant changes in dietary intake during the past decades have been associated with the increase in incidence of UC. The relationship between diet and UC development has been indicated in several epidemiological studies [4]. Two recent meta-analysis studies showed that soft drink consumption and sucrose intake were associated with 69% and 10% increased risk of UC development, respectively [5,6]. Consumption of fruits (odds ratio: 0.57) and vegetables (odds ratio: 0.71) was related to decreased odds of UC development in another meta-analysis study [7]. A significant association between meat intake (red meat in particular) and UC risk was found in a meta-analysis of seven epidemiological studies (summary relative risk: 1.47) [8]. Furthermore, whereas *n*-3 polyunsaturated fatty acids (PUFAs) content of diet was related to decreased odds of UC development (odds ratio:

0.56) [9], dietary arachidonic acid (an n-6 PUFA) as measured in adipose tissue increased risk of UC development (relative risk: 4.16) in a large prospective cohort study among Danish adults [10]. Although the exact pathophysiological mechanisms in which diet plays a role in IBD development remain unknown, several plausible explanations including its effects on composition of gut microbiota, production of microbial metabolites, alterations in mucosal immunity, and mucosal barrier function have been proposed [11] (Figure 1).

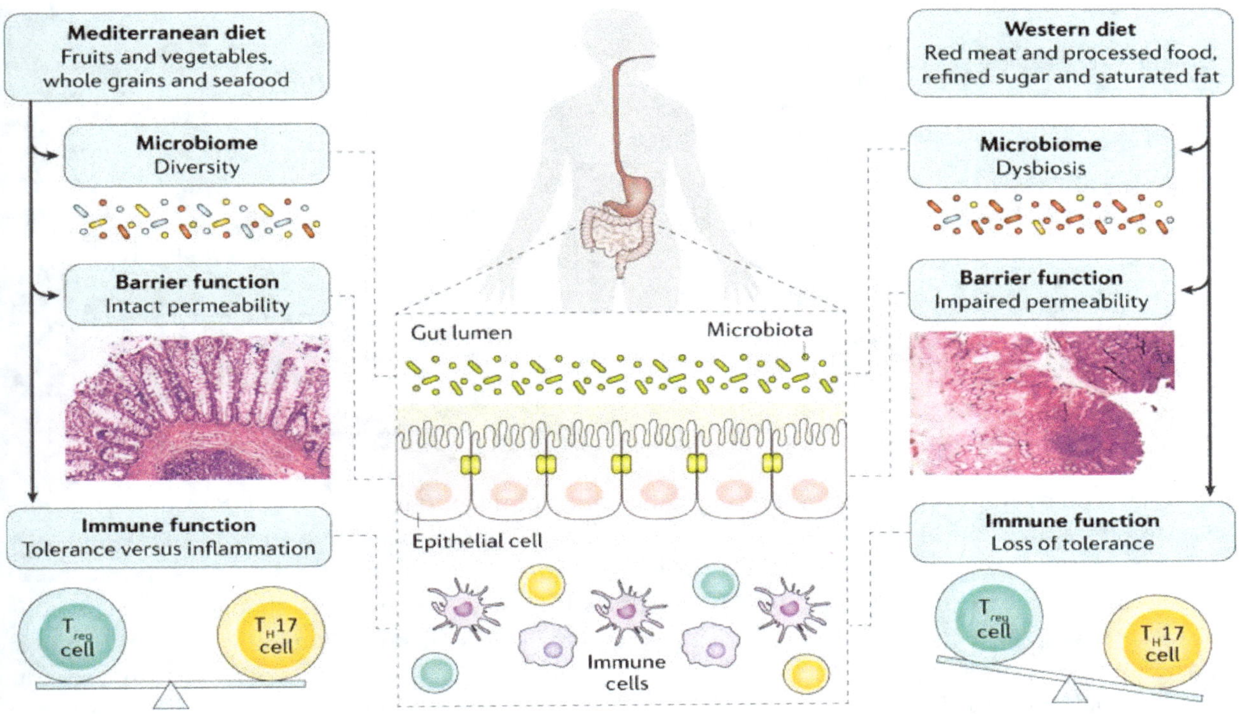

Figure 1. Although the exact mechanisms responsible for the association between diet and development of inflammatory bowel disease is unknown, several mechanisms have been suggested. An unhealthy dietary pattern such as a Western diet has been linked to changes in the gut microbiome and epithelial barrier function and seems to have a direct influence on immune function, triggering a pro-inflammatory environment characterized by an imbalance in the T helper 17 (T_H17) cell to regulatory T (T_{reg}) cell ratio [Adapted with permission [11]].

Abnormalities in the intestinal microbiota have been reported in some, but not all UC patients [1,12–14]. In some studies, UC patients have been shown to have decreased bacterial diversity, characterized by a decreased Firmicutes and increased *Gammaproteobacteria* and *Enterobacteriaceae* [15]. However, it is not clear if bacterial dysbiosis is the cause or effect of mucosal inflammation in UC [1,13] (Figure 2).

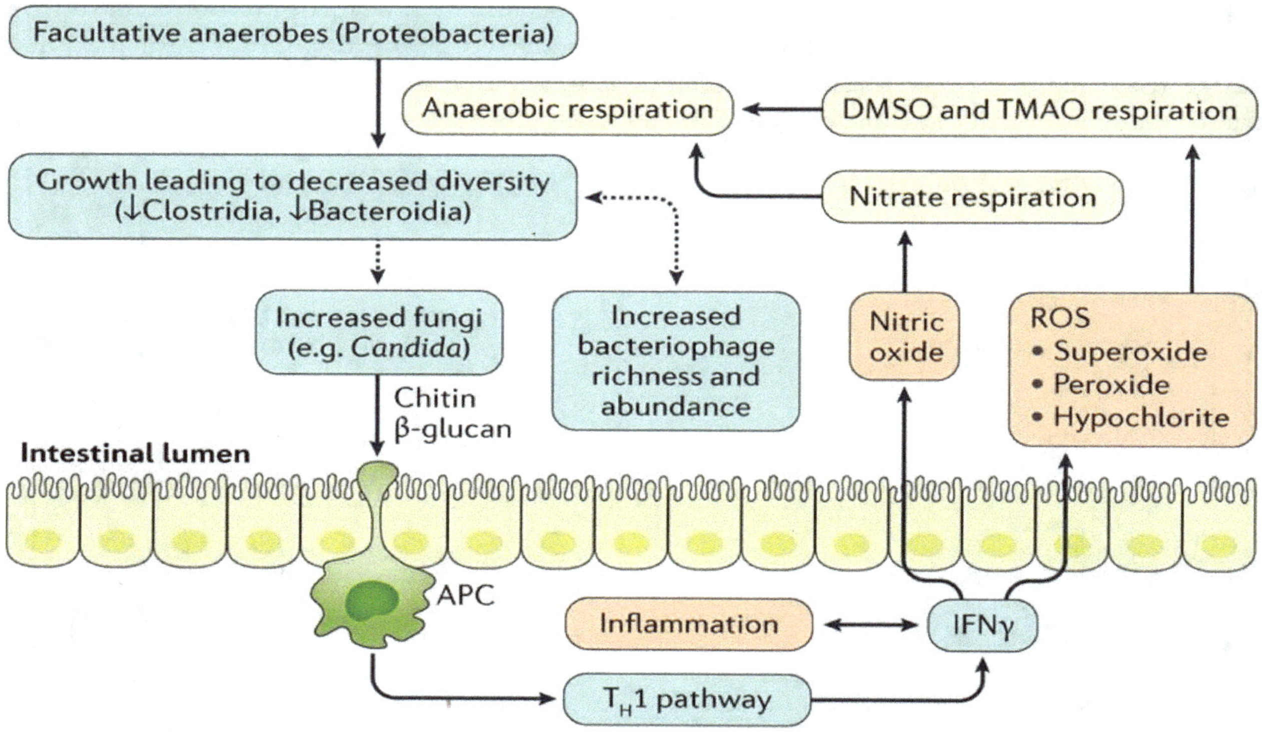

Figure 2. The relationship between gut microbiota and colonic inflammation in inflammatory bowel disease. Inflammation in colon stimulates production of Interferon gamma (IFN-γ) that eventually generates reactive oxygen species (ROS). ROS make products for anaerobic respiration. These products can be used by facultative anaerobes to outgrow, which leads to decreased bacterial diversity. The dysbiotic microbiota may further stimulate the growth of fungi that can worsen inflammation via chitin and β -glucan antigen-presenting cell (APC) activation of the type 1 T helper (T_H1) pathway. In addition, the microbial dysbiosis is associated with increased bacteriophage richness and abundance, which can affect the bacterial microbiota via gene transfer. DMSO, dimethyl sulfoxide; TMAO, trimethylamine N-oxide. [Adapted with permission [13]].

Dietary factors can be related to UC pathogenesis or disease course through direct effects on the host or indirect effects through modulations of composition or function of gut microbiota. Diet has a major role in shaping gut microbial composition [16]. For instance, increased *Bacteroidetes* and decreased *Firmicutes* and *Enterobacteriaceae* in rural African children in comparison to European children were mainly attributed to differences in dietary patterns between the two populations [17]. Therefore, it has been suggested that diet-induced changes in microbiota may transform healthy gut microbiota into a disease-inducing entity that could either initiate or perpetuate inflammation in patients with IBD [16]. Agus et al. [18] indicated that a high fat/high sugar diet resulted in intestinal mucosal dysbiosis characterized by an overgrowth of pro-inflammatory proteobacteria and a decrease in protective bacteria. In addition, they showed that the transplantation of feces from high fat/high sugar fed mice to germ-free mice increased susceptibility to adherent-invasive *Escherichia coli* infection.

In addition to their significant effects on microbial composition, dietary factors can also affect the metabolic functions of gut microbiota. Short chain fatty acids (SCFA), which are defined as the groups of fatty acids with fewer than six carbons including formic acid (C1), acetic acid (C2), propionic acid (C3), butyric acid (C4), and valeric acid (C5), are derived from commensal bacterial fermentation of indigestible dietary fibers in both the small and large intestines [19,20]. Acetate, propionate and butyrate account for more than 95 % of all the SCFA content in the gut [19]. Acetate and butyrate in particular have an essential role in maintaining mucosal barrier function and modulating immune function [21,22] (Figure 3). SCFA regulate the functions of epithelial and/or immune cells through altering gene expression, cellular differentiation, chemotaxis, proliferation, and apoptosis [19].

The number of SCFA-producing bacteria such as *Faecalibacterium prausnitzii* is decreased in some UC patients, and these are inversely correlated with disease activity [23]. Moreover, a western diet characterized by high intake of sugar [18,24] and fat [18] and decreased amount of dietary fiber was associated with decreased SCFAs and increased susceptibility to colitis in experimental studies.

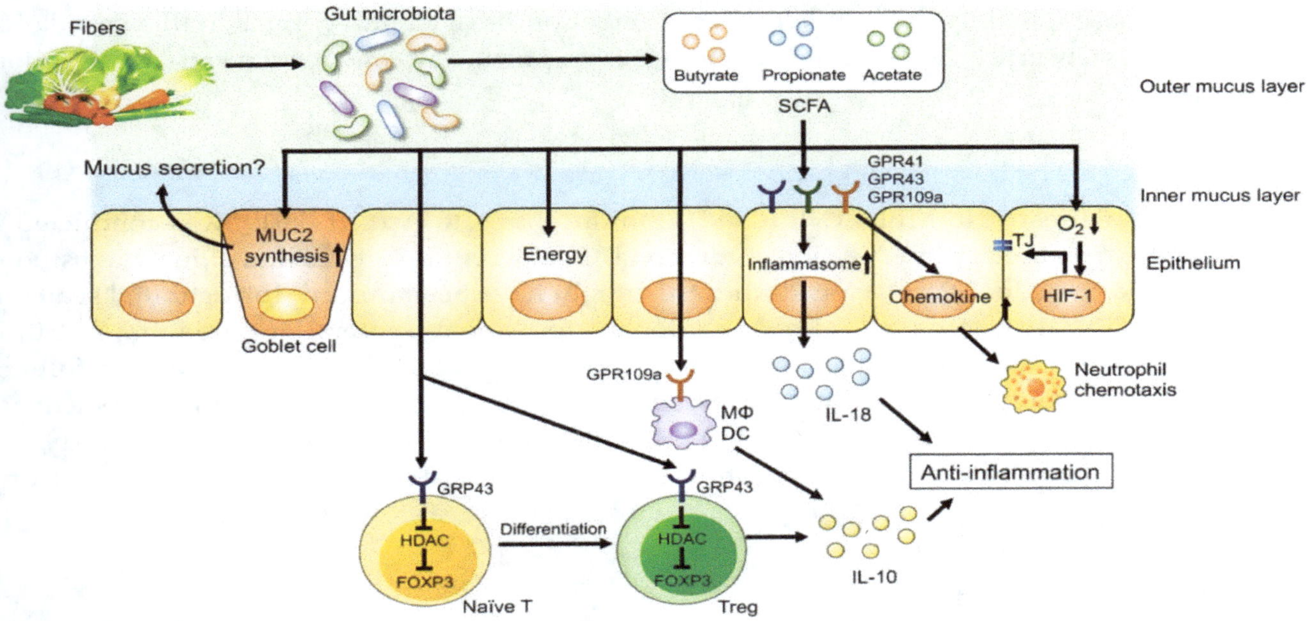

Figure 3. The role of fiber-derived short chain fatty acids (SCFAs) in regulation of intestinal homeostasis. SCFAs serve as energy substrates for colonocytes. In addition, SCFAs regulate intestinal barrier function and immune system through G-protein-coupled receptors (GPRs) signaling. SCFAs promote the differentiation of regulatory T (Treg) cells and the production of interleukin (IL)-10 through GPR43. Furthermore, SCFA facilitate inflammasome activation in colonic epithelial cells through GPR43, stimulating IL-18 production that is critical for anti-inflammation and epithelial repair. SCFAs also regulate intestinal barrier function via enhancing the expression of tight junction proteins and the synthesis of mucin (MUC)2. DC, dendritic cells; FOXP3, forkhead box P3; HDAC, histone deacetylases; Mϕ, macrophages; TJ, tight junctions. [Adapted with permission [22]].

The mucus layer and intestinal epithelium are the first physical and chemical barriers against intestinal bacteria, pathogens, and food antigens. A dysregulated mucosal immune response characterized by alterations in the innate immune system, activation of effector T-cells, increased presence of B-cells and antibody production, and increased production of pro-inflammatory mediators have a major role in the pathogenesis of IBD [1,25]. Dietary factors can have direct effects on host cells. For instance, it was shown that luminal iron may directly affect function of intestinal epithelial cells and T cells in addition to triggering epithelial cell stress-associated apoptosis [26]. Zinc is an important cofactor for various intestinal metalloproteinases, and zinc deficiency has been associated with reduced barrier integrity and increased permeability in IBD patients [27]. There is also increasing evidence for a role of vitamin D in strengthening the innate immune system and reducing inflammation in experimental and human IBD [28]. Relationships between PUFAs content of diet and inflammatory processes in IBD have also been shown [29,30]. Eicosapentaenoic acid and docosahexaenoic acid that are long chain dietary *n*-3 PUFAs inhibit genes that are involved in inflammatory process and alter the composition of cell membranes by displacing *n*-6 PUFAs, influencing lipid raft formation in cell signaling [30]. Dietary amino acids act as key regulatory factors in cellular and microbial metabolic pathways and play important roles in gut homeostasis. Intestinal inflammation as seen in IBD affects several metabolic pathways related to metabolism of amino acids [22]. It has been reported that several food additives, such as maltodextrin, emulsifying agents, or thickeners such as carboxymethyl cellulose, carrageenan, and xanthan gum, may also have detrimental effects on intestinal homeostasis as well [31]. A complete review of all dietary factors and host interactions is beyond the scope of this review; however, those interactions have been described comprehensively in other recent review articles [11,21,22,31–34].

Currently, dietary recommendations for management of IBD-related symptoms are scarce and non-evidence-based, mainly due to the limited number of dietary interventions in this population. In the present review article, we summarize findings from previously conducted dietary interventions in UC patients.

2. Methods

An electronic search in MEDLINE (Ovid) from inception to April 1, 2019, was conducted in order to identify any dietary intervention studies on UC subjects). Reference lists of included studies were also checked to identify relevant studies that might have been missed during initial search in MEDLINE. Studies that only focused on nutritional supplements, enteral or parenteral nutrition, or were published in languages other than English were not included. A comprehensive full-text review of identified studies was conducted after the title screening and abstract screening of potentially relevant articles. Collected data included journal name, publication year, design of the study, age, sex, sample size, disease condition, intervention and comparator(s) of interest, outcome(s), outcome measures, and main findings. The MEDLINE search strategy was as follows:

1. randomized controlled trial/
2. clinical trial.pt.
3. randomi?ed.ti,ab.
4. placebo.ti,ab.
5. randomly.ti,ab.
6. trial.ti,ab.
7. 1 or 2 or 3 or 4 or 5 or 6
8. Inflammatory Bowel Diseases/
9. inflammatory bowel disease.tw.
10. ibd.tw.
11. ulcerative colitis.tw.
12. colitis.tw.
13. 8 or 9 or 10 or 11 or 12
14. Diet/
15. diet*.tw.
16. food.tw.
17. 14 or 15 or 16
18. 7 and 13 and 17

3. Results

Our primary electronic search yielded 424 unique references. After title and abstract screening, nine studies were selected for full-text review. Following the full-text review, seven randomized controlled trials that met the inclusion and exclusion criteria were selected for this review [35–41]. The general characteristics of the included studies are summarized in Table 1.

Table 1. General characteristics of studies examining the role of diet for maintenance of remission in ulcerative colitis patients.

First Author (Year)	Country	Study Design	Population	Intervention/Comparator(s) (Sample Size [1])	Duration	Outcomes and Assessment Tools
Wright (1965) [35]	UK	Randomized controlled clinical trial	Adult UC patients in clinical remission after induction of remission	Milk-free diet (n = 26)/gluten-free plus milk-free diet (n = 27)/"dummy diet" as control (n = 24)	12 months	Relapse: Symptoms + sigmoidoscopy, biopsy, dietary adherence: interview
Candy (1995) [36]	South Africa	Randomized, controlled clinical trial	Adult UC patients with mild to moderate disease activity	Symptoms-guided elimination diet (n = 11)/normal diet as control (n = 7)	6 weeks	Induction of clinical remission, sigmoidoscopy, histopathology, dietary adherence: interview
Strisciuglio (2013) [37]	Italy	Single-center, randomized, controlled clinical trial	Pediatric newly diagnosed UC patients	Cow's milk protein elimination diet (n = 14)/normal diet as control (n = 15)	12 months	Induction of clinical remission, clinical relapse: PUCAI, Physician global assessment, serum C-reactive protein, erythrocyte sedimentation rate, fecal calprotectin, endoscopic evaluation, histological evaluation, dietary adherence: food diaries
Kyaw (2014) [38]	UK	Randomized, controlled clinical trial	Adult UC patients	Comprehensive dietary advices (n = 61)/general dietary recommendations +normal diet as control (n = 51)	24 weeks	Disease activity: SCCAI, quality of life: IBDQ, dietary adherence: food frequency questionnaire
Bhattacharyya (2017) [39]	USA	Randomized, double-blind, placebo-controlled, multicenter, clinical trial	Adult UC patients in clinical remission	No-carrageenan diet + carrageenan-containing capsules (200 mg/d) (n = 7)/no-carrageenan diet + placebo (dextrose) (n = 7)	12 months	Clinical relapse: SCCAI, quality of life: SIBDQ, serum cytokines, fecal calprotectin, dietary adherence: 24 h dietary recalls
Pedersen (2017) [40]	Denmark	Randomized, open-label, controlled clinical trial	Adult UC patients in remission, or mild to moderate disease activity and coexisting IBS-like symptoms	Low FODMAP diet (n = 44)/normal habitual diet as control (n = 45)	6 weeks	Disease activity: SCCAI, Severity of IBS symptoms: IBS-SSS, quality of life: SIBDQ, C-reactive protein, fecal calprotectin, dietary adherence: food frequency questionnaire
Jian (2018) [41]	China	Randomized, open-label, stratified clinical trial	Adult UC patients in remission, or mild to moderate disease activity	Immunoglobulin G-guided exclusion diet (n = 49)/normal diet as control (n = 48)	6 months	Disease activity: Mayo score, quality of life: IBDQ, body mass index, albumin, transferrin, prealbumin, extraintestinal manifestation of the disease, food-specific IgG antibodies, dietary adherence: food diaries

UC: ulcerative colitis; PUCAI: Pediatric Ulcerative Colitis Activity Index; SCCAI: Simple Clinical Colitis Activity Index; SIBDQ: Short Inflammatory Bowel Disease Questionnaire; IBS: Irritable bowel syndrome; FODMAP: Fermentable, Oligosaccharides, Disaccharides, Monosaccharides and Polyols; IBS-SSS: IBS symptom severity system; IBDQ: Inflammatory Bowel Disease Questionnaire. [1] Number of patients used for statistical analysis.

Wright et al. [35] randomly allocated UC patients with disease relapse into a milk-free diet (n = 26) (all milk and milk products, whether in the form of dairy products such as fresh milk and cheese or as powdered milk, were excluded, and butter was permitted), a gluten-free plus milk-free diet (n = 27), or a control group (n = 24). Patients were asked to follow the diets for one year after the induction of remission, and they were followed monthly to assess if they experienced disease relapse, which was defined as diarrhea with an average of four or more stools a day for at least a week and with macroscopic blood present, together with sigmoidoscopic evidence of inflammation. Although the relapse rate was higher in patients randomized to the control group in comparison to those on a milk-free diet (79.2% vs. 61.5%), it did not reach statistical significance (p = 0.2). In addition, the relapse rate in the gluten-free plus milk-free diet was 70.4%, which was comparable to that in the other two groups.

In a small randomized controlled trial for 6 weeks [36], 18 adult UC patients with mild to moderate disease activity were randomized to a symptoms-guided elimination diet (n = 11) or a control group (n = 7). Patients in the control group were asked to document but not alter their dietary intake. However, patients in the experimental group were instructed to exclude foods that appeared to provoke their symptoms. Fried foods were prohibited. In addition, refined sugars, additives and preservatives, all condiments and spices other than salt, and beverages other than boiled water were prohibited during the 6-week trial for patients randomized to the elimination diet group. In the first week, dairy products were excluded from the diet, but were introduced over the next weeks in the following order: Skim milk, yogurt, skim-milk cheese, full-cream milk, cream, and full-cream cheese. Each week, subjects in the intervention group were interviewed in person, and their symptoms were reviewed in relation to the foods eaten during the previous week. The food menu was expanded over the 6-week trial to include as more variety of foods that each participant could tolerate. The induction of clinical remission rate (the passage of normal stools with absence of rectal bleeding) 6 weeks after the baseline visit was significantly higher in patients who received the symptoms-guided diet (36.3% vs. 0.0%). However, the endoscopic and histologic improvement was comparable between the two groups.

In another study [37], children with newly diagnosed UC were randomly assigned to a cow's milk protein (CMP) elimination diet (n = 14) or a normal diet as the control group (n = 15). The study aimed to compare the clinical remission rate between the two groups following the IBD induction therapy and the rate of clinical relapse (defined as the occurrence or worsening of symptoms accompanied by an increase of Pediatric Ulcerative Colitis Activity Index > 10 points which required treatment with corticosteroids, immunosuppressive agents, or surgery) between the two groups during the one-year trial. The authors reported that the clinical response rate four weeks after the initiation of the induction therapy was not different between the two groups (92.8% in CMP elimination diet vs. 80.0% in the control group, p = 0.6). In addition, clinical relapse rate was comparable between the two groups (53.8% in CMP elimination diet group vs. 53.3% in the control group). In addition, they found no significant changes in serum C-reactive protein (CRP), erythrocyte sedimentation rate or fecal calprotectin (FCP) in the two diet groups from baseline to the last visit.

Kyaw et al. [38] recruited 112 adult UC patients and randomly assigned them to a dietary intervention and a control group. Patients in the intervention group were given an educational booklet that contained dietary recommendations to eat little and often (four to six times a day), drink adequate fluids, decrease excess intake of fat, decrease simple carbohydrates, and decrease high-fiber foods during flare. Patients were also advised to increase intake of "good-quality protein" during flare and eliminate dairy products if they were lactose intolerant. Patients randomized to the control group were provided with a booklet that included general recommendations on healthy eating (e.g., to choose higher fiber or whole grain carbohydrates, to eat lots of fruits and vegetables) and were assigned to follow their usual diet. At 24 weeks, there was a significant reduction in the Simple Clinical Colitis Activity Index (SCCAI) score in the intervention group compared with an increase in the score in the control group. However, there was no statistically significant change in quality of life scores from baseline to week 24 in the two groups.

Bhattacharyya et al. [39] conducted a small, randomized, double-blind, placebo-controlled, multicenter, clinical trial on UC patients to investigate the effect of the common food additive carrageenan on clinical relapse rates. The authors recruited UC patients over the age of 18 in clinical remission (SCCAI ≤ 2). Patients randomized to the carrageenan group ($n = 5$) received the carrageenan-containing capsules (200 mg/day). Patients randomized to the placebo group received similar-appearing dextrose-containing capsules ($n = 7$). The study duration was 12 months, and participants were instructed to follow a carrageenan-free diet during that period. The primary outcome measure was occurrence of clinical relapse, which was defined as an increase of two (or more) points on the SCCAI in association with an increase in treatment. The Short Inflammatory Bowel Disease Questionnaire was used to assess changes in quality of life. In addition, blood and stool samples were collected to measure inflammatory markers. They found that UC patients who were on a carrageenan-free diet plus placebo had a lower relapse rate in comparison to patients who were on a similar diet plus two oral capsules of carrageenan per day (0.0% vs. 60.0%, $p = 0.05$). In addition, they reported that carrageenan consumption aggravated disease activity as indicated by increase in FCP ($p = 0.06$) and interleukin-6 ($p = 0.02$). However, there was no statistically significant difference between the two groups in terms of changes in quality of life scores.

Pedersen et al. [40] conducted an open-label trial of patients with IBD (61 UC and 28 CD) in remission or with mild-to-moderate disease and coexisting IBS-like symptoms. Patients were randomly assigned to a low Fermentable, Oligosaccharides, Disaccharides, Monosaccharides and Polyols (FODMAP) diet ($n = 44$) or a normal diet ($n = 45$) for 6 weeks. In UC patients, there was a significant decrease in severity of IBS-related symptoms (assessed by IBS symptom Severity System) in both diet groups, and this response was not different between the two groups. However, the authors reported a significant decrease in disease activity assessed by SCCAI but only in patients randomized to the low-FODMAP diet. In addition, low-FODMAP diet increased quality of life of IBD patients (assessed by SIBDQ). However, low-FODMAP diet did not change CRP and FCP levels significantly.

In a recent open-label, stratified study, Jian et al. [41] randomly allocated 97 UC patients who were in remission or had mild to moderate disease activity to a food exclusion group versus a sham diet group. At baseline, the presence of blood IgG antibodies specific to egg, wheat, milk, corn, tomato, crab, rice, soybean, cod, shrimp, mushrooms, beef, chicken, and pork antigens were tested. Based on IgG antibody titers, patients randomized to the exclusion diet group were instructed to stop or reduce taking specific food items. Patients in the control group were asked to follow their routine diet. The duration of the trial was 6 months. They reported that in comparison to the control diet, following the exclusion diet was associated with a significant decrease in Mayo scores and improvement in quality of life.

4. Discussion

It has been suggested that environmental factors including diet play an important role in the pathophysiology of IBD and especially in UC, a chronic colonic inflammation. In the present article, after a brief overview of potential mechanisms in which diet plays a role in the pathogenesis of IBD, we then reviewed dietary intervention studies in UC patients.

The three randomized controlled trials that have been performed to assess the efficacy of dietary interventions for maintenance of remission in UC [35,37,39] were all focused on complete exclusion of one or more food items that were hypothesized to trigger IBD symptoms. Two of these studies [35,37] aimed to eliminate milk or dairy products; however, they failed to show a significant decrease in relapse rate in patients randomized to the elimination diet group in comparison to those randomized to the control diet. This finding is important as unnecessary dietary restrictions that lack supporting scientific evidence may result in several nutritional deficiencies (e.g., calcium due to exclusion of milk and dairy products) in IBD patients [42]. Therefore, patients should be informed by their health care team about the possible harmful effects of food elimination diets.

In the present review, the only elimination diet that was associated with a reduction in clinical relapse rate in UC patients who were in remission at baseline was a carrageenan-free diet [39]. Carrageenan belongs to a family of sulfated polysaccharides and are extracted from seaweeds. It is approved as "generally recognized as safe" by the United States Food and Drug Administration and is used in the food industry for its gelling, thickening, and stabilizing properties. It has been suggested that carrageenan may reduce protein and peptide bioaccessibility, disrupt normal epithelial function, and promote intestinal inflammation [43]. However, others have been skeptical about these findings, which are mainly derived from experimental animal studies [44]. The results from the randomized clinical trial in which a carrageenan-free diet was found to be related to lower relapse rate and decreased inflammation (as assessed by decreased serum interleukin-6 and FCP) should be interpreted with caution as the sample size of this multi-center trial was very small ($n = 12$) and the reported p-values obtained from parametric tests were marginally significant. Therefore, these interesting findings need to be confirmed in future well-powered randomized controlled studies.

We identified only two studies [36,37] that tested the efficacy of diet for induction of remission in UC patients. In the first study, exclusion of food items that were found to trigger UC-related symptoms was associated with higher clinical remission rate in comparison to a normal diet [36]. Although the elimination of foods was based on each participant's self-reported food intolerance, there were some general recommendations regarding specific food groups/items such as dairy products, refined sugar, and beverages. However, the study was performed on a small number of patients ($n = 18$), and the duration of follow-up was short (6 weeks). In addition, the intervention did not result in endoscopic or histologic improvement in that time period. Furthermore, patients in the intervention group experienced a mean weight loss of 2.5 kg that was not explained in the study. The authors also reported that there was no food that triggered symptoms in all patients. However, spicy and curried foods and fruits (specially grapes, melon, and citruses) were commonly reported to provoke symptoms. In the second study, which was performed in pediatric UC patients with active disease, elimination of cow milk protein from diet was not beneficial neither for induction or for maintenance of remission during a one-year follow-up in comparison to a control diet [37]. As mentioned by the authors, the dietary restrictions that many IBD patients follow often are not supported by scientific evidence. These inappropriate diets reduce caloric intake and may contribute to malnutrition and micronutrient deficiencies, especially in pediatric patients. Whether a subgroup of patients with UC (e.g., patients with lactose intolerance or atopy) will benefit from elimination diets or not needs to be explored in future clinical trials.

In this review, we also included three other studies that recruited patients with active disease and UC remission concurrently. They reported the effectiveness of comprehensive dietary advices [38], low FODMAP [40] or IgG-guided exclusion diets [41] in reduction of disease activity in UC patients. Although these findings are encouraging, one of the major limitations of these studies is that they did not report their findings for patients with active disease versus patients in UC remission separately to allow meaningful interpretations [45]. Therefore, we suggest that in future studies the dietary interventions be focused on clearly specified groups of patients (e.g., active disease or in remission) or study outcomes to be reported for different groups of participants separately.

Diet is of major interest for IBD patients, and they use a variety of dietary strategies to manage their underlying disease and related symptoms [34]. Despite the significant role of diet in the development of IBD or management of gastrointestinal symptoms in these patients, we could identify only a few randomized controlled trials that assessed the efficacy of diet for induction of remission, maintenance of remission, or improvement of gastrointestinal symptoms in UC patients. In addition, in the previous studies, the underlying mechanisms in which diet may prevent increases in colonic or systemic inflammation and ultimately help patients to maintain remission have not been investigated. There are many omics fields involved in the study of pathogenesis of IBD such as genomics, metagenomics, transcriptomics, proteomics, and metabolomics [32]. As dietary factors have a significant impact on some of these key players of IBD development, investigating the changes in this multi-omic network of IBD during a controlled dietary intervention has the potential to elucidate the underlying mechanisms of diet-IBD interactions. High quality, well-powered human dietary intervention studies for management of IBD may include the following: Quantification of baseline habitual diet using appropriate tools such as food frequency questionnaires, monitoring of adherence to the diet using food recalls/records, large long-term controlled trials, use of a control diet to determine the specificity of observed effects to the intervention, use of a variety of subjective and objective endpoints (e.g., symptoms, quality of life, clinical biomarkers, endoscopic and histological evaluations) to monitor response to dietary interventions [34], and consider the use of omic-based assessments of serum, urine, stool, and/or intestinal biopsies to investigate underlying protective mechanisms. Considering findings from previous observational studies and clinical trials, investigating the potential benefits of following a healthy dietary pattern, such as experimental anti-inflammatory diets that incorporate several dietary recommendations, is of great value in the management of UC-related symptoms and inflammation. Furthermore, as indicated in elimination diet studies, food intolerances are individual-based, and not all patients will benefit from excluding certain food items/groups. Therefore, personalized dietary recommendations that take into account each patient's food intolerances and food preferences should be the subject of future well-designed dietary trials in IBD patients.

5. Conclusions

In conclusion, we found that there have been few well-designed and/or adequately powered randomized clinical trials to investigate the role of diet in maintenance of remission in UC patients. As suggested in a recent Cochrane systematic review [45], consensus on the composition of evidence-based dietary interventions in IBD patients is required and there is a need for more high-quality, well-powered, randomized, controlled trials to assess the efficacy of these interventions.

References

1. Ungaro, R.; Mehandru, S.; Allen, P.B.; Peyrin-Biroulet, L.; Colombel, J.F. Ulcerative colitis. *Lancet* **2017**, *389*, 1756–1770. [CrossRef]
2. Ramos, G.P.; Papadakis, K.A. Mechanisms of Disease: Inflammatory Bowel Diseases. *Mayo Clin. Proc.* **2019**, *94*, 155–165. [CrossRef] [PubMed]
3. Ananthakrishnan, A.N. Debate session: So what causes inflammatory bowel disease? It's all in the environment. *J. Gastroenterol. Hepatol.* **2018**, *33*, 24. [CrossRef] [PubMed]
4. Hou, J.K.; Abraham, B.; El-Serag, H. Dietary Intake and Risk of Developing Inflammatory Bowel Disease: A Systematic Review of the Literature. *Am. J. Gastroenterol.* **2011**, *106*, 563–573. [CrossRef] [PubMed]
5. Nie, J.Y.; Zhao, Q. Beverage consumption and risk of ulcerative colitis: Systematic review and meta-analysis of epidemiological studies. *Medicine (Baltimore)* **2017**, *96*, e9070. [CrossRef] [PubMed]
6. Wang, F.; Feng, J.; Gao, Q.; Ma, M.; Lin, X.; Liu, J.; Li, J.; Zhao, Q. Carbohydrate and protein intake and risk of ulcerative colitis: Systematic review and dose-response meta-analysis of epidemiological studies. *Clin. Nutr.* **2017**, *36*, 1259–1265. [CrossRef]
7. Li, F.; Liu, X.; Wang, W.; Zhang, D. Consumption of vegetables and fruit and the risk of inflammatory bowel disease: a meta-analysis. *Eur. J. Gastroenterol. Hepatol.* **2015**, *27*, 623–630. [CrossRef] [PubMed]
8. Ge, J.; Han, T.-J.; Liu, J.; Li, J.-S.; Zhang, X.-H.; Wang, Y.; Li, Q.-Y.; Zhu, Q.; Yang, C.-M. Meat intake and risk of inflammatory bowel disease: A meta-analysis. *Turk. J. Gastroenterol.* **2015**, *26*, 492–497. [CrossRef] [PubMed]
9. John, S.; Luben, R.; Shrestha, S.S.; Welch, A.; Khaw, K.-T.; Hart, A.R. Dietary *n*-3 polyunsaturated fatty acids and the aetiology of ulcerative colitis: A UK prospective cohort study. *Eur. J. Gastroenterol. Hepatol.* **2010**, *22*, 602–606. [CrossRef]
10. De Silva, P.S.; Olsen, A.; Christensen, J.; Schmidt, E.B.; Overvaad, K.; Tjonneland, A.; Hart, A.R. An association between dietary arachidonic acid, measured in adipose tissue, and ulcerative colitis. *Gastroenterology* **2010**, *139*, 1912–1917. [CrossRef] [PubMed]
11. Khalili, H.; Chan, S.S.M.; Lochhead, P.; Ananthakrishnan, A.N.; Hart, A.R.; Chan, A.T. The role of diet in the aetiopathogenesis of inflammatory bowel disease. *Nat. Rev. Gastroenterol. Hepatol.* **2018**, *15*, 525–535. [CrossRef] [PubMed]
12. McIlroy, J.; Ianiro, G.; Mukhopadhya, I.; Hansen, R.; Hold, G.L. Review article: the gut microbiome in inflammatory bowel disease-avenues for microbial management. *Aliment. Pharmacol. Ther.* **2018**, *47*, 26–42. [CrossRef] [PubMed]

13. Ni, J.; Wu, G.D.; Albenberg, L.; Tomov, V.T. Gut microbiota and IBD: causation or correlation? *Nat. Rev. Gastroenterol. Hepatol.* **2017**, *14*, 573–584. [CrossRef] [PubMed]
14. Nishida, A.; Inoue, R.; Inatomi, O.; Bamba, S.; Naito, Y.; Andoh, A. Gut microbiota in the pathogenesis of inflammatory bowel disease. *Clin. J. Gastroenterol.* **2018**, *11*, 1–10. [CrossRef] [PubMed]
15. Frank, D.N.; Amand, A.L.S.; Feldman, R.A.; Boedeker, E.C.; Harpaz, N.; Pace, N.R. Molecular-phylogenetic characterization of microbial community imbalances in human inflammatory bowel diseases. *Proc. Natl. Acad. Sci. USA* **2007**, *104*, 13780–13785. [CrossRef] [PubMed]
16. Brown, K.; DeCoffe, D.; Molcan, E.; Gibson, D.L. Diet-Induced Dysbiosis of the Intestinal Microbiota and the Effects on Immunity and Disease. *Nutrients* **2012**, *4*, 1095–1119. [CrossRef] [PubMed]
17. De Filippo, C.; Cavalieri, D.; Di Paola, M.; Ramazzotti, M.; Poullet, J.B.; Massart, S.; Collini, S.; Pieraccini, G.; Lionetti, P. Impact of diet in shaping gut microbiota revealed by a comparative study in children from Europe and rural Africa. *Proc. Natl. Acad. Sci. USA* **2010**, *107*, 14691–14696. [CrossRef]
18. Agus, A.; Denizot, J.; Thévenot, J.; Martinez-Medina, M.; Massier, S.; Sauvanet, P.; Bernalier-Donadille, A.; Denis, S.; Hofman, P.; Bonnet, R.; et al. Western diet induces a shift in microbiota composition enhancing susceptibility to Adherent-Invasive *E. coli* infection and intestinal inflammation. *Sci. Rep.* **2016**, *6*, 19032. [CrossRef] [PubMed]
19. Sun, M.; Wu, W.; Liu, Z.; Cong, Y. Microbiota metabolite short chain fatty acids, GPCR, and inflammatory bowel diseases. *J. Gastroenterol.* **2017**, *52*, 1–8. [CrossRef]
20. Neis, E.P.; van Eijk, H.M.; Lenaerts, K.; Olde Damink, S.W.; Blaak, E.E.; Dejong, C.H.; Rensen, S.S. Distal versus proximal intestinal short-chain fatty acid release in man. *Gut* **2019**, *68*, 764–765. [CrossRef]
21. Reddavide, R.; Rotolo, O.; Caruso, M.G.; Stasi, E.; Notarnicola, M.; Miraglia, C.; Nouvenne, A.; Meschi, T.; De' Angelis, G.L.; Di Mario, F.; et al. The role of diet in the prevention and treatment of Inflammatory Bowel Diseases. *Acta Biomed.* **2018**, *89*, 60–75. [PubMed]
22. Sugihara, K.; Morhardt, T.L.; Kamada, N. The Role of Dietary Nutrients in Inflammatory Bowel Disease. *Front. Immunol.* **2019**, *9*, 3183. [CrossRef] [PubMed]
23. Machiels, K.; Joossens, M.; Sabino, J.; De Preter, V.; Arijs, I.; Eeckhaut, V.; Ballet, V.; Claes, K.; Van Immerseel, F.; Verbeke, K.; et al. A decrease of the butyrate-producing species *Roseburia hominis* and *Faecalibacterium prausnitzii* defines dysbiosis in patients with ulcerative colitis. *Gut* **2014**, *63*, 1275–1283. [CrossRef] [PubMed]
24. Koleva, P.; Ketabi, A.; Valcheva, R.; Gänzle, M.G.; Dieleman, L.A. Chemically defined diet alters the protective properties of fructo-oligosaccharides and isomalto-oligosaccharides in HLA-B27 transgenic rats. *PLoS ONE* **2014**, *9*, e111717. [CrossRef] [PubMed]
25. Ahluwalia, B.; Moraes, L.; Magnusson, M.K.; Ohman, L. Immunopathogenesis of inflammatory bowel disease and mechanisms of biological therapies. *Scand. J. Gastroenterol.* **2018**, *53*, 379–389. [CrossRef] [PubMed]
26. Werner, T.; Wagner, S.J.; Martínez, I.; Walter, J.; Chang, J.S.; Clavel, T.; Kisling, S.; Schuemann, K.; Haller, D. Depletion of luminal iron alters the gut microbiota and prevents Crohn's disease-like ileitis. *Gut* **2011**, *60*, 325–333. [CrossRef]
27. Sturniolo, G.C.; Di Leo, V.; Ferronato, A.; D'Odorico, A.; D'Incà, R. Zinc Supplementation Tightens "Leaky Gut" in Crohn's Disease. *Inflamm. Bowel Dis.* **2001**, *7*, 94–98. [CrossRef]
28. Reich, K.M.; Fedorak, R.N.; Madsen, K.; I Kroeker, K. Vitamin D improves inflammatory bowel disease outcomes: Basic science and clinical review. *World J. Gastroenterol.* **2014**, *20*, 4934–4947. [CrossRef]
29. Scoville, E.A.; Allaman, M.M.; Adams, D.W.; Motley, A.K.; Peyton, S.C.; Ferguson, S.L.; Horst, S.N.; Williams, C.S.; Beaulieu, D.B.; Schwartz, D.A.; et al. Serum Polyunsaturated Fatty Acids Correlate with Serum Cytokines and Clinical Disease Activity in Crohn's Disease. *Sci. Rep.* **2019**, *9*, 2882. [CrossRef]
30. Scaioli, E.; Liverani, E.; Belluzzi, A. The Imbalance between n-6/n-3 Polyunsaturated Fatty Acids and Inflammatory Bowel Disease: A Comprehensive Review and Future Therapeutic Perspectives. *Int. J. Mol. Sci.* **2017**, *18*, 2619. [CrossRef]
31. Ruemmele, F.M. Role of Diet in Inflammatory Bowel Disease. *Ann. Nutr. Metab.* **2016**, *68*, 33–41. [CrossRef] [PubMed]
32. Ananthakrishnan, A.N.; Bernstein, C.N.; Iliopoulos, D.; Macpherson, A.; Neurath, M.F.; Ali, R.A.R.; Vavricka, S.R.; Fiocchi, C. Environmental triggers in IBD: A review of progress and evidence. *Nat. Rev. Gastroenterol. Hepatol.* **2018**, *15*, 39–49. [CrossRef] [PubMed]
33. Levine, A.; Boneh, R.S.; Wine, E. Evolving role of diet in the pathogenesis and treatment of inflammatory bowel diseases. *Gut* **2018**, *67*, 1726–1738. [CrossRef] [PubMed]

34. Haskey, N.; Gibson, D.L. An Examination of Diet for the Maintenance of Remission in Inflammatory Bowel Disease. *Nutrients* **2017**, *9*, 259. [CrossRef] [PubMed]
35. Wright, R.; Truelove, S.C. A Controlled Therapeutic Trial of Various Diets in Ulcerative Colitis. *BMJ* **1965**, *2*, 138–141. [CrossRef] [PubMed]
36. Candy, S.; Borok, G.; Wright, J.P.; Boniface, V.; Goodman, R. The value of an elimination diet in the management of patients with ulcerative colitis. *South Afr. Med. J.* **1995**, *85*, 1176–1179.
37. Strisciuglio, C.; Giannetti, E.; Martinelli, M.; Sciorio, E.; Staiano, A.; Miele, E. Does cow's milk protein elimination diet have a role on induction and maintenance of remission in children with ulcerative colitis? *Acta Paediatr.* **2013**, *102*, e273–e278. [CrossRef]
38. Kyaw, M.H.; Moshkovska, T.; Mayberry, J. A prospective, randomized, controlled, exploratory study of comprehensive dietary advice in ulcerative colitis: Impact on disease activity and quality of life. *Eur. J. Gastroenterol. Hepatol.* **2014**, *26*, 910–917. [CrossRef]
39. Bhattacharyya, S.; Shumard, T.; Xie, H.; Dodda, A.; Varady, K.A.; Feferman, L.; Halline, A.G.; Goldstein, J.L.; Hanauer, S.B.; Tobacman, J.K. A randomized trial of the effects of the no-carrageenan diet on ulcerative colitis disease activity. *Nutr. Healthy Aging* **2017**, *4*, 181–192. [CrossRef]
40. Pedersen, N.; Ankersen, D.V.; Felding, M.; Wachmann, H.; Végh, Z.; Molzen, L.; Burisch, J.; Andersen, J.R.; Munkholm, P. Low-FODMAP diet reduces irritable bowel symptoms in patients with inflammatory bowel disease. *World J. Gastroenterol.* **2017**, *23*, 3356–3366. [CrossRef]
41. Jian, L.; Anqi, H.; Gang, L.; Litian, W.; Yanyan, X.; Mengdi, W.; Tong, L. Food Exclusion Based on IgG Antibodies Alleviates Symptoms in Ulcerative Colitis: A Prospective Study. *Inflamm. Bowel Dis.* **2018**, *24*, 1918–1925. [CrossRef] [PubMed]
42. Lim, H.-S.; Kim, S.-K.; Hong, S.-J. Food Elimination Diet and Nutritional Deficiency in Patients with Inflammatory Bowel Disease. *Clin. Nutr. Res.* **2018**, *7*, 48–55. [CrossRef] [PubMed]
43. Fahoum, L.; (Moscovici), A.J.; David, S.; Shaoul, R.; Rozen, G.; Meyron-Holtz, E.G.; Lesmes, U.; Meyron-Holtz, E.G. Digestive fate of dietary carrageenan: Evidence of interference with digestive proteolysis and disruption of gut epithelial function. *Mol. Nutr. Food Res.* **2017**, *61*, 1600545. [CrossRef] [PubMed]
44. Weiner, M.L.; McKim, J.M. Comment on "Revisiting the carrageenan controversy: Do we really understand the digestive fate and safety of carrageenan in our foods?". *Food Funct.* **2019**, *10*, 1760–1762. [CrossRef] [PubMed]
45. Limketkai, B.N.; Iheozor-Ejiofor, Z.; Gjuladin-Hellon, T.; Parian, A.; Matarese, L.E.; Bracewell, K.; Macdonald, J.K.; Gordon, M.; Mullin, G.E. Dietary interventions for induction and maintenance of remission in inflammatory bowel disease. *Cochrane Database Syst. Rev.* **2019**, *2*, CD012. [CrossRef]

13

Implications of the Westernized Diet in the Onset and Progression of IBD

Fernando Rizzello [1,†], Enzo Spisni [2,*,†], Elisabetta Giovanardi [1], Veronica Imbesi [1], Marco Salice [1], Patrizia Alvisi [3], Maria Chiara Valerii [1,2,†] and Paolo Gionchetti [1,†]

1. Department of Medical and Surgical Sciences, University of Bologna, Via Massarenti 9, 40138 Bologna, Italy; fernando.rizzello@unibo.it (F.R.); elisabett.giovanardi@studio.unibo.it (E.G.); veronica.imbesi@studio.unibo.it (V.I.); marco.salice@hotmail.com (M.S.); chiaravalerii@hotmail.it (M.C.V.); paolo.gionchetti@unibo.it (P.G.)
2. Department of Biological, Geological and Environmental Sciences, University of Bologna, Via Selmi 3, 40126 Bologna, Italy
3. Pediatric Unit, Maggiore Hospital, Largo Bartolo Nigrisoli, 2, 40133 Bologna, Italy; Patrizia.alvisi@ausl.bologna.it

* Correspondence: enzo.spisni@unibo.it

† F.R., E.S., M.C.V. and P.G. equally contributed.

Abstract: Inflammatory bowel diseases (IBD) are currently considered multifactorial pathologies in which various combined environmental factors act on a genetic background, giving rise to a chronic inflammation of the gastrointestinal tract. Among the various environmental factors, it now seems clear that the diet plays the major role in IBD onset and progression. Several clinical studies have attempted to understand the impact of diet in the development and progression of these diseases in order to establish useful guidelines for their management. However, the modest and sometimes contradictory results did not lead to the definition of shared dietary suggestions. On the other hand, food fads and recommendations based on anecdotal episodes are often followed by IBD patients to improve their diet. This review provides a critical overview of existing data on the role of diet as a risk factor for IBD. The methodology used was that of analyzing the results of clinical studies conducted on diet and IBD over the last 12 years through PubMed, as well as analyzing the most relevant studies on nutrients and their possible roles in IBD through the knowledge of the mechanisms by which they can modulate the microbiota or the intestinal physiology.

Keywords: Inflammatory Bowel Disease (IBD); Mediterranean Diet; Western-style Diet (WSD); Nutritional Approach

---

1. IBD and Environmental Risk Factors

The etiology of inflammatory bowel disease (IBD) remains unclear. The most accredited theory is the interplay between genetic susceptibility and exposure to environmental risk factors, such as pollution, stress, diet, pathogen infections, antibiotic treatment and cigarette smoking, also known as the exposome paradigm [1]. Many studies evidence a rise in both the incidence and prevalence of IBD in traditionally low-incidence areas, such as southern Europe, Asia and most developing countries where Western lifestyle and nutritional habits are progressively being adopted [2]. The prevalence of IBD has also increased significantly in the pediatric population [3].

Many studies have concluded that people emigrating from low-prevalence regions, such as Asia, to high-prevalence countries like northern Europe are at greater risk of developing IBD. This is especially true for first-generation immigrant children who show similar IBD incidence and prevalence patterns to the indigenous population [4].

These findings would seem to reduce the importance of a genetic predisposition to IBD and incriminate major lifestyle changes for the rising IBD rates observed in developing countries, in immigrant populations moving to high-prevalence countries, and children in developed countries. These considerations suggest that environmental factors significantly modify the expression of Crohn's Disease (CD) and Ulcerative Colitis (UC). IBD would therefore appear to be a worldwide disease linked to environmental factors such as the diet, lifestyle and pollutants prevalent in industrialized urban societies [4,5].

Diet is a key environmental factor. It plays a major role in the homeostasis of the gut microenvironment, influencing the gut's microbial composition and functioning, the gut barrier, host immunity and the gut physiology by regulating gut hormone release [6,7]. The diet in the developed "Western" world is very different from the traditional diet of previous generations when the prevalence of IBD was considerably lower. The most radical change has been the switch from a plant-based to an animal-sourced diet. This radically modified the gut microbiota and microbiome decreasing the amount of bacteria involved in fiber degradation, such as *Prevotella and Treponema*. [8,9]. Another important change is the increased presence of xenobiotics in food and especially in meat. Xenobiotics are chemical substance that are not naturally produced or expected to be present within the organism and that mainly derive from environmental pollution or from pesticide, widely used in conventional agriculture. Xenobiotics can undergo the bio-magnification process in intensively farmed animal meat. In fact, changes in the gut microbiome and xenobiotic metabolism have been found in children with Crohn's disease [10].

Recent data suggest that another important change brought about by the Western diet is an overall higher calorie intake, especially from sugar, refined carbohydrates, animal proteins and ultra-processed foods. The role of these latter in gut homeostasis is still under investigation [11], and there are not in-depth studies linking ultra-processed foods and IBD, however, it is becoming increasingly evident that some food additives have negative effects on the gut microbiota.

In conclusion, diet may well play a key role in both the pathogenesis and clinical course of IBD. As a result, diet should become an effective tool to optimize the efficacy of the conventional treatment of these diseases.

2. The Microbiota and IBD

The human gut is colonized by a specific and dynamic subset of trillions of microorganisms. Fundamental for our body functions, these microorganisms weigh about 1 kg—significantly more than all the cells of the human body—and contain more than 100 times as many genes as the human genome. They constitute the so-called 'gut microbiota' of the host's gastrointestinal tract [12].

The human microbiota comprises different types of microorganisms, including bacteria (prokaryotes), archaea, fungi, protists, and viruses. Its composition differs significantly in the different regions of the gut. Indeed, the displacement of microbial communities within the intestinal tract can sometimes give rise to pathologies such as the small intestinal bacterial overgrowth (SIBO) syndrome [13].

The gut microbiota and its host exist in a symbiotic relationship. Together they form a sort of "super-organism" with a wide range of functions. These include digesting substrates, producing nutrients, developing and regulating the immune system, preventing the growth of harmful microorganisms by forming a barrier against colonization or invasion, and detoxifying certain xenobiotics [14]. An adequate biodiversity of the microbiota plays an important role not only for the correct functions of the intestine but also in other organs and systems, such as the enteric and central nervous system [15]. Brain and microbiota interactions have led to the recognition of a new term called "microbiota-gut-brain axis". This term refers to a two-way communication system that allows intestinal microbes to change the physiology of the brain and the brain to modulate the intestinal functions. The evidence of this two-way communication comes from multiple studies that have shown that stressful events in an individual's life can alter the composition of the intestinal microbiota, as well as reciprocally, the infection of intestinal pathogenic bacteria can induce anxiogenic behavior in mice [16,17]. Moreover, impaired responses of the central nervous system to stressors have also been clearly demonstrated in patients with microbiota alterations due to active Crohn's disease [18].

Another characteristic of the gut microbiota is its inter-individual variability due to genetic predisposition and factors such as environmental microbes, geography, climate, sanitation, pollution, diet and lifestyle (Figure 1). It follows that the composition of an individual's microbiota changes continuously in a mutualistic response to extrinsic and intrinsic variables. Excessive alterations of the gut microbiota lead to an intestinal imbalance between protective and harmful bacteria, called dysbiosis. This condition seems to be responsible for the inadequate response of the immune system to both external and intestinal epitopes, and may contribute to the loss of oral tolerance. This imbalance can have serious effects during infancy and early childhood when the microbiota is still maturing [19]. Dysbiosis may also be a leading contributory cause of several gut microbiota-related diseases, including IBD [20,21].

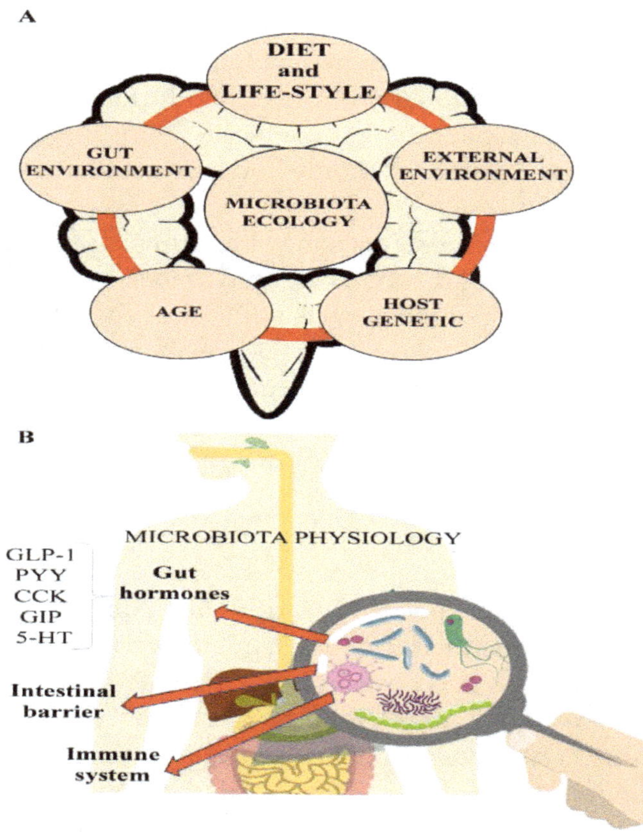

Figure 1. Factors implicated in the modulation of the microbiota ecology (**A**) and complex microbiota interactions with the gastrointestinal physiology (**B**). PYY, Peptide YY; GLP-1, Glucagon-like peptide-1; CCK, Cholecystokinin; GIP, Gastric inhibitory polypeptide; 5-HT, 5-hydroxytryptamine or Serotonin.

While many studies have clearly demonstrated the presence of severe intestinal permeability alterations during the active phases of IBD, permeability seems to recover during the remission phase. It should be noted, however, that modest alterations in intestinal permeability are difficult to be measured *in vivo* [22].

IBD are associated with alterations in the composition of the intestinal microbiota, namely a significant reduction of bacterial diversity, an increase in several pro-inflammatory components called "pathobionts", such as Proteobacteria and Actinobacteria, and the depletion of "health-promoting" anti-inflammatory bacterial genus, such as *Faecalibacterium* and *Roseburia* [23].

During the acute phases of IBD, altered intestinal permeability causes commensal bacteria and microbial antigens to translocate from the lumen to the submucosa, giving rise to local and systemic inflammation. These translocations activate the immune cells, which in turn release numerous pro-inflammatory cytokines, activating an inflammatory loop and inducing chronic intestinal inflammation [24].

The microbiota's plasticity allows the gut microbiome to respond rapidly to changes in dietary patterns. The fermentable carbohydrates, protein, fat, and sugars ingested modulate the levels of beneficial and harmful microbes, toxic microbial metabolites and protective metabolites, such as short-chain fatty acids (SCFAs) [25].

Dietary fibers, polysaccharides, sugars (i.e. lactose) and peptides that are not digested by host enzymes in the upper gut are partly degraded by the gut microbiota in the cecum and colon through a process called fermentation. The major products of fiber fermentation are SCFAs, in particular, acetate, propionate, and butyrate [26]. SCFAs play important multifactorial roles in energy homeostasis, host immune function [25,27] and general gut physiology [25,28] (Table 1). As a result, the amount of SCFAs synthesized, especially in the colon, has been adopted as an indirect measure of microbiota health [28]. High salt consumption also affects the gut microbiome of both mice and humans by lowering the intestinal survival of Lactobacillaceae [29].

Table 1. The multifactorial role of the SCFAs in energy homeostasis in host immune function and host physiology [25,27,28]. GABA, gamma-Aminobutyric acid; CNS, Central Nervous System; ENS, Enteric Nervous system; PYY, Peptide YY; GLP-1, Glucagon-like peptide-1.

CNS Activity	Metabolic Regulations	Immune Homeostasis
GABA production in CNS Modulation of ENS and CNS function Serotonin biosynthesis	Energy source Intestinal gluconeogenesis Antilipolytic activity (WAT) Lepitin production (WAT) Release of major appetite and glucose regulatory peptides (PYY, GPL1) (L-cell)	Enhancement of IL-10 (DC) IL-18 biosynthesis (IEC) Treg polarization Reduction of TNF, IL-6, IFN (DC) IEC barrier fortification IgA promotion

The modulation of intestinal microbiota can be also implemented through probiotics. Probiotics have been defined by the World Health Organization (WHO) as "live microorganisms which, when administered in adequate quantities, confer health benefits to the host". They can play beneficial effects on the digestive system, through multiple mechanisms including interference with potential pathogenic microorganisms, improvement of the barrier function, immunomodulation and the modulation of neurotransmitter synthesis [30,31]. The impact of probiotics on IBD has been the subject of numerous studies. Data derived from studies on animal IBD models showed a high potential of different bacterial strains in modulating the clinical course of experimental IBD. Instead, on humans the experimental results showed little evidence of efficacy on Crohn's disease (CD), modest data on Ulcerative Colitis (UC) but a good support for patients affected by pouchitis, the inflammation of the ileal pouch which is created in the management of IBD patients [32].

It has recently been demonstrated that several dietary components can alter the intestinal microbiota. These include xenobiotics belonging to the group of environmental contaminants, but also additives normally used for the preparation of ultra-processed foods. The xenobiotics capable to have negative effects on the microbiota include organochlorine pesticides [33], glyphosate [34] and perfluorooctanesulfonic acid [35]. All these components have been found in human breast milk, and may therefore negatively modulate the microbial ecology of babies whose unstable microbiota could rapidly develop into a permanently altered gut environment [35]. The effect of food additives added to ultra-processed foods will be discussed in detail below.

Studies of IBD-associated microbiome have evidenced the important role played by the gut environment in the manifestation of IBD. It has also been observed that among the environmental factors associated with microbiota development and alterations, diet plays a key role in modulating the composition and functions of the microbiome and epithelial barrier, and may even influence epigenetic changes. It follows that the food may deeply modulate the microbiome-gut axis and therefore it may represent an important therapeutic tool to counteract dysbiosis and modify the natural history of IBD, bearing out the motto *"We are what we eat"* [7].

3. Evolution of the Human Diet

The first dramatic change in human nutrition occurred about 10,000 years ago during the Neolithic age with the transition of the hunter/gatherer society to one based on agriculture and livestock farming. This change profoundly modified man's diet. Instead of a wide range of different foods that changed with the seasons and with the migratory patterns of animals, our diet became restricted to a few domesticated plants and farmed animal species. For the human metabolism this meant a dramatic change in glycemic load, fatty acid composition, macro- and micro-nutrient concentration and total fiber content. Indeed, in evolutionary terms, this dietary change is so recent that the human species has not had enough time to adapt its gastro-intestinal physiology [36]. Many foods common in the new diet were completely absent in the hunter/gatherer society. Milk, for example, was consumed only during breastfeeding, and dairy products were completely absent [37]. The first evidence of dairy milk consumption has been dated to about 6,000 years ago [2,38]. Cereals are another interesting example. At the beginning of the Holocene age (12,000–10,000 years ago), cereals—always unrefined—were still rarely eaten. The first evidence of white flour production has been traced back to around 3500 Before Christ (BC) in ancient Egypt [39], but the widespread consumption of highly refined flours began only 150–200 years ago [40].

The second truly revolutionary change in the human diet was the introduction of industrialized food following the Second World War. Driven by the so-called "green revolution", which made widespread use of agricultural chemicals, industrialized food production led to a huge rise in the availability of refined cereals, sugar, cheese, butter and coffee (Figure 2). Before this, sugar had been a rare component of the human diet. The first evidence of crystallized sugar can be traced back to 500 BC in India [41]. Before that, the only source of sugar had been honey, available in very limited amounts and only at certain times of the year. Even subsequently, sugar remained a rare commodity. Before the industrial revolution, the annual average sugar consumption in the United States was 6.8 kg per person while in 1970 it exceeded 55 kg, and in 2000 stood at 69 kg [42].

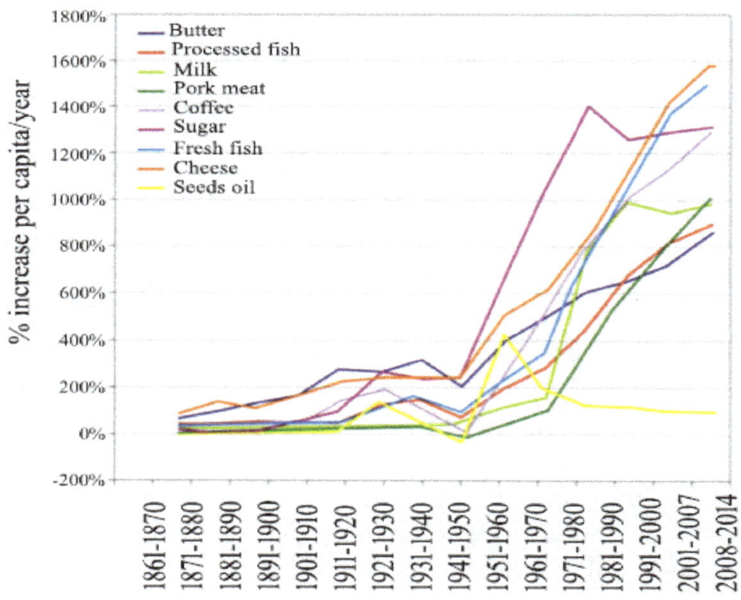

Figure 2. Variation in average food consumption of the population in Italy, one of the countries where the Mediterranean diet was initially discovered, from the end of the 1800s to the early 2000s. The basis of comparison (100%) is the period 1861–1871. Data source: Italian National Research Institute for Food and Nutrition (INRAN), 2013.

Industrialization and the advent of intensive farming also involved a change in farmed animal feed. As a result, the quality of farmed meat, and especially its fat content, is today completely different from the wild animal meat consumed by hunter/gatherers. This is because mammal fat stores are localized in subcutaneous and abdominal adipose tissue in the form of saturated fatty acids (SFAs), while polyunsaturated and monounsaturated fatty acids (PUFAs and MUFAs) prevail in the muscles. It has been estimated that prior to domestication, wild animals consumed most of their subcutaneous and abdominal fat reserves, with the result that our hunter ancestors ate meat with high levels of muscle-stored PUFAs and MUFAs and little or no SFAs [43–46]. Industrial farming, on the other hand, has led to hyper-fed animals with high percentages of accumulated SFAs [45,46].

First extracted around 5000 years ago, vegetable oils were not initially used as a food. It was only with industrialization and the introduction of new extraction techniques that seed oils became products for human consumption (Figure 2). With the advent of hydrogenation in 1980, hydrogenated vegetable fats suddenly became part of our daily diet. Overall, the increase in dietary fat has certainly had an impact on the microbiota and GI diseases [47].

Salt consumption seems to have started at the beginning of the Neolithic age, although its massive consumption only began with the industrial revolution. This has led to an inversion of our ingested sodium/potassium ratio compared to the Neolithic diet. Today, 90% of the salt in the Western-style diet (WSD) comes from processed foods [36]. Food industrialization has also caused a sharp drop in the consumption of fruits and vegetables, and therefore fibers, vitamins and potassium [44,48]. In conclusion, industrialization and the resultant change in diet caused a sudden rise in man's net acid load after digestion, also known as the Potential Renal Acid Load, PRAL. This is because staple WSD foods like cheese, refined cereals and meat are net acid producers while the vegetable-rich diet of our pre-agricultural ancestors was a net base producer [49].

The dramatic change in man's diet is still ongoing. Ultra-processed foods, recently classified as the NOVA-4 group [50], are now readily available and today account for over 50% of the total energy intake of the United States population [11,51].

4. The Western-Style Diet and Its Pro-Inflammatory Foods

Compared to traditional regional diets, such as Mediterranean, Indian, Japanese and South East Asian, the WSD contains significantly higher amounts of simple refined carbohydrates, saturated fats, red meat, dairy products and industrialized foods, and a concomitantly lower quantity of vegetables, fruits, legumes, whole cereals, raw foods and fibers in general (Figure 3). In fact, the WSD consists mainly of calorie-dense foods high in saturated fats, glycemic carbohydrates and animal proteins. Many studies have looked at the association between WSD and obesity, hypertension [52], chronic kidney disease [53] and other non-communicable diseases [54]. Their findings clearly show that the WSD may promote intestinal inflammation through various mechanisms, including alterations of the microbiota [55–58]. Although the relationship between the WSD and IBD has been only partially investigated [59,60], it is nonetheless true that the WSD contains nutrients able to elicit a direct or indirect pro-inflammatory effect on the intestine through one of the three components involved in gut physiology: the immune system, the microbiota, and the intestinal barrier. Moreover, the WSD is low in nutrients and micronutrients with anti-inflammatory and anti-oxidant proprieties. It is therefore not unreasonable to consider the transition to the WSD, also defined as diet westernization, as one of the major environmental factors responsible for the rising incidence and prevalence of IBD. A very interesting in-depth study on the effects of this dietary switch on the intestinal microbiota of children has been recently published [61]. The authors clearly demonstrate that the gradual increase of animal proteins (meat and dairy products), saturated fats, and processed and refined foods to the rural vegetarian diet of urban African children drastically changed their microbial profiles and gut functioning. The sharp drop in fiber intake as a result of the dietary change was found to lead to a concomitant fall in microbial populations able to ferment dietary fibers and a sharp rise in other bacterial groups able to metabolize animal proteins, animal fats and sugars. The westernization of the diet has involved and overwhelmed even the traditional oriental diets, such as the Japanese or that of South East Asia, which are diets geographically associated with a low prevalence of IBD [62]. The potential implications of WSD components on the gut immune system, the microbiota and the intestinal permeability will be analyzed in detail in the following sections of this review.

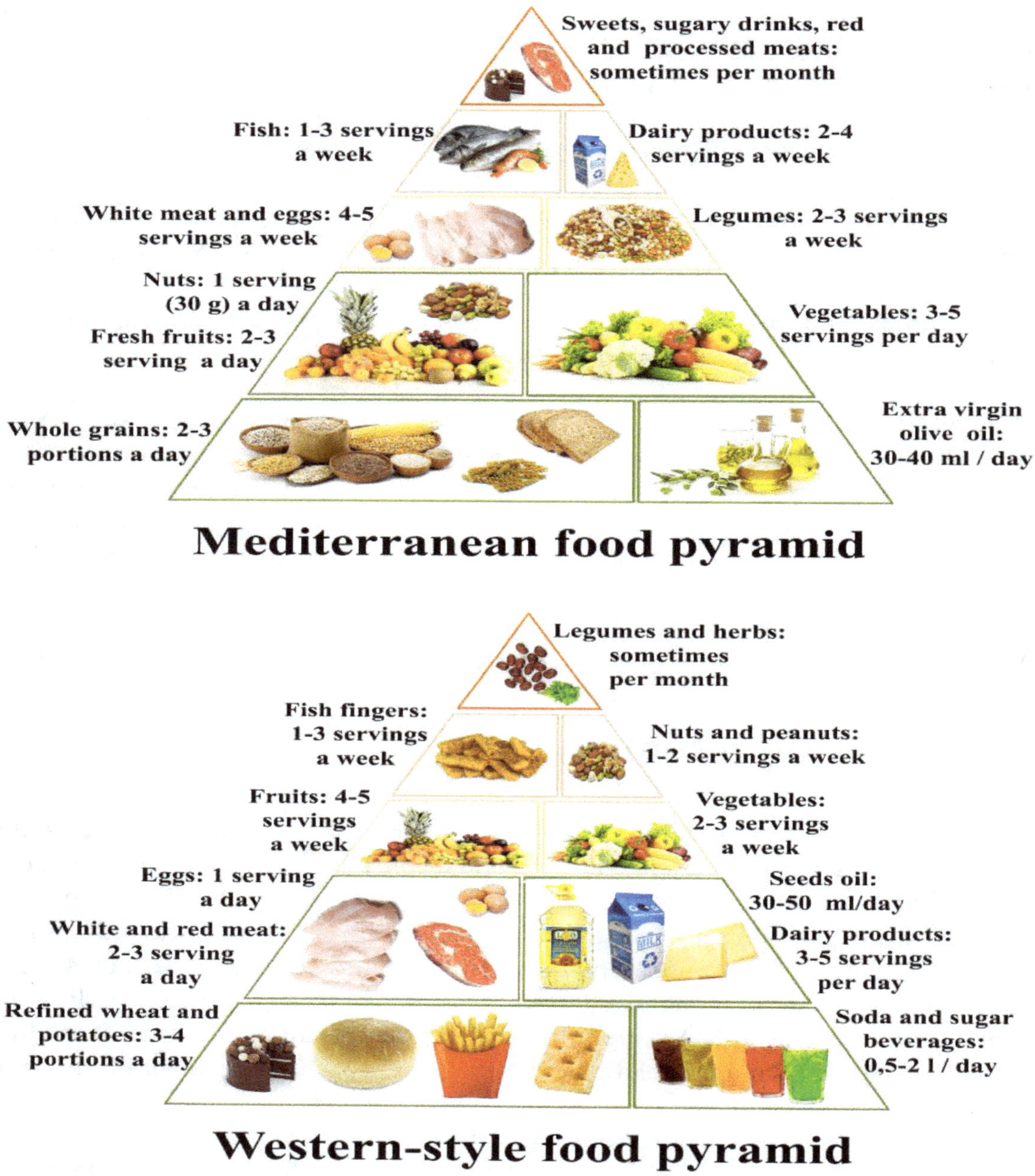
Sweets, sugary drinks, red and processed meats: sometimes per month
Fish: 1-3 servings a week
Dairy products: 2-4 servings a week
White meat and eggs: 4-5 servings a week
Legumes: 2-3 servings a week
Nuts: 1 serving (30 g) a day
Fresh fruits: 2-3 serving a day
Vegetables: 3-5 servings per day
Whole grains: 2-3 portions a day
Extra virgin olive oil: 30-40 ml / day
Mediterranean food pyramid
Legumes and herbs: sometimes per month
Fish fingers: 1-3 servings a week
Nuts and peanuts: 1-2 servings a week
Fruits: 4-5 servings a week
Vegetables: 2-3 servings a week
Eggs: 1 serving a day
White and red meat: 2-3 serving a day
Seeds oil: 30-50 ml/day
Dairy products: 3-5 servings per day
Refined wheat and potatoes: 3-4 portions a day
Soda and sugar beverages: 0,5-2 l / day
Western-style food pyramid

Figure 3. Comparison between the Mediterranean diet (upper) and the Western-style diet (lower) pyramids. The Mediterranean diet pyramid is inspired by the eating habits of Greece, Southern Italy, and Spain before 1950s. The principal aspects of this diet include high consumption of fruits, vegetables, unrefined cereals, legumes and olive oil, moderate to high consumption of fish, moderate consumption of dairy products and low consumption of non-fish meat.

5. Carbohydrates

Carbohydrates are classified on the basis of their chemical structure into mono- and di-saccharides (simple sugars, such as glucose, fructose, sucrose), oligosaccharides (fructo- and galacto-oligosaccharides), and polysaccharides (starch, cellulose, inulin). A fraction of the carbohydrates ingested remains undigested in the small intestine and passes to the large intestine to be fermented and/or excreted. For this reason, carbohydrates are also classified according to their absorbability in the small intestine. For example, simple sugars and starches are hydrolyzed and absorbed in the small intestine and are therefore known as *available carbohydrates*. Inulin, fructo-oligosaccharides and galacto-oligosaccharides, known as *resistant starches*, are not hydrolyzed in the small intestine but fermented by the large bowel microbiota, and are therefore called *unavailable carbohydrates*. Finally, insoluble fibers including plant cell-wall polysaccharides, such as cellulose and pectin, and some storage polysaccharides, such as inulin and oligosaccharides, are also called *non-digestible* components because they pass through the digestive tract largely intact, exerting a laxative effect by changing the osmotic properties of the luminal content and by increasing the intestinal fecal mass. The quality of the carbohydrate ingested, for example, whether mono-, di- or oligo-saccharides, also seems to impact the clinical course of IBD. In fact, a correlation has been observed between fructose and lactose malabsorption and IBD severity [59,63]. In light of this evidence, a fructose- and lactose-free diet has been proposed for IBD patients [59].

Lactose malabsorption is frequently detected in IBD, especially in CD patients. However, prevalence is ethnicity dependent, being higher among Asian populations. Moreover, although lactose avoidance may improve symptoms in patients with lactose intolerance, evidence of objective disease improvement is currently lacking. Studies of a lactose-free diet in IBD patients are currently underway [59].

High consumption of fermentable carbohydrates such as glucose, fructose, sucrose, lactose or polyols (sorbitol, mannitol, xylitol and maltitol) has been shown to exceed the intestine's absorptive ability, increasing dysbiosis and gut permeability, thus promoting inflammation. These fermentable carbohydrates, which include oligo-, di-, and monosaccharides and polyol, are known as FODMAPs (Table 2). Being poorly absorbed, they are rapidly fermented by bacteria in the gut, giving rise to a high osmotic load. This is the rationale behind the FODMAP-exclusion diet. Firstly proposed for Irritable Bowel Syndrome (IBS) patients, the FODMAP-exclusion diet was applied for a limited period to a few IBD patients [64] in an attempt to alleviate their IBS-like symptoms, such as bloating, flatulence, crampy pain, and diarrhea, but proved very limited benefit. Moreover, since undernutrition is a common feature of IBD, the use of this very restrictive diet should be carefully considered [64].

Table 2. Carbohydrates included or excluded in the low-FODMAPs diet.

Food Group	Include	Exclude
Fruit	Bananas, strawberry, raspberry, blueberry, orange, mandarin, clementine, cantaloupe, grapes, melons, lemon, lime, kiwi, passion fruit	Apple, applesauce, apricots, blackberries, cherries, nectarines, pears, peach, plum, prune, watermelon, grapefruit, dried fruit
Vegetables	Carrots, celery, corn, alfalfa, bean sprouts, bell pepper, broccoli (<1/2 cup), bok choy, cucumber, eggplant, green bean, kale, lettuce, potato, spinach, spring onion (green top), squash, tomato, turnip, zucchini	Brussels sprouts, asparagus, avocado, beetroot, cauliflower, cabbage, garlic, leek, mushroom, onion, pea shallot, snow pea, sweet corn, sweet potato
Grains	Rice, oats	Wheat, rye
Legumes	Certain legumes (soya)	Many legumes (chickpeas, lentils, beans)
Dairy	Lactose-free yoghurt and milk; almond, coconut, rice or soy "milk", hard cheese, low-lactose cheese	Cow, goat, sheep milk, buttermilk, soymilk, soft cheese cream and ice cream
Beverage	Fruit juice and vegetable juices from permitted foods, wine	Soft drinks, sports drinks, fruit juice and vegetable juices from unpermitted foods, alcohol
Other	Maple syrup	Honey and sweeteners

Turning to complex carbohydrates, several epidemiological studies have observed associations between the consumption of refined carbohydrates and the risk of developing IBD. However, these data are not sufficiently statistically significant to allow confirmation of this hypothesis [7]. Nonetheless, the WSD contains many different refined carbohydrates, such as sucrose and starch found especially in soft drinks, white bread, cakes, and desserts, all high-density energy-rich but nutrient-poor products. In the long term, they may cause alterations of the gut microbiota and immune system, increasing the risk for many diseases including IBD [65]. Other dietary approaches have been proposed in an attempt to improve IBD symptoms. These include the "specific carbohydrate diet" (SCD), first described by Haas and co-workers in 1924 to treat celiac disease, and subsequently applied to IBD patients [66,67]. The SCD excludes gluten and complex carbohydrates since they are poorly absorbed and lead to bacterial fermentation, which in turn induces dysbiosis in the gut lumen due to pathobiont expansion (Table 3). Only monosaccharides such as glucose, fructose and galactose are permitted. Clinical trials, albeit involving very few patients, reported improvements in bowel symptoms, with some patients able to discontinue at least one of their IBD medications at the end of the SCD trial period [67].

Table 3. Carbohydrates included or excluded in the Specific Carbohydrate Diet (SCD).

Food Group	Include	Exclude
Fruit	All fresh fruit	Canned fruit (because of possible added sugars and starches)
Vegetables	Fresh vegetables	Canned or frozen vegetables (because of possible added sugars and starches), potatoes and yams
Grains	None	All cereal grain
Legumes	Certain legumes (lentils, split pea)	Certain legumes (chickpeas, soybeans) and soybean "milk"
Dairy	Lactose-free dairy (milk, cheese and yogurt)	Milk and all dairy products
Beverage	Wine	Instant tea, coffee and beer
Other	Honey,	Corn syrup, chocolate

In conclusion, if poorly absorbed, all carbohydrates may be fermented, promoting dysbiosis and inflammation. An excess of any kind of carbohydrate in IBD patients with intestinal malabsorption may easily exacerbate existing intestinal dyshomeostasis, which in turn may contribute to dysmetabolism of other nutrients, such as fats.

It is therefore reasonable to conclude that IBD diets should carefully monitor the intake of simple and complex carbohydrates and strictly limit lactose, especially in patients intolerant to this sugar. In fact, exclusion of specific carbohydrates (known as carbohydrate monotony) is a common feature of the different diet-based IBD therapies, in light of the suggestion that carbohydrate variation could be linked to IBD pathogenesis [68]. It does, however, seem unlikely that a single sub-group of foods could be the cause of IBD.

6. Proteins

Several mechanisms of action have been postulated to explain the possible negative impact of high protein (HP) consumption in IBD patients. One hypothesis is that the intestine's limited capacity to assimilate proteins, especially in IBD patients, leads to non-absorbed proteins to reach the colonic lumen where they alter microbiota composition by reducing the abundance of bacteria like *Roseburia/E.Rectale*, considered health-promoting microorganisms for their ability to produce butyrate [69]. In fact, HP diets appear to induce IBD-like dysbiosis [70]. Rats fed a HP diet showed increased prokaryotic protease activity, a phenomenon apparently linked to the pathogenesis of IBD [71]. HP diets may also lead to an imbalance of metabolites of protein catabolism by colonic bacteria (ammonium, hydrogen sulfide, p-cresol and phenol), which could damage colonocytes and the intestinal barrier [72,73]. Several animal studies on colitis have also demonstrated that proteins derived from red meat, milk and dairy products can exacerbate colitis. However, human epidemiological data only partially support these findings. This is probably due to the complexity of the human diet and diverging nutritional data collection methods [70]. In fact, two epidemiological studies have shown a correlation between IBD and high animal protein intake derived from meat and fish but not from eggs or dairy products, while no correlation was found with the consumption of vegetable proteins [74,75]. Two meta-analyzes conducted in 2011 and 2015 also indicate that the consumption of red, white and processed meat may be considered risk factors for the development of IBD [6,76]. Conversely, two more recent studies have produced conflicting results as to a correlation between meat consumption and IBD activity. The first, by Opstelten et al. [77] involving 165 patients with IBD in remission and 1469 healthy controls, indicated that although IBD patients eat more meat than controls, there was no correlation with disease exacerbation. The second study on 53 patients with active disease and 50 in remission concluded that meat is a risk factor for active disease [77,78]. In addition to the protein metabolism mechanism already discussed, it has also been hypothesized that the effect of meat consumption on the onset and course of these diseases could be linked to the cooking process, which notoriously leads to the formation of carcinogenic or mutagenic molecules such as heterocyclic amines, acrylamide and polycyclic aromatic hydrocarbon, associated with endothelial damage and altered immune responses [79]. However, the most convincing studies on meat and IBD have focused on the risk of high saturated and high n-6 polyunsaturated fatty acid (PUFA) intake as a consequence of high meat (especially red meat) consumption.

Gastro-resistant proteins are another point of attention when structuring an IBD diet since the abundance of gastro-resistant proteins in some foods can alter intestinal permeability. Gluten is a gastro-resistant protein complex. Its digestion gives rise to toxic and antigenic peptides (especially alpha-gliadin peptides), which may not only interfere with the tight junction between enterocytes but also with enterocyte survival, affecting the intestinal barrier. This, together with strong evidence of gluten sensitivity in IBD patients [80], has led to the gluten-free diet being recommended for IBD sufferers. Indeed, a gluten-free diet is often self-imposed by patients in an attempt to alleviate symptoms. Ancient wheat varieties, although seemingly giving rise to similar amounts of toxic and antigenic gluten peptides [81], have been shown to ameliorate gut and systemic inflammation in a range of patients, including IBS sufferers [82]. For this reason, ancient varieties of low immunogenic impact grains, such as Senatore Cappelli (*Triticum turgidum durum*) and Enkir (*Triticum monococcum*), or a novel grain variety with low gluten immunogenicity like Tritordeum [83] should be considered for inclusion in the IBD diet. Being gluten-free, rice has also been suggested as a complex carbohydrate suitable for the IBD diet. This includes whole grain rice, provided it is cooked at length [84].

Milk and dairy products contain large quantities of caseins, gastro-resistant proteins known to increase dysbiosis, inflammation and intestinal permeability in the mouse gut [85]. For this reason, milk and dairy foods are excluded in most IBD diets and indeed, commonly restricted by IBD patients themselves [86]. On the other hand, fermented milk products have shown positive effects on IBD patients. Kefir was administered in a randomized controlled trial to 25 IBD patients with positive effects on clinical parameters, such as erythrocyte sedimentation rate, C-reactive protein, bloating, general-feeling scores, and the *Lactobacillus* bacterial load evaluated in patient feces [87]. Yogurt was administered to IBD patients in a double-blind placebo-controlled clinical trial with beneficial effects on the mean numbers of *Lactobacillus*, *Bifidobacterium*, and *Bacteroides* in the feces of the treated group [88].

In conclusion, although performed with only a few patients, the studies conducted so far would seem to suggest that the IBD diet should reduce the overall amount of meat, eliminate red and processed meat, and eliminate or greatly reduce gluten and dairy products (caseins), with the sole exception of yogurt and kefir.

7. Fats

Recent epidemiological data attribute a protective effect to n-3 PUFAs in UC prevention and therapy [89,90]. Conversely, consumption of higher ratios of n-6/n-3 PUFAs has been associated with increased UC incidence. The role of n-3 PUFAs in CD prevention and therapy, however, appears complex and controversial [89]. The physiological basis for PUFAs' role in IBD is that the eicosanoids produced by n-3 and n-6 PUFA are key immune response regulators, being precursors of several pro-inflammatory (n-6 PUFA) and anti-inflammatory (n-3 PUFA) molecules. It has been demonstrated that n-6 PUFAs are more available than n-3 PUFA for eicosanoid metabolism in the UC colon mucosa. For this reason, dietary supplementation with n-3 PUFA, and especially eicosapentaenoic acid (EPA), can reduce the production of prostaglandin E2, thromboxane B2 and hydroxyeicosatetraenoic acid inflammatory mediators [91–93]. The anti-inflammatory effects of n-3 PUFA have also been linked to the synthesis of molecules like resolvins, protectins and maresins, which counteract IBD-related dysbiosis [94], and the down-regulation of pro-inflammatory genes [95]. However, two IBD studies have indicated that PUFA intake may have a different impact in CD compared to UC patients. In their study on 137 UC patients and 38 healthy controls, Wiese and collaborators [96] showed that the concentration of inflammatory tissue cytokines in UC patients was directly related to the amount of serum SFAs and inversely related to total PUFAs, EPA and docosahexaenoic acid (DHA), confirming the protective role of n-3 PUFAs in UC. But a recent study by Scoville and collaborators [97] on 116 CD patients and 27 healthy controls showed that n-3 PUFA serum concentrations were directly related to disease severity. In particular, the authors found EPA concentration to be strongly related to pro-inflammatory serum cytokine concentrations. This datum not only suggests that fatty acid dysmetabolism occurs in patients with CD but also that n-3 PUFA and EPA serum levels may also have a negative effect in CD patients. Conversely, no correlation with SFA concentration was observed in UC patients [97]. Interestingly, both studies, which administered the same amounts of meat, total fat, and SFA to IBD patients and healthy controls, found that n-6 PUFA/n-3 PUFA ratios were similar in CD patients and healthy subjects, despite higher respect the WHO recommendations.

In summary, we may conclude that high fat intake should be avoided in IBD sufferers since high fat diets may lead to an accumulation of secondary bile acids, such as deoxycholic acid, which can inhibit Bacteroidetes and Firmicutes phyla growth, leading to IBD-like dysbiosis [7]. However, a prospective study carried on 170,805 women showed no correlation between fat consumption and IBD risk, but rather a positive correlation between high trans-unsaturated fat intake and UC risk [89]. In addition, the intake of n-3 PUFA and EPA in particular, within foods or supplements, may have positive effects on health, but only for UC patients.

8. Dietary Fibers

Dietary fibers are non-digestible complex carbohydrates present in plants. They are grouped according to their solubility or insolubility in water. Since humans lack fiber-specific enzymes, fibers remain mainly undigested and are therefore not absorbed by the gastrointestinal tract. However, small amounts of the ingested fibers are fermented by the bacteria in the gut, especially in the colon. Present in fruits, vegetables, cereals and legumes, dietary fibers can exert a protective role against IBD through four independent mechanisms [90]:

Reducing intestinal transit time;

Increasing the synthesis of SCFAs such as acetate, butyrate and propionate, which may positively modulate intestinal inflammation;

Improving gut microbiota composition, thus counteracting IBD-related dysbiosis;

Contributing to the maintenance of intestinal barrier functions.

No conclusive studies exist evidencing the efficacy of dietary fibers in slowing IBD progression [98]. A study conducted by Andersen and collaborators [90] showed no association between average fiber intake (total fiber, fiber from fruit, vegetables and cereals) and the subsequent development of CD or UC. Moreover, it has been shown that fibers may exacerbate gastrointestinal (GI) symptoms, such as abdominal distension, flatulence, constipation, and diarrhea in IBD patients during remission periods [99]. It is therefore reasonable to postulate that a high fiber diet is not beneficial for individuals with insufficient "fiber-degrading bacteria" in their gut microbiota [100]. However, while this type of diet may be contraindicated for patients during disease flares, it is nonetheless highly recommended, with appropriate adjustments, after remission in an attempt to approximate the 30g/die WHO recommended intake.

As suggested by Eswaran and collaborators [99], patients in remission should receive a diet with low levels of insoluble fibers, such as those in skinned vegetables like zucchini, carrots, eggplants, green beans and chards. The vegetables should be very well cooked and consumed as a cream, at least initially. Peeled fresh fruit is another option, providing small quantities of insoluble fiber. Putting ingredients through a juice extractor will further reduce the amount of insoluble fiber present in fruit, vegetables and legumes while maintaining most of the soluble fiber fraction, vitamin and mineral content. There is also some unsubstantiated evidence that fruit and vegetable consumption may have a protective immune-modulating effect on IBD patients since they contain protective compounds that may help to prevent disease flares [101]. Another source of insoluble fibers is whole grain cereals. Here too, it seems appropriate to include cereals in the diet only after remission, doing it gradually to avoid worsening of the disease-related GI symptoms [84,99]. Although many IBD patients avoid foods containing fibers, this may lead to micronutrient deficiency and aggravate the malnutrition often presented by sufferers of this disease.

9. Micronutrients

IBD patients tend to suffer from nutrient malabsorption and/or have erroneous nutritional patterns [102], with the result that many are likely to present micronutrient, vitamin and mineral deficiencies. Since micronutrient deficiency may affect immune system physiology and thus facilitate disease relapse, diet or supplementation adjustment strategies could be a key to improove patients' quality of life [103]. The main vitamin deficiencies found in IBD-patients are of fat-soluble vitamins A (retinol and retinoids) and D, and water-soluble vitamins B12 and B9 (folic acid). Experimental models have provided some evidence that vitamin A (provided as retinol) supplementation attenuates intestinal inflammation and improves the gut environment, with significant benefits to health [65]. As antioxidants, vitamins A have a probable protective role against free radicals and oxidative damage, both of which are increased in these patients [104].

As well as regulating bone, calcium, and phosphorus metabolism, Vitamin D has a key role in intestinal defense mechanisms, regulating the adaptive and innate immune systems and suppressing microbial invasion of the epithelium [105,106]. Vitamin D deficiency has been detected in 16% to 95% of IBD sufferers, mainly in CD patients [107]. This may be due to several factors, such as intestinal malabsorption, low exposure to sunlight, lack of physical activity, or insufficient dietary intake. Therapy targeting the vitamin D3 signaling pathway has been suggested in IBD since it may regulate both innate and adaptive immune functions. However, the overall effect of vitamins on IBD is still not well understood, and the clinical studies performed have shown contrasting results. A Danish study conducted between 2005 and 2008 randomized 94 IBD patients to receive oral vitamin D3 or placebo. Although patients receiving vitamin D3 showed a reduced risk of clinical relapse (from 29% to 13%), this was not statistically significant [108]. Similarly, a more recent Iranian study on 108 IBD patients found that oral vitamin D3 supplementation gave rise to lower serum TNF levels, which, however, were also not statistically significant [109].

Folic acid, or folate, is available in several vegetables and is absorbed in the duodenum and proximal jejunum. Both micronutrients are essential for cell metabolism, and folate deficiency is often correlated with vitamin B12 deficiency, this latter mainly available in animal products. Despite their ample availability in food, folate and vitamin B12 absorption occurs in areas often damaged by phlogosis, which may be the cause of impaired uptake in IBD-patients [110].

Trace elements are another important avenue of ongoing research into the prevention and control of IBD. Iron deficiency is very frequent in IBD and the leading cause of anemia among IBD patients. In a recent study, 27% of all CD and 21% of all UC patients were found to have anemia [111]. An iron-, heme- and nonheme-rich diet or oral/parenteral supplementation is therefore mandatory. However, iron—and especially ferrous sulfate—is a known pro-oxidative agent, raising concern that oral iron may increase oxidative stress in patients with colitis [112].

Zinc is an essential micronutrient, an enzyme co-factor involved in cellular immunity, cell growth and wound healing. Zinc deficiency has been associated with excessive loss of GI secretions due to chronic diarrhea or fistula drainage in IBD patients. Prevalent in 15% to 40% of IBD patients, it has also been associated with hospitalization, surgery and other disease complications [113].

Selenium is a non-metal trace element existing in both the inorganic and organic form. It is translationally incorporated as selenocysteine into selenoproteins, which can modulate various cellular pathways involved in inflammation. Adequate selenium intake is thus essential for normal immune functions [114]. In fact, selenium deficiency has been correlated with gastrointestinal inflammation and altered gut microbiota composition [115]. Epidemiological studies suggest that selenium serum levels are inversely correlated with IBD incidence. Moreover, selenium blood concentrations were found to be significantly lower in Caucasians and Asiatic IBD patients, especially in CD [116,117]. Although further studies are necessary to assess the mechanism underlying the effect of selenium deficiency in IBD, it would seem important to ensure adequate selenium intake in all IBD patients.

10. Food Additives and Ultra-Processed Food

Ultra-processed foods (NOVA 4 classification) are the result of a series of industrial processes, many requiring sophisticated equipment and technology. Ultra-processed food manufacture entails fractioning whole foods into different substances, their chemical modification and subsequent assembly with other modified and unmodified food products. The industrial techniques used include extrusion, molding, pre-frying, and the addition of "cosmetic" palatability additives [50]. The presence of high levels of ultra-processed food in the diet has already been linked to a number of non-communicable diseases including cancer, obesity and type 1 and 2 diabetes [118–120]. Despite this, however, the role of these foods on the intestinal microbiota, and on IBD in particular, has never been investigated. However, there is well-documented scientific evidence of the negative effects on the microbiota of food additives typically present in a considerable number of ultra-processed foods. Various studies have clearly shown the negative effect of non-caloric artificial sweeteners often present in carbonated soft drinks on microbiome composition and functioning [121]. The sweetener sucralose has been shown to reduce the relative amount of *Clostridium* cluster XIVa in mice feces [122]. Dietary emulsifiers have also been shown to directly alter human microbiota composition and gene expression in an ex vivo model [123], while maltodextrins, commonly used for the production of soft drinks, candy and sport energy products, have been found to cause microbiota alterations [124] and affect gut epithelial cells, reducing mucus production and exacerbating gut inflammation [125].

The commonly used food additive carrageenan has been shown to induce intestinal inflammation in animal models. Although there is little evidence of the role carrageenan may play in the development of IBD since direct carrageenan assessment trials in man are unethical, animal studies have clearly demonstrated that this additive induces IBD-like histopathological features, alters the microbiome, and disrupts the intestinal epithelial barrier [126]. Red meat, eggs naturally contain high levels of sulfites due to their high cysteine content, which can become a substrate for the production of hydrogen sulfide (H_2S) by sulfate-reducing bacteria. However, sulfites are also abundantly used as food additives to limit bacterial contamination. Generally considered safe for human consumption, they are present in food and alcoholic beverages in quantities up to 5000 parts per million (ppm). However, even at lower concentrations, sulfites have been shown to damage beneficial bacteria, such as *Lactobacillus* and *S. thermophilus* in the human gut [127]. Sulfites can be produced by intestinal microbiota even starting from taurine (from the bacterium *B. wadsworthia*) which is a typical ingredient of energy drinks or from chondroitin sulfate, a widely used food supplement in the treatment of osteoarthritis [128]. Some studies have found that patients with UC show a higher production of H_2S in the gut, but it is not clear whether this increased synthesis is simply linked to the increased intestinal inflammation [128].

11. Alcohol

Small quantities of alcohol are first metabolized in the stomach. Larger amounts are absorbed in the small intestine and may reach the large bowel from the bloodstream where it is metabolized by luminal bacterial alcohol dehydrogenase, producing the toxic compound acetaldehyde [129,130]

Severe dysbiosis has been associated with chronic alcohol abuse. In addition, the high sugar content of some alcoholic drinks may be associated with osmotic diarrhea [131]. A study of 52 Crohn's and 38 UC patients with an alcohol consumption pattern similar to the general population found that although 75% of the IBD patients reported worsening of their symptoms, this could not be related to alcohol intake [132]. In 2018, a prospective cohort study of 262,451 subjects enrolled in six countries showed no association between alcohol use and the onset of IBD [133]. Interestingly, two studies have found a correlation between UC disease activity and sulfite, an additive commonly used also in processed alcoholic drinks [134,135]. In conclusion, although there are insufficient data to define alcohol as a risk factor for IBD, its toxic effect on colon mucosa strongly suggests limiting alcohol intake in IBD sufferers.

12. Nutritional approach in IBD

Recently, numerous new dietary philosophies have become popular. These include the paleo and the vegan diets, often recommended in the management of gastrointestinal diseases such as IBD. However, there is no clinical evidence to support their use in IBD [113]. The only nutritional approach with strong evidence of efficacy is Exclusive Enteral Nutrition (EEN), a diet based on foods classified according to their nitrogen content as: elemental (amino acid based), semi-elemental (oligopeptide based) and polymeric (whole protein based). EEN has proved as efficacious as steroid treatment in inducing remission of CD in children and adults but not of UC [136]. Although the above-mentioned low FODMAPs diet has been mainly used to alleviate symptoms in IBS patients, there are currently no consistent data supporting its use in IBD. A pilot study conducted on 52 CD and 20 UC patients showed that 50% of patients had an improvement in abdominal pain, bloating, and diarrhea [137]. A double-blind controlled placebo cross-over trial was conducted with 32 patients with quiescent disease and IBS-like symptoms that had proved responsive to a Low-FODMAP diet. Patients were randomly assigned to receive fructans, galacto-oligosaccharides, sorbitol, glucose or placebo. The study found that only fructans exacerbated symptoms in patients, which casts into question the real usefulness of the low FODMAPs diet in IBD [138]. Another uncontrolled clinical trial included a semi-vegetarian diet as an "add-on therapy" to the biological drugs used to induce remission. 26 adults and 11 children with recently diagnosed CD and 9 adults with relapsing CD received a lacto-ovo semi-vegetarian diet that included fish once a week and meat once every 2 weeks. Results showed an increase of the expected remission rate in all patients [139]. Yet another study of CD patients on a semi-vegetarian diet for two years reported the absence of CD relapse in 15 of the 16 patients treated [140]. The IgG exclusion diet, on the other hand, is a personalized regime based on preliminary blood titration of food IgG. Two studies conducted by the same research group have demonstrated the efficacy of this diet. The first, an open-label pilot study, was conducted on 40 symptomatic CD patients [141] while the second was a randomized study enrolling 76 subjects with active CD. In this second study, the foods most frequently excluded were milk, beef, pork and eggs. The personalized diet significantly improved patients' quality of life and disease activity, measured using the Crohn's Disease Activity Index (CDAI) and Harvey-Bradshaw Index (HBI) [142].

Although SCD diet is one of the most popular among IBD patients, it has many restrictions making compliance difficult. Obih and collaborators [143] conducted a retrospective study on 26 IBD children who had followed the SCD for 3–48 months, 18 of whom were receiving concomitant medication therapy. 12 of the 26 patients showed improvements in their clinical and inflammatory markers. It should, however, be noted that in the medium and long term the SCD diet may cause adverse effects, such as weight loss and nutritional deficiencies. Patients following this diet must therefore be carefully monitored.

Another study on the SCD, involving 50 adult IBD (mainly colonic CD) patients, obtained a better symptom score and a higher quality of life. Some patients were even able to maintain clinical remission without medication [144]. The fecal microbiota of patients on the SCD was observed to have a higher biodiversity index compared to matched patients eating a WSD [144]. These data suggest that the SCD may be a good starting point from which to plan a dietary regime for IBD patients, especially in the maintenance phase.

13. Conclusions

Although the study data are still often unsubstantiated, it is important not to underestimate the role diet can play in supporting conventional IBD therapies, not only helping to induce and maintain clinical remission, but above all, improving patient quality of life.

While controversy still surrounds the exact role played by diet in the development of IBD, there are indications that diet may significantly modulate disease onset and activity. No formal dietary guidelines exist, however, for patients with IBD. The wide variability of study results is due in part to the design limitations of what are largely underpowered, retrospective studies, and in part to the heterogeneous disease subtypes (UC, CD) recruited to the studies.

The complexity of the human diet makes it very difficult to identify individual foods as risk factors. It is in fact more likely that complex nutritional patterns very different from either the traditional Mediterranean diet or other traditional diets matching our evolutionary status may impact pathogenesis and the clinical course of IBD. In evolutionary terms, in fact, people in industrialized countries can be described as nutritionally mismatched and more susceptible - to degrees depending on their genetic background - the many non-communicable diet-related diseases, including IBD.

We now know the mechanisms of action whereby certain food groups may have a negative impact on the microbiota, triggering intestinal inflammation or intestinal permeability. We also know that the Western population tends to eat excessive amounts of "dangerous" foodstuffs. As mentioned above, the reason why studies have failed to provide strong evidence of dietary efficacy could be due to individual variability as well the small patient series studied. However, as one of the factors involved in the onset and progression of IBD, diet requires further in-depth study, especially since IBD patients tend to have disordered and unbalanced eating patterns. Although guidelines on IBD prevention and treatment are starting to appear (Figure 4) [60], it must be remembered, however, that they are based more on logical assumptions and animal models than on evidence provided by broad controlled human clinical studies.

	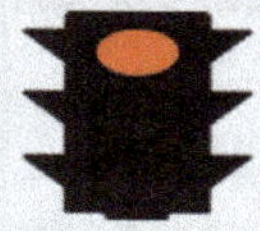
Carbohydrates: White rice, basmati rice, rice noodles, oats, ancients grains bread and pasta, fresh potatoes (frozen potatoes or chips are not allowed) Fresh chicken, fresh fish, eggs. Once a week fresh unprocessed beef steak (lean meat) Peeled fruit and vegetables: tomatoes, cucumbers, carrot fresh spinach (side portion), zucchini, apple (if no tight stricture), bananas, few strawberry, kiwi, slice melon Fresh onion or garlic or ginger Condiments: Olive oil, canola oil, pepper, paprika, cinnamon stick Fresh herbs: mint leaves, oregano, coriander, rosemary, sage, basil, thyme Beverages: water, herbal tea, freshly squeezed orange or lemon juice daily (not from cartons or bottles), and vegetables drinks and Lactose-free or fermented dairy products (kefir, yoghurt and low amount of milk), vegetal milks (almond, coconut, rice, or oat), low amounts of hard (goat or sheep) cheese Sugars : true hard honey	Refined carbohydrates: Wheat, breakfast cereals, bread for toast of any kind, pizza , gluten-free industrial products Processed or smoked meats and fish: sausages, lunched meats, salami, fish sticks Dairy products: Cow, goat, sheep milk, cow cheese, buttermilk, soft cheese, cream and ice cream. Legumes: Beans, chickpeas, soybeans and soymilk Condiments: salt, margarine sauces, salad dressing, syrup, jam of any kind Canned products, canned fruits and canned or frozen vegetables Packaged snacks: potato snacks, popcorn, nuts snacks. Candies, cake and dessert, milk-chocolate Beverages: all soft drinks, all sport energy drinks, beer, alcoholic drinks, fruit juices, instant tea and coffee preparations Sugars: sorbitol, mannitol, xylitol and maltitol , corn syrup Food additives: sucralose, emulsifiers, maltodextrins, carrageenan, sulfites
	Carbohydrates: Whole rice, whole red and black rice Legumes: lentils, split peas, soybean sprouts Beverages: Espresso or American coffee, wine Sugars: table sugar (max 2-3 teaspoons a day for permitted beverages) Dark chocolate (Cocoa minimum 80%)

Figure 4. A possible diet for IBD: dietary foods and factors potentially affecting positively or negatively host intestinal barrier, immunity and microbioma in IBD patients.

Author Contributions: Writing—original draft preparation, F.R., E.S., M.C.V. and P.G.; writing—review and editing, E.S., M.C.V., V.I., E.G., M.S. and P.A.

References

1. Leso, V.; Ricciardi, W.; Iavicoli, I. Occupational risk factors in inflammatory bowel disease. *Eur. Rev. Med. Pharmacol. Sci.* **2015**, *19*, 2838–2851.
2. Loftus, E.V., Jr. Clinical epidemiology of inflammatory bowel disease: Incidence, prevalence, and environmental influences. *Gastroenterology* **2004**, *126*, 1504–1517. [CrossRef] [PubMed]
3. Benchimol, E.I.; Bernstein, C.N.; Bitton, A.; Carroll, M.W.; Singh, H.; Otley, A.R.; Vutcovici, M.; El-Matary, W.; Nguyen, G.C.; Griffiths, A.M.; et al. Trends in epidemiology of pediatric inflammatory bowel disease in Canada: Distributed network analysis of multiple population-based provincial health administrative databases. *Am. J. Gastroenterol.* **2017**, *112*, 1120–1134. [CrossRef] [PubMed]
4. Molodecky, N.A.; Panaccione, R.; Ghosh, S.; Barkema, H.W.; Kaplan, G.G. Alberta Inflammatory Bowel Disease Consortium. Challenges associated with identifying the environmental determinants of the inflammatory bowel diseases. *Inflamm. Bowel Dis.* **2011**, *17*, 1792–1799. [CrossRef]
5. Ng, S.C.; Bernstein, C.N.; Vatn, M.H.; Lakatos, P.L.; Loftus, E.V., Jr.; Tysk, C.; O'Morain, C.; Moum, B.; Colombel, J.F. Epidemiology and Natural History Task Force of the International Organization of Inflammatory Bowel Disease (IOIBD). Geographical variability and environmental risk factors in inflammatory bowel disease. *Gut* **2013**, *62*, 630–649. [CrossRef] [PubMed]
6. Hou, J.K.; Abraham, B.; El-Serag, H. Dietary intake and risk of developing inflammatory bowel disease: A systematic review of the literature. *Am. J. Gastroenterol.* **2011**, *106*, 563–573. [CrossRef]
7. Levine, A.; Sigall Boneh, R.; Wine, E. Evolving role of diet in the pathogenesis and treatment of inflammatory bowel diseases. *Gut* **2018**, *67*, 1726–1738. [CrossRef] [PubMed]
8. Zuo, T.; Kamm, M.A.; Colombel, J.F.; Ng, S.C. Urbanization and the gut microbiota in health and inflammatory bowel disease. *Nat. Rev. Gastroenterol. Hepatol.* **2018**, *15*, 440–452. [CrossRef]
9. David, L.A.; Maurice, C.F.; Carmody, R.N.; Gootenberg, D.B.; Button, J.E.; Wolfe, B.E.; Ling, A.V.; Devlin, A.S.; Varma, Y.; Fischbach, M.A.; et al. Diet rapidly and reproducibly alters the human gut microbiome. *Nature* **2014**, *505*, 559–563. [CrossRef]
10. Dunn, K.A.; Moore-Connors, J.; MacIntyre, B.; Stadnyk, A.; Thomas, N.A.; Noble, A.; Mahdi, G.; Rashid, M.; Otley, A.R.; Bielawski, J.P.; et al. The Gut microbiome of pediatric Crohn's disease patients differs from healthy controls in genes that can influence the balance between a healthy and dysregulated immune response. *Inflamm. Bowel Dis.* **2016**, *22*, 2607–2618. [CrossRef] [PubMed]
11. Martínez Steele, E.; Baraldi, L.G.; Louzada, M.L.; Moubarac, J.C.; Mozaffarian, D.; Monteiro, C.A. Ultra-processed foods and added sugars in the US diet: Evidence from a nationally representative cross-sectional study. *BMJ.* **2016**, *6*, e009892. [CrossRef] [PubMed]
12. Rajilić-Stojanović, M.; De Vos, W.M. The first 1000 cultured species of the human gastrointestinal microbiota. *FEMS Microbiol. Rev.* **2014**, *38*, 996–1047. [CrossRef]
13. Human Microbiome Project Consortium. Structure, function and diversity of the healthy human microbiome. *Nature* **2012**, *486*, 207–214. [CrossRef] [PubMed]
14. Aleksandrova, K.; Romero-Mosquera, B.; Hernandez, V. Diet, Gut microbiome and epigenetics: Emerging links with inflammatory bowel diseases and prospects for management and prevention. *Nutrients* **2017**, *9*, E962. [CrossRef] [PubMed]
15. Dinan, T.G.; Cryan, J.F. The microbiome-gut-brain axis in health and disease. *Gastroenterol. Clin. North Am.* **2017**, *46*, 77–89. [CrossRef]
16. Mukhtar, K.; Nawaz, H.; Abid, S. Functional gastrointestinal disorders and gut-brain axis: What does the future hold? *Wolrd J. Gastroenterol.* **2019**, *25*, 552–566. [CrossRef] [PubMed]
17. Goehler, L.E.; Park, S.M.; Opitz, N.; Lyte, M.; Gaykema, R.P. Campylobacter jejuni infection increases anxiety-like behavior in the holeboard: Possible anatomical substrates for viscerosensory modulation of exploratory behavior. *Brain Behav. Immun.* **2008**, *22*, 354–366. [CrossRef]
18. Agostini, A.; Ballotta, D.; Righi, S.; Moretti, M.; Bertani, A.; Scarcelli, A.; Sartini, A.; Ercolani, M.; Nichelli, P. Campieri, M.; et al. Stress and brain functional changes in patients with Crohn's disease: A functional magnetic resonance imaging study. *Neurogastroenterol. Motil.* **2017**, *29*, 1–10. [CrossRef]

19. Frolkis, A.; Dieleman, L.A.; Barkema, H.W.; Panaccione, R.; Ghosh, S.; Fedorak, R.N.; Madsen, K.; Kaplan, G.G.; Alberta IBD Consortium. Environment and the inflammatory bowel diseases. *Can. J. Gastroenterol.* **2013**, *27*, e18–e24. [CrossRef]
20. Viggiano, D.; Ianiro, G.; Vanella, G.; Bibbò, S.; Bruno, G.; Simeone, G.; Mele, G. Gut barrier in health and disease: Focus on childhood. *Eur. Rev. Med. Pharmacol. Sci.* **2015**, *19*, 1077–1085.
21. Lopetuso, L.R.; Scaldaferri, F.; Bruno, G.; Petito, V.; Franceschi, F.; Gasbarrini, A. The therapeutic management of gut barrier leaking: The emerging role for mucosal barrier protectors. *Eur. Rev. Med. Pharmacol. Sci.* **2015**, *19*, 1068–1076.
22. Carrière, J.; Darfeuille-Michaud, A.; Nguyen, H.T. Infectious etiopathogenesis of Crohn's disease. *World J. Gastroenterol* **2014**, *20*, 12102–12117. [CrossRef]
23. Kostic, A.D.; Xavier, R.J.; Gevers, D. The microbiome in inflammatory bowel diseases: Current status and the future ahead. *Gastroenterology* **2014**, *146*, 1489–1499. [CrossRef] [PubMed]
24. De Souza, H.S.; Fiocchi, C. Immunopathogenesis of IBD: Current state of the art. *Nat. Rev. Gastroenterol Hepatol.* **2016**, *13*, 13–27. [CrossRef]
25. Koh, A.; De Vadder, F.; Kovatcheva-Datchary, P.; Bäckhed, F. From Dietary Fiber to Host Physiology: Short-Chain Fatty Acids as Key Bacterial Metabolites. *Cell* **2016**, *165*, 1332–1345. [CrossRef]
26. Macfarlane, G.T.; Macfarlane, S. Bacteria, colonic fermentation, and gastrointestinal health. *J. AOAC Int.* **2012**, *95*, 50–60. [CrossRef] [PubMed]
27. Tilg, H.; Moschen, A. Microbiota and diabetes: An evolving relationship. *Gut* **2014**, *63*, 1513–1521. [CrossRef]
28. Nastasi, C.; Candela, M.; Bonefeld, C.M.; Geisler, C.; Hansen, M.; Krejsgaard, T.; Biagi, E.; Andersen, M.H.; Brigidi, P.; Ødum, N.; et al. The effect of short-chain fatty acids on human monocyte-derived dendritic cells. *Sci. Rep.* **2015**, *5*, 16148. [CrossRef]
29. Wilck, N.; Matus, M.G.; Kearney, S.M.; Olesen, S.W.; Forslund, K.; Bartolomaeus, H.; Haase, S.; Mähler, A.; Balogh, A.; Markó, L.; et al. Salt-responsive gut commensal modulates TH17 axis and disease. *Nat. Cell Boil.* **2017**, *551*, 585–589. [CrossRef]
30. Ritchie, M.L.; Romanuk, T.N. A meta-analysis of probiotic efficacy for gastrointestinal diseases. *PLOS ONE* **2012**, *7*, e34938. [CrossRef] [PubMed]
31. Sánchez, B.; Delgado, S.; Blanco-Míguez, A.; Lourenço, A.; Gueimonde, M.; Margolles, A. Probiotics, gut microbiota, and their influence on host health and disease. *Mol. Nutr. Food Res.* **2017**, *61*. [CrossRef]
32. Abraham, B.P.; Quigley, E.M.M. Probiotics in inflammatory bowel disease. *Gastroenterol. Clin. North Am.* **2017**, *46*, 769–782. [CrossRef] [PubMed]
33. Liu, Q.; Shao, W.; Zhang, C.; Xu, C.; Wang, Q.; Liu, H.; Sun, H.; Jiang, Z.; Gu, A. Organochloride pesticides modulated gut microbiota and influenced bile acid metabolism in mice. *Environ. Pollut.* **2017**, *226*, 268–276. [CrossRef]
34. Mao, Q.; Manservisi, F.; Panzacchi, S.; Mandrioli, D.; Menghetti, I.; Vornoli, A.; Bua, L.; Falcioni, L.; Lesseur, C.; Chen, J.; et al. The Ramazzini Institute 13-week pilot study on glyphosate and Roundup administered at human-equivalent dose to Sprague Dawley rats: Effects on the microbiome. *Environ. Health.* **2018**, *17*, 50. [CrossRef] [PubMed]
35. Iszatt, N.; Janssen, S.; Lenters, V.; Dahl, C.; Stigum, H.; Knight, R.; Mandal, S.; Peddada, S.; González, A.; Midtvedt, T.; et al. Environmental toxicants in breast milk of Norwegian mothers and gut bacteria composition and metabolites in their infants at 1 month. *Microbiome* **2019**, *7*, 34. [CrossRef] [PubMed]
36. Cordain, L.; Eaton, S.B.; Sebastian, A.; Mann, N.; Lindeberg, S.; Watkins, B.A.; O'Keefe, J.H.; Brand-Miller, J. Origins and evolution of the Western diet: Health implications for the 21st century. *Am. J. Clin. Nutr.* **2005**, *81*, 341–354. [CrossRef]
37. Zeder, M.A.; Hesse, B. The initial domestication of goats (Capra hircus) in the Zagros mountains 10,000 years ago. *Science* **2000**, *287*, 2254–2257. [CrossRef] [PubMed]
38. Copley, M.S.; Berstan, R.; Dudd, S.N.; Docherty, G.; Mukherjee, A.J.; Straker, V.; Payne, S.; Evershed, R.P. Direct chemical evidence for widespread dairying in prehistoric Britain. *Proc. Natl. Acad. Sci. USA* **2003**, *100*, 1524–1529. [CrossRef]
39. Cleave, T.L. *The Saccharine Disease*; Stonebridge Press: Bristol, UK, 1974; pp. 6–27.

40. Storck, J.; Teague, W.D. *Flour for Man's Bread, a History of Milling*; University of Minnesota Press: Minneapolis, MS, USA, 1952.
41. Galloway, P.J.; Thomson, G.A.; Fisher, B.M.; Semple, C.G. Insulin-induced hypoglycemia induces a rise in C-reactive protein. *Diabetes Care.* **2000**, *23*, 861–862. [CrossRef]
42. Food Availability (Per Capita) Data System (Table: Sugar and sweeteners). Available online: https://www.ers.usda.gov/data-products/food-availability-per-capita-data-system/ (accessed on 6 May 2019).
43. Cordain, L.; Watkins, B.A.; Florant, G.L.; Kelher, M.; Rogers, L.L.; Li, Y. Fatty acid analysis of wild ruminant tissues: Evolutionary implications for reducing diet-related chronic disease. *Eur. J. Clin. Nutr.* **2002**, *56*, 181–191. [CrossRef]
44. Cordain, L. The nutritional characteristics of a contemporary diet based upon Paleolithic food groups. *JANA* **2002**, *5*, 15–24.
45. Stahl, W.R. Organ weights in primates and other mammals. *Science* **1965**, *150*, 1039–1042. [CrossRef] [PubMed]
46. Rule, D.C.; Broughton, K.S.; Shellito, S.M.; Maiorano, G. Comparison of muscle fatty acid profiles and cholesterol concentrations of bison, beef cattle, elk, and chicken. *J. Anim. Sci.* **2002**, *80*, 1202–1211. [CrossRef]
47. Zhang, M.; Yang, X.J. Effects of a high fat diet on intestinal microbiota and gastrointestinal diseases. *World J. Gastroenterol* **2016**, *28*, 8905–8909. [CrossRef]
48. Frassetto, L.; Morris, R.C., Jr.; Sellmeyer, D.E.; Todd, K.; Sebastian, A. Diet, evolution and aging—The pathophysiologic effects of the post-agricultural inversion of the potassium-to-sodium and base-to-chloride ratios in the human diet. *Eur. J. Nutr.* **2001**, *40*, 200–213. [CrossRef] [PubMed]
49. Cordain, L.; Gotshall, R.; Eaton, S.B.; Eaton, S.B., 3rd. Physical activity, energy expenditure and fitness: An evolutionary perspective. *Int. J. Sports Med.* **1998**, *19*, 328–335. [CrossRef]
50. Monteiro, C.A.; Cannon, G.; Levy, R.B.; Moubarac, J.C.; Louzada, M.L.; Rauber, F.; Khandpur, N.; Cediel, G.; Neri, D.; Martinez-Steele, E.; et al. Ultra-processed foods: What they are and how to identify them. *Public. Health. Nutr.* **2019**, *22*, 936–941. [CrossRef]
51. Kim, H.; Hu, E.A.; Rebholz, C.M. Ultra-processed food intake and mortality in the USA: Results from the Third National Health and Nutrition Examination Survey (NHANES III, 1988-1994). *Public Health Nutr.* **2019**, *21*, 1–9. [CrossRef]
52. Rai, S.K.; Fung, T.T.; Lu, N.; Keller, S.F.; Curhan, G.C.; Choi, H.K. The dietary approaches to stop hypertension (DASH) diet, Western diet, and risk of gout in men: Prospective cohort study. *BMJ* **2017**, *357*, j1794. [CrossRef]
53. Hariharan, D.; Vellanki, K.; Kramer, H. The Western diet and chronic kidney disease. *Curr. Hypertens. Rep.* **2015**, *17*, 16. [CrossRef]
54. Melaku, Y.A.; Renzaho, A.; Gill, T.K.; Taylor, A.W.; Dal Grande, E.; De Courten, B.; Baye, E.; Gonzalez-Chica, D.; Hyppönen, E.; Shi, Z.; et al. Burden and trend of diet-related non-communicable diseases in Australia and comparison with 34 OECD countries, 1990–2015: Findings from the Global Burden of Disease Study 2015. *Eur. J. Nutr.* **2018**, *58*, 1299–1313. [CrossRef]
55. Smith, P.M.; Howitt, M.R.; Panikov, N.; Michaud, M.; Gallini, C.A.; Bohlooly-Y, M.; Glickman, J.N.; Garrett, W.S. The microbial metabolites, short chain fatty acids, regulate colonic Treg cell homeostasis. *Science* **2013**, *341*, 569–573. [CrossRef]
56. Devkota, S.; Wang, Y.; Musch, M.W.; Leone, V.; Fehlner-Peach, H.; Nadimpalli, A.; Antonopoulos, D.A.; Jabri, B.; Chang, E.B. Dietary-fat-induced taurocholic acid promotes pathobiont expansion and colitis in Il10-/- mice. *Nature* **2012**, *487*, 104–108. [CrossRef]
57. Chassaing, B.; Koren, O.; Goodrich, J.K.; Poole, A.C.; Srinivasan, S.; Ley, R.E.; Gewirtz, A.T. Dietary emulsifiers impact the mouse gut microbiota promoting colitis and metabolic syndrome. *Nature. Cell Biol.* **2015**, *519*, 92–96. [CrossRef] [PubMed]
58. Zinöcker, M.K.; Lindseth, I.A. The Western diet–microbiome-host interaction and its role in metabolic disease. *Nutrients* **2018**, *10*, E365. [CrossRef] [PubMed]
59. Limdi, J.K. Dietary practices and inflammatory bowel disease. *Indian. J. Gastroenterol.* **2018**, *37*, 284–292. [CrossRef]
60. Marion-Letellier, R.; Savoye, G.; Ghosh, S. IBD: In food we trust. *J. Crohns Colitis* **2016**, *10*, 1351–1361. [CrossRef]

61. De Filippo, C.; Di Paola, M.; Ramazzotti, M.; Albanese, D.; Pieraccini, G.; Banci, E.; Miglietta, F.; Cavalieri, D.; Lionetti, P. Diet, Environments, and gut microbiota: A preliminary investigation in children living in rural and urban burkina faso and italy. *Front. Microbiol.* **2017**, *8*, 1979. [CrossRef]
62. Chiba, M.; Nakane, K.; Komatsu, M. Westernized diet is the most ubiquitous environmental factor in inflammatory bowel disease. *Perm. J.* **2019**, *23*, 18–107. [CrossRef] [PubMed]
63. Dixon, L.J.; Kabi, A.; Nickerson, K.P.; McDonald, C. Combinatorial effects of diet and genetics on inflammatory bowel disease pathogenesis. *Inflamm. Bowel Dis.* **2015**, *21*, 912–922. [CrossRef] [PubMed]
64. Gibson, P.R. Use of the low-FODMAP diet in inflammatory bowel disease. *J. Gastroenterol. Hepatol.* **2017**, *32*, 40–42. [CrossRef]
65. Statovci, D.; Aguilera, M.; MacSharry, J.; Melgar, S. The Impact of Western diet and nutrients on the microbiota and immune response at mucosal interfaces. *Front. Immunol.* **2017**, *8*, 838. [CrossRef]
66. Hou, J.K.; Lee, D.; Lewis, J. Diet and inflammatory bowel disease: Review of patient-targeted recommendations. *Clin. Gastroenterol Hepatol.* **2014**, *12*, 1592–1600. [CrossRef]
67. Olendzki, B.C.; Silverstein, T.D.; Persuitte, G.M.; Ma, Y.; Baldwin, K.R.; Cave, D. An anti-inflammatory diet as treatment for inflammatory bowel disease: A case series report. *Nutr. J.* **2014**, *13*, 5. [CrossRef] [PubMed]
68. Britto, S.; Kellermayer, R. Carbohydrate monotony as protection and treatment for inflammatory bowel disease. *J. Crohns Colitis* **2019**. [CrossRef]
69. Russell, W.R.; Gratz, S.W.; Duncan, S.H.; Holtrop, G.; Ince, J.; Scobbie, L.; Duncan, G.; Johnstone, A.M.; Lobley, G.E.; Wallace, R.J.; et al. High-protein, reduced-carbohydrate weight-loss diets promote metabolite profiles likely to be detrimental to colonic health. *Am. J. Clin. Nutr.* **2011**, *93*, 1062–1072. [CrossRef] [PubMed]
70. Vidal-Lletjós, S.; Beaumont, M.; Tomé, D.; Benamouzig, R.; Blachier, F.; Lan, A. Dietary protein and amino acid supplementation in inflammatory bowel disease course: What impact on the colonic mucosa? *Nutrients* **2017**, *9*, 310. [CrossRef]
71. Steck, N.; Hoffmann, M.; Sava, I.G.; Kim, S.C.; Hahne, H.; Tonkonogy, S.L.; Mair, K.; Krueger, D.; Pruteanu, M.; Shanahan, F.; et al. Enterococcus faecalis metalloprotease compromises epithelial barrier and contributes to intestinal inflammation. *Gastroenterology* **2011**, *141*, 959–971. [CrossRef]
72. Blachier, F.; Beaumont, M.; Andriamihaja, M.; Davila, A.-M.; Lan, A.; Grauso, M.; Armand, L.; Benamouzig, R.; Tomé, D. Changes in the luminal environment of the colonic epithelial cells and physiopathological consequences. *Am. J. Pathol.* **2017**, *187*, 476–486. [CrossRef]
73. Blachier, F.; Beaumont, M.; Kim, E. Cysteine-derived hydrogen sulfide and gut health: A matter of endogenous or bacterial origin. *Curr. Opin. Clin. Nutr. Metab. Care* **2019**, *22*, 68–75. [CrossRef]
74. Shoda, R.; Matsueda, K.; Yamato, S.; Umeda, N. Epidemiologic analysis of Crohn disease in Japan: Increased dietary intake of n-6 polyunsaturated fatty acids and animal protein relates to the increased incidence of Crohn disease in Japan. *Am. J. Clin. Nutr.* **1996**, *63*, 741–745. [CrossRef] [PubMed]
75. Jantchou, P.; Morois, S.; Clavel-Chapelon, F.; Boutron-Ruault, M.C.; Carbonnel, F. Animal protein intake and risk of inflammatory bowel disease: The E3N prospective study. *Am. J. Gastroenterol.* **2010**, *105*, 2195–2201. [CrossRef] [PubMed]
76. Ge, J.; Wang, D.; Fan, L. Effect of personalized nutrition guidance on the birth rate of fetal macrosomia in Chinese population: A meta-analysis of nine randomized controlled trials. *Cell Biochem. Biophys.* **2015**, *72*, 669–674. [CrossRef] [PubMed]
77. Opstelten, J.L.; De Vries, J.H.M.; Wools, A.; Siersema, P.D.; Oldenburg, B.; Witteman, B.J.M. Dietary intake of patients with inflammatory bowel disease: A comparison with individuals from a general population and associations with relapse. *Clin. Nutr.* **2018**, *S0261–5614*, 31202–31203. [CrossRef] [PubMed]
78. Tasson, L.; Canova, C.; Vettorato, M.G.; Savarino, E.; Zanotti, R. Influence of diet on the course of inflammatory bowel disease. *Dig. Dis. Sci.* **2017**, *62*, 2087–2094. [CrossRef]
79. Wang, Z.W.; Ji, F.; Teng, W.J.; Yuan, X.G.; Ye, X.M. Risk factors and gene polymorphisms of inflammatory bowel disease in population of Zhejiang, China. *World J. Gastroenterol.* **2011**, *17*, 118–122. [CrossRef] [PubMed]
80. Limketkai, B.N.; Sepulveda, R.; Hing, T.; Shah, N.D.; Choe, M.; Limsui, D.; Shah, S. Prevalence and factors associated with gluten sensitivity in inflammatory bowel disease. *Scand. J. Gastroenterol.* **2018**, *53*, 147–151. [CrossRef] [PubMed]

81. Bianca, D.; Ficco, M.; Prandi, B.; Amaretti, A.; Anfelli, I.; Leonardi, A.; Raimondi, S.; Pecchioni, N.; De Vita, P.; Faccini, A.; et al. Comparison of gluten peptides and potential prebiotic carbohydrates in old and modern Triticum turgidum ssp. genotypes. *Food Res. Int.* **2018**, *120*, 568–576.
82. Dinu, M.; Whittaker, A.; Pagliai, G.; Benedettelli, S.; Sofi, F. Ancient wheat species and human health: Biochemical and clinical implications. *J. Nutr. Biochem.* **2018**, *52*, 1–9. [CrossRef]
83. Vaquero, L.; Comino, I.; Vivas, S.; Rodríguez-Martín, L.; Giménez, M.J.; Pastor, J.; Sousa, C.; Barro, F. Tritordeum: A novel cereal for food processing with good acceptability and significant reduction in gluten immunogenic peptides in comparison with wheat. *J. Sci. Food Agric.* **2018**, *98*, 2201–2209. [CrossRef]
84. Reddavide, R.; Rotolo, O.; Caruso, M.G.; Stasi, E.; Notarnicola, M.; Miraglia, C.; Nouvenne, A.; Meschi, T.; De' Angelis, G.L.; Di Mario, F.; et al. The role of diet in the prevention and treatment of inflammatory bowel diseases. *Acta Biomed.* **2018**, *89*, 60–75. [PubMed]
85. Llewellyn, S.R.; Britton, G.J.; Contijoch, E.J.; Vennaro, O.H.; Mortha, A.; Colombel, J.F.; Grinspan, A.; Clemente, J.C.; Merad, M.; Faith, J.J. Interactions between diet and the intestinal microbiota alter intestinal permeability and colitis severity in mice. *Gastroenterology* **2018**, *154*, 1037–1046. [CrossRef]
86. Lim, H.-S.; Kim, S.-K.; Hong, S.-J. Food elimination diet and nutritional deficiency in patients with inflammatory bowel disease. *Clin. Nutr. Res.* **2018**, *7*, 48–55. [CrossRef]
87. Yılmaz, İ.; Dolar, M.E.; Özpınar, H. Effect of administering kefir on the changes in fecal microbiota and symptoms of inflammatory bowel disease: A randomized controlled trial. *Turk. J. Gastroenterol.* **2019**, *30*, 242–253. [CrossRef] [PubMed]
88. Shadnoush, M.; Hosseini, R.S.; Khalilnezhad, A.; Navai, L.; Goudarzi, H.; Vaezjalali, M. Effects of probiotics on gut microbiota in patients with inflammatory bowel disease: A double-blind, placebo-controlled clinical trial. *Korean J. Gastroenterol.* **2015**, *65*, 215. [CrossRef] [PubMed]
89. Ananthakrishnan, A.N.; Khalili, H.; Konijeti, G.G.; Higuchi, L.M.; de Silva, P.; Fuchs, C.S.; Willett, W.C.; Richter, J.M.; Chan, A.T. Long-term intake of dietary fat and risk of ulcerative colitis and Crohn's disease. *Gut* **2014**, *63*, 776–784. [CrossRef]
90. Andersen, V.; Chan, S.; Luben, R.; Khaw, K.T.; Olsen, A.; Tjonneland, A.; Kaaks, R.; Grip, O.; Bergmann, M.M.; Boeing, H.; et al. Fiber intake and the development of inflammatory bowel disease: A European prospective multi-centre cohort study (EPIC-IBD). *J. Crohns Colitis* **2018**, *12*, 129–136. [CrossRef] [PubMed]
91. Scaioli, E.; Sartini, A.; Bellanova, M.; Campieri, M.; Festi, D.; Bazzoli, F.; Belluzzi, A. Eicosapentaenoic acid reduces fecal levels of calprotectin and prevents relapse in patients with ulcerative colitis. *Clin. Gastroenterol. Hepatol.* **2018**, *16*, 1268–1275.e2. [CrossRef] [PubMed]
92. Calder, P.C. Marine omega-3 fatty acids and inflammatory processes: Effects, mechanisms and clinical relevance. *Biochim. Biophys. Acta* **2015**, *1851*, 469–484. [CrossRef]
93. Lee, T.H.; Hoover, R.L.; Williams, J.D.; Sperling, R.I.; Ravalese, J., 3rd; Spur, B.W.; Robinson, D.R.; Corey, E.J.; Lewis, R.A.; Austen, K.F. Effect of dietary enrichment with eicosapentaenoic and docosahexaenoic acids on in vitro neutrophil and monocyte leukotriene generation and neutrophil function. *New Engl. J. Med.* **1985**, *312*, 1217–1224. [CrossRef] [PubMed]
94. Serhan, C.N. Pro-resolving lipid mediators are leads for resolution physiology. *Nature* **2014**, *510*, 92–101. [CrossRef]
95. Scaioli, E.; Liverani, E.; Belluzzi, A. The imbalance between n-6/n-3 polyunsaturated fatty acids and inflammatory bowel disease: A comprehensive review and future therapeutic perspectives. *Int. J. Mol. Sci.* **2017**, *18*, 2619. [CrossRef] [PubMed]
96. Wiese, D.M.; Horst, S.N.; Brown, C.T.; Allaman, M.M.; Hodges, M.E.; Slaughter, J.C.; Druce, J.P.; Beaulieu, D.B.; Schwartz, D.A.; Wilson, K.T.; et al. Serum fatty acids are correlated with inflammatory cytokines in ulcerative colitis. *PLOS ONE* **2016**, *11*, e0156387. [CrossRef]
97. Scoville, E.A.; Allaman, M.M.; Adams, D.W.; Motley, A.K.; Peyton, S.C.; Ferguson, S.L.; Horst, S.N.; Williams, C.S.; Beaulieu, D.B.; Schwartz, D.A.; et al. Serum polyunsaturated fatty acids correlate with serum cytokines and clinical disease activity in Crohn's disease. *Sci. Rep.* **2019**, *9*, 2882. [CrossRef] [PubMed]
98. Benjamin, J.L.; Hedin, C.R.H.; Koutsoumpas, A.; Ng, S.C.; McCarthy, N.E.; Hart, A.L.; Kamm, M.A.; Sanderson, J.D.; Knight, S.C.; Forbes, A.; et al. Randomised, double-blind, placebo-controlled trial of fructo-oligosaccharides in active Crohn's disease. *Gut* **2011**, *60*, 923–929. [CrossRef]
99. Eswaran, S.; Muir, J.; Chey, W.D. Fiber and functional gastrointestinal disorders. *Am. J. Gastroenterol.* **2013**, *108*, 718–727. [CrossRef]

100. Sugihara, K.; Morhardt, T.L.; Kamada, N. The role of dietary nutrients in inflammatory bowel disease. *Front. Immunol.* **2019**, *9*, 3183. [CrossRef] [PubMed]
101. Boeing, H.; Bechthold, A.; Bub, A.; Ellinger, S.; Haller, D.; Kroke, A.; Leschik-Bonnet, E.; Müller, M.J.; Oberritter, H.; Schulze, M.B.; et al. Critical review: Vegetables and fruit in the prevention of chronic diseases. *Eur. J. Nutr.* **2012**, *51*, 637–663. [CrossRef]
102. Taylor, L.; Almutairdi, A.; Shommu, N.; Fedorak, R.; Ghosh, S.; Reimer, R.A.; Panaccione, R.; Raman, M. Cross-sectional analysis of overall dietary intake and Mediterranean dietary pattern in patients with Crohn's disease. *Nutrients* **2018**, *10*, 1761. [CrossRef] [PubMed]
103. Malavia, D.; Crawford, A.; Wilson, D. Nutritional immunity and fungal pathogenesis: The struggle for micronutrients at the host-pathogen interface. *Adv. Microb. Physiol.* **2017**, *70*, 85–103.
104. Soares-Mota, M.; Silva, T.A.; Gomes, L.M.; Pinto, M.A.; Mc Mendonça, L.; Farias, M.L.F.; Nunes, T.; Ramalho, A.; Zaltman, C. High prevalence of vitamin A deficiency in Crohn's disease patients according to serum retinol levels and the relative dose-response test. *World J. Gastroenterol.* **2015**, *21*, 1614–1620. [CrossRef] [PubMed]
105. Ardesia, M.; Ferlazzo, G.; Fries, W. Vitamin D and inflammatory bowel disease. *BioMed Res. Int.* **2015**, *2015*, 1–16. [CrossRef]
106. Ooi, J.H.; Li, Y.; Rogers, C.J.; Cantorna, M.T. Vitamin D regulates the gut microbiome and protects mice from dextran sodium sulfate–induced colitis. *J. Nutr.* **2013**, *143*, 1679–1686. [CrossRef] [PubMed]
107. Ko, K.H.; Kim, Y.S.; Lee, B.K.; Choi, J.H.; Woo, Y.M.; Kim, J.Y.; Moon, J.S. Vitamin D deficiency is associated with disease activity in patients with Crohn's disease. *Intest. Res.* **2018**, *17*, 70–77. [CrossRef] [PubMed]
108. Jørgensen, S.P.; Agnholt, J.; Glerup, H.; Lyhne, S.; Villadsen, G.E.; Hvas, C.L.; Bartels, L.E.; Kelsen, J.; Christensen, L.A.; Dahlerup, J.F. Clinical trial: Vitamin D3 treatment in Crohn's disease - a randomized double-blind placebo-controlled study. *Aliment. Pharmacol. Ther.* **2010**, *32*, 377–383. [CrossRef] [PubMed]
109. Dadaei, T.; Safapoor, M.H.; Asadzadeh Aghdaei, H.A.; Balaii, H.; Pourhoseingholi, M.A.; Naderi, N.; Zojaji, H.; Azimzadeh, P.; Mohammadi, P.; Zali, M.R. Effect of vitamin D3 supplementation on TNF-α serum level and disease activity index in Iranian IBD patients. *Gastroenterol. Hepatol. Bed Bench* **2015**, *8*, 49–55. [PubMed]
110. Pan, Y.; Liu, Y.; Guo, H.; Jabir, M.S.; Liu, X.; Cui, W.; Li, D. Associations between folate and vitamin B12 levels and inflammatory bowel disease: A meta-analysis. *Nutrients* **2017**, *9*, E382. [CrossRef] [PubMed]
111. Madanchi, M.; Fagagnini, S.; Fournier, N.; Biedermann, L.; Zeitz, J.; Battegay, E.; Zimmerli, L.; Vavricka, S.R.; Rogler, G.; Scharl, M.; et al. The relevance of vitamin and iron deficiency in patients with inflammatory bowel diseases in patients of the swiss IBD cohort. *Inflamm. Bowel Dis.* **2018**, *24*, 1768–1779. [CrossRef]
112. Goldsmith, J.R.; Sartor, R.B. The role of diet on intestinal microbiota metabolism: Downstream impacts on host immune function and health, and therapeutic implications. *J. Gastroenterol.* **2014**, *49*, 785–798. [CrossRef]
113. Kakodkar, S.; Mutlu, E.A. Diet as a therapeutic option for adult inflammatory bowel disease. *Gastroenterol. Clin. North Am.* **2017**, *46*, 745–767. [CrossRef]
114. Stoffaneller, R.; Morse, N.L. A review of dietary selenium intake and selenium status in Europe and the Middle East. *Nutrients* **2015**, *7*, 1494–1537. [CrossRef]
115. Kudva, A.K.; Shay, A.E.; Prabhu, K.S. Selenium and inflammatory bowel disease. *Am. J. Physiol. Gastrointest. Liver Physiol.* **2015**, *309*, G71–G77. [CrossRef]
116. Reimund, J.-M.; Hirth, C.; Koehl, C.; Baumann, R.; Duclos, B. Antioxidant and immune status in active Crohn's disease. A possible relationship. *Clin. Nutr.* **2000**, *19*, 43–48. [CrossRef]
117. Han, Y.M.; Yoon, H.; Lim, S.; Sung, M.-K.; Shin, C.M.; Park, Y.S.; Kim, N.; Lee, D.H.; Kim, J.S. Risk factors for vitamin D, zinc, and selenium deficiencies in Korean patients with inflammatory bowel disease. *Gut Liver* **2017**, *11*, 363–369. [CrossRef]
118. Costa, C.S.; Rauber, F.; Leffa, P.S.; Sangalli, C.N.; Campagnolo, P.D.B.; Vitolo, M.R. Ultra-processed food consumption and its effects on anthropometric and glucose profile: A longitudinal study during childhood. *Nutr. Metab. Cardiovasc. Dis.* **2019**, *29*, 177–184. [CrossRef]
119. Fiolet, T.; Srour, B.; Sellem, L.; Kesse-Guyot, E.; Allès, B.; Méjean, C.; Deschasaux, M.; Fassier, P.; Latino-Martel, P.; Beslay, M.; et al. Consumption of ultra-processed foods and cancer risk: Results from NutriNet-Santé prospective cohort. *BMJ* **2018**, *360*, k322. [CrossRef] [PubMed]

120. Aguayo-Patrón, S.V.; Calderón de la Barca, A.M. Old Fashioned vs. Ultra-Processed-Based current diets: Possible Implication in the increased susceptibility to type 1 diabetes and celiac disease in childhood. *Foods* **2017**, *6*, E100. [CrossRef]
121. Rother, K.I.; Conway, E.M.; Sylvetsky, A.C. How non-nutritive sweeteners influence hormones and health. *Trends. Endocrinol. Metab.* **2018**, *29*, 455–467. [CrossRef]
122. Uebanso, T.; Ohnishi, A.; Kitayama, R.; Yoshimoto, A.; Nakahashi, M.; Shimohata, T.; Mawatari, K.; Takahashi, A. Effects of low-dose non-caloric sweetener consumption on gut microbiota in mice. *Nutrients* **2017**, *9*, 560. [CrossRef]
123. Chassaing, B.; Van De Wiele, T.; De Bodt, J.; Marzorati, M.; Gewirtz, A.T. Dietary emulsifiers directly alter human microbiota composition and gene expression ex vivo potentiating intestinal inflammation. *Gut* **2017**, *66*, 1414–1427. [CrossRef]
124. Baer, D.J.; Stote, K.S.; Henderson, T.; Paul, D.R.; Okuma, K.; Tagami, H.; Kanahori, S.; Gordon, D.T.; Rumpler, W.V.; Ukhanova, M.; et al. The metabolizable energy of dietary resistant maltodextrin is variable and alters fecal microbiota composition in adult men. *J. Nutr.* **2014**, *144*, 1023–1029. [CrossRef]
125. Laudisi, F.; Di Fusco, D.; DiNallo, V.; Stolfi, C.; Di Grazia, A.; Marafini, I.; Colantoni, A.; Ortenzi, A.; Alteri, C.; Guerrieri, F.; et al. The food additive maltodextrin promotes endoplasmic reticulum stress–driven mucus depletion and exacerbates intestinal inflammation. *Cell. Mol. Gastroenterol. Hepatol.* **2019**, *7*, 457–473. [CrossRef] [PubMed]
126. Martino, J.V.; Van Limbergen, J.; Cahill, L.E. The role of carrageenan and carboxymethylcellulose in the development of intestinal inflammation. *Front. Pediatr.* **2017**, *5*, 96. [CrossRef]
127. Irwin, S.V.; Fisher, P.; Graham, E.; Malek, A.; Robidoux, A. Sulfites inhibit the growth of four species of beneficial gut bacteria at concentrations regarded as safe for food. *PLOS ONE* **2017**, *12*, e0186629. [CrossRef]
128. Lewis, J.D.; Abreu, M.T. Diet as a trigger or therapy for inflammatory bowel diseases. *Gastroenterology* **2017**, *152*, 398–414.e6. [CrossRef]
129. Bode, C.; Bode, J.C. Effect of alcohol consumption on the gut. *Best Pr. Clin. Gastroenterol.* **2003**, *17*, 575–592. [CrossRef]
130. Salaspuro, M. Bacteriocolonic pathway for ethanol oxidation: Characteristics and implications. *Ann. Med.* **1996**, *28*, 195–200. [CrossRef] [PubMed]
131. Mantzouranis, G.; Fafliora, E.; Saridi, M.; Tatsioni, A.; Glanztounis, G.; Albani, E.; Katsanos, K.H.; Christodoulou, D.K. Alcohol and narcotics use in inflammatory bowel disease. *Ann. Gastroenterol.* **2018**, *31*, 649–658. [CrossRef]
132. Swanson, G.R.; Sedghi, S.; Farhadi, A.; Keshavarzian, A. Pattern of alcohol consumption and its effect on gastrointestinal symptoms in inflammatory bowel disease. *Alcohol* **2010**, *44*, 223–228. [CrossRef]
133. Bergmann, M.M.; Hernandez, V.; Bernigau, W.; Boeing, H.; Chan, S.S.; Luben, R.; Khaw, K.T.; Van Schaik, F.; Oldenburg, B.; Bueno-De-Mesquita, B.; et al. No association of alcohol use and the risk of ulcerative colitis or Crohn's disease: Data from a European Prospective cohort study (EPIC). *Eur. J. Clin. Nutr.* **2017**, *71*, 512–518. [CrossRef]
134. Magee, E.A.; Edmond, L.M.; Tasker, S.M.; Kong, S.C.; Curno, R.; Cummings, J.H. Associations between diet and disease activity in ulcerative colitis patients using a novel method of data analysis. *Nutr. J.* **2005**, *4*, 7. [CrossRef] [PubMed]
135. Jowett, S.L.; Seal, C.J.; Pearce, M.S.; Phillips, E.; Gregory, W.; Barton, J.R.; Welfare, M.R. Influence of dietary factors on the clinical course of ulcerative colitis: A prospective cohort study. *Gut* **2004**, *53*, 1479–1484. [CrossRef] [PubMed]
136. Zachos, M.; Tondeur, M.; Griffiths, A.M. Enteral nutritional therapy for induction of remission in Crohn's disease. *Cochrane Database Syst. Rev.* **2007**, CD000542. [CrossRef]
137. Gearry, R.B.; Irving, P.M.; Barrett, J.S.; Nathan, D.M.; Shepherd, S.J.; Gibson, P.R. Reduction of dietary poorly absorbed short-chain carbohydrates (FODMAPs) improves abdominal symptoms in patients with inflammatory bowel disease-a pilot study. *J. Crohns Colitis* **2009**, *3*, 8–14. [CrossRef]
138. Cox, S.R.; Prince, A.C.; Myers, C.E.; Irving, P.M.; Lindsay, J.O.; Lomer, M.C.; Whelan, K. Fermentable carbohydrates [FODMAPs] exacerbate functional gastrointestinal symptoms in patients with inflammatory bowel disease: A randomised, double-blind, placebo-controlled, cross-over, re-challenge trial. *J. Crohns Colitis* **2017**, *11*, 1420–1429. [CrossRef]

139. Chiba, M.; Abe, T.; Tsuda, H.; Sugawara, T.; Tsuda, S.; Tozawa, H.; Fujiwara, K.; Imai, H. Lifestyle-related disease in Crohn's disease: Relapse prevention by a semi-vegetarian diet. *World J. Gastroenterol.* **2010**, *16*, 2484–2495. [CrossRef] [PubMed]
140. Chiba, M.; Nakane, K.; Tsuji, T.; Tsuda, S.; Ishii, H.; Ohno, H.; Watanabe, K.; Ito, M.; Komatsu, M.; Yamada, K.; et al. Relapse prevention in ulcerative colitis by plant-based diet through educational hospitalization: A single-group trial. *Perm. J.* **2018**, *22*, 17–167. [CrossRef]
141. Rajendran, N.; Kumar, D. Food-specific IgG4-guided exclusion diets improve symptoms in Crohn's disease: A pilot study. *Colorectal Dis.* **2011**, *13*, 1009–1013. [CrossRef]
142. Gunasekeera, V.; Mendall, M.A.; Chan, D.; Kumar, D. treatment of Crohn's disease with an IgG4-guided exclusion diet: A randomized controlled trial. *Dig. Dis. Sci.* **2016**, *61*, 1148–1157. [CrossRef]
143. Obih, C.; Wahbeh, G.; Lee, D.; Braly, K.; Giefer, M.; Shaffer, M.L.; Nielson, H.; Suskind, D.L. Specific carbohydrate diet for pediatric inflammatory bowel disease in clinical practice within an academic IBD center. *Nutrition* **2016**, *32*, 418–425. [CrossRef] [PubMed]
144. Kakodkar, S.; Farooqui, A.J.; Mikolaitis, S.L.; Mutlu, E.A. The specific carbohydrate diet for inflammatory bowel disease: A case series. *J. Acad. Nutr. Diet.* **2015**, *115*, 1226–1232. [CrossRef] [PubMed]

14

Exclusive Enteral Nutrition: Clinical Effects and Changes in Mucosal Cytokine Profile in Pediatric New Inflammatory Bowel Disease

Helena Rolandsdotter [1,2,*], Kerstin Jönsson-Videsäter [3,4], Ulrika L. Fagerberg [5,6], Yigael Finkel [1,2] and Michael Eberhardson [7,8]

1 Department of Clinical Science and Education, Södersjukhuset, Karolinska Institutet, 11883 Stockholm, Sweden; Yigael.finkel@sll.se
2 Department of Gastroenterology, Sachs' Children and Youth Hospital, Södersjukhuset, 11883 Stockholm, Sweden
3 Clinical Immunology and Transfusion Medicine, Karolinska University Hospital, 14157 Huddinge, Sweden; kerstin.jonsson-videsater@sll.se
4 Department of Medicine, Huddinge, Karolinska Institutet, 14157 Huddinge, Sweden
5 Department of Women's and Children's Health, Karolinska Institutet, 17177 Stockholm, Sweden; ulrika.fagerberg@ki.se
6 Center for Clinical Research, Västmanland Hospital, Uppsala University, 72189 Västerås, Sweden
7 Department of Gastroenterology, Karolinska University Hospital, 17177 Stockholm, Sweden; Michael.eberhardson@ki.se
8 Department of Medicine Solna, Karolinska Institutet, 17176 Stockholm, Sweden
* Correspondence: helena.jonsson.rolandsdotter@ki.se

Abstract: Exclusive Enteral Nutrition (EEN) is the first-line treatment in children with Crohn's disease (CD) for induction of remission. However, the mode of action remains conjectural. The aim of this study was to investigate whether the effect of EEN is paralleled by changes in the mucosal cytokine profiles (MCP). Twelve children with new onset inflammatory bowel disease (IBD) received induction treatment with a polymeric EEN. We assessed clinical, endoscopic and histologic scoring before and after EEN. Twelve colonic cytokines were analyzed by Polymerase Chain Reaction (PCR) in six of the IBD patients at onset and after EEN as well as in six non-IBD control children at the diagnostic colonoscopy. Twelve children completed 6 weeks of EEN, except from one child who completed 4 weeks. At the control colonoscopy, 83% were in complete clinical remission. Changes were found in the MCPs of individual patients after EEN. In particular, children with IBD showed significantly higher values of Interleukin (IL)-12β ($p = 0.008$) and IL-23α ($p = 0.02$) compared to non-IBD controls at the diagnostic colonoscopy. Furthermore, an overall change in proinflammatory cytokines was noted in the IBD-group after treatment. Further studies are warranted to understand the role of EEN in MCP.

Keywords: exclusive enteral nutrition; children; IBD; remission; mucosal cytokines

---

1. Introduction

Crohn's disease (CD) and Ulcerative Colitis (UC), the major entities of pediatric IBD, are chronic inflammatory conditions of the gastrointestinal tract. Childhood IBD is characterized by more severe symptoms and wider disease extension at diagnosis compared to adults [1]. Abdominal pain, nausea and bloody diarrhea are common symptoms in both children and adults while growth retardation is frequently seen in pediatric patients [2]. EEN is the first-line treatment for remission induction of CD in pediatric patients. The clinical remission rate is 73–80% and it effectively induces mucosal healing

(MH) at a rate that is superior to corticosteroids [3–7]. EEN consists of high energy liquid formulas, which are either elemental, semi-elemental or polymeric based. EEN is recommended to all children with luminal disease, including those with colonic involvement [3].

The immunological effects driven by EEN that contribute to mucosal healing (MH) are not yet fully understood [7]. The intestine hosts a majority of the body's immune cells (70–80%) [8] and the interactions between a disrupted microbial composition, an impaired intestinal mucosal barrier and the mucosal immune system are considered to play an important role in the IBD development and its chronicity [7]. Some studies suggest that a deficiency of host immunity also contributes to the pathogenesis of IBD [9]. The cytokines, small immune-regulating messenger proteins, play a crucial part in the inflammatory response by regulating cell differentiation, producing proinflammatory cytokines and recruiting white blood cells from the bone marrow [10]. There are only a few studies that show that EEN seems to affect the expression of cytokines in the mucosa [11–13].

The aim of this study was to investigate the clinical effect of EEN as induction therapy and whether the effect of EEN is paralleled by changes in the mucosal cytokine profiles (MCP).

2. Materials and Methods

We conducted a prospective cohort study of children with new onset symptoms of possible IBD between August 2013 and September 2016. The inclusion criterion was previously healthy children up to 18 years of age with signs of IBD and the exclusion criterion was any use of immunosuppressive drugs within 6 months prior to inclusion. Thirteen children who fulfilled the ECCO/ESPGHAN consensus criteria for pediatric CD (14) entered the EEN study but one patient immediately left the study after the diagnostic endoscopy. One child received concomitant medication with mesalazine (53 mg/kg/day). Six patients who did not receive any IBD diagnosis were included as non-IBD controls. Demographic data are presented in Table 1.

Table 1. Demography and Paris classification of 13 IBD patients at inclusion.

Sex (Girls/Boys)	6/7
Age in years, median (IQR) range	12.5 (10.5–14.5) 7.8–16.4
Symptom duration in months, median (IQR) range	6 (3.1–11.1) 1.5–12
Paris classification	No (=13)
A1aL1B1G1	1
A1bL1B1G0	4
A1bL2B1G0	4
A1bL2L4bB3G1	1
A1bL3L4aB1G0	1
A1bL2L4aB1G0	1
A1bL3L4aB1G0p	1

2.1. Examinations and Tests

The patients were investigated according to the ECCO/ESPGHAN guidelines for pediatric IBD with initial laboratory investigations: peripheral blood count, liver enzymes, albumin, erythrocyte sedimentation rate (ESR), iron status, C-reactive protein (CRP), fecal calprotectin and stool cultures to exclude infectious etiology. In line with the guidelines, all patients were investigated with upper endoscopy and ileocolonoscopy under general anesthesia with multiple mucosal biopsies for histopathological evaluation [14]. For the study, four mucosal biopsies were obtained from the most inflamed site in the ileum or colon. The endoscopies were documented by a still picture system integrated in the computerized medical record program (Picsara, Mawell, Solna, Sweden). A control upper and lower endoscopy with biopsy harvesting at the same site as the diagnostic endoscopy was performed shortly after completion of EEN remission treatment in children with CD. No CC was performed in the six non-IBD controls. The body weight of study patients was obtained before and after the EEN treatment.

2.2. *Clinical Assessment of Disease Activity and Disease Extension*

We used the validated disease activity scoring PCDAI (Pediatric CD Activity Index) with <10 points for remission, 10–27.5 for mild disease, >27.5–37.5 moderate disease and >37.5–100 for severe disease. A PCDAI decrease of >12.5 points was regarded as a clinically significant response to treatment [15]. PCDAI score was assessed at inclusion and at CC. Disease extension was assessed by Paris classification [16].

2.3. *Endoscopic Scoring*

Simple Endoscopic Score for Crohn's disease (SES-CD) was used to assess the mucosal inflammation in the CD patients [17] and was evaluated either by the endoscopist or by the investigator from the charts (the endoscopy history and endoscopy imaging). SES-CD describes the presence and size of ulcers, extent of the ulcerated surface, extent of the affected surface and the presence and type of narrowing scored with 0–3 points in rectum, sigmoid and left colon, transverse colon, right colon and ileum. Remission is equal to 0–2 points, mild disease to 3–6 points, moderate to 7–15 points and severe disease to $\geq$16 points.

2.4. *Histopathology Scoring*

The mucosal biopsies were reviewed by the validated histological Geboes scoring [18]. Grades < 3 were regarded as the absence of IBD inflammation, while grades $\geq$3 were regarded as the presence of IBD inflammation of varying degrees (3:1–3:7) with the following subgroups: a = basal plasmacytosis, b = lymphoid nodules, c = Paneth cell hyperplasia, d = eosinophils in the lamina propria, e = histiocytic cell proliferation, f = giant cells, g = granuloma, h = vasculitis and i = dysplasia.

2.5. *Exclusive Enteral Nutrition (EEN)*

Fortimel Energy®, a polymeric formula, was prescribed to meet a daily energy intake estimated at 120% of recommended daily allowance (RDA). Fortimel Energy® contains 625 kJ, 5.8 g of fat and 5.9 g of protein/100 mL (Nutricia Advanced Medical Nutrition, Solna, Sweden). The EEN treatment was introduced by a daily step-wise increase by 25% of full daily intake for three days, which was followed by six weeks of EEN and rounded off by a step-wise decrease by 25% of full daily intake for 3 days. The children were allowed to drink clear beverages, eat a few popsicles and a few hard mints per day during the EEN treatment. Patients were allowed additional formula at their own discretion for daily satiation. At de-escalation, the patients were advised to avoid large amounts of dairy products, spicy food and large amount of legumes. The children and caregivers had one introductory session with a dietitian. Thereafter, the dietitian had weekly phone calls to monitor intake and motivate the patients and caregivers to complete the whole EEN treatment period. Scheduled clinical assessments were arranged after two weeks of EEN.

2.6. *Cytokine-Selection*

A panel of cytokines that are known to participate in chronic intestinal inflammation were selected for testing. We investigated Colony Stimulating Factor(CSF)-2, Interferon(IFN)-γ, Tumor Necrosis Factor(TNF)-α, Interleukin(IL)-1β, IL-4, IL-6, IL-10, IL-12β, IL-22, IL-23α, IL-36γ, Tumor Growth factor(TGF)-β1 and a control gene ABL. The amount of messenger-RNA (m-RNA) in the different proinflammatory mediators was compared to the signal from the ABL-gene and the result is presented as the cytokine/ABL ratio. We used TaqMan® Gene Expression Assays, applied biosystems (Thermo Fischer Scientific®, Waltham, MA, USA)

2.7. *RNA Extraction and Gene Expression by Quantitative Real-Time PCR*

Biopsies for MCP were put into the RNA-later (Invitrogen, Waltham, MA USA) and kept at +6 °C for 24 h and then frozen (−20 °C) until analysis. Total RNA was isolated by utilizing the

Fibrous tissue kit (Qiagen, Hilden, Germany) with slight modification. Defrosted and minced biopsies (3 mm) were homogenized with a pestle motor (WVR®, Radnor, PA, USA) for 30–60 s in 350 μL of RLT-buffer and 350 μL of 70% ethanol was added. The homogenates were loaded into spin columns and centrifuged before the columns were washed with 350 μL of RW1-buffer. Samples in the columns were treated by DNase I and washed with 350 μL of RW1-buffer, with the remainder handled according to the manufacturer protocol. cDNA was obtained by reverse transcription. Quantitative real-time PCR (qPCR) was performed using the 7500 Fast Real Time PCR System (Applied Biosystems, Foster City, CA, USA) for quantification. Probes were obtained from Applied Biosystems, TaqMan® MGB probes, FAM™ dye-labeled: IL-1β (Hs00174097_m1), IL-4 (Hs00174122_m1), IL-6 (Hs00985639_m1), IL-10 (Hs00961622_m1), IL-12β (Hs001011518_m1), IL-22 (Hs01574154_m1), IL-23 (Hs00900828_g1), IL-36γ (Hs00219742_m1), TGF-β1 (Hs00998133_m1), TNF-α (Hs01113624_g1), IFN-γ (Hs00989291_m1), GM-CSF-2 (Hs00929873_m1) and ABL1 (Hs01104728_m1) according to the manufacturer protocol. Fold increases of mRNA transcripts were calculated as follows: $\Delta Ct = Ct$ (gene of interest) − Ct (ABL1), $\Delta\Delta Ct = \Delta Ct$ sample − average ΔCt control group and fold difference $= 2 - \Delta\Delta Ct$. For technical reasons, CMCP was not analyzed in all children with IBD both at diagnosis and at CC. No active selection was performed.

2.8. Ethical Approval

The study was approved by the local Ethics Committee in Stockholm, Sweden (No. 2010/1252-31/1). Informed written consents were obtained from legal guardians for patients and also from all patients over 15 years of age before any study-related procedures were initiated in accordance with the Helsinki II Declaration.

2.9. Statistics

The comparisons between clinical chemistry values, SES-CD and disease activity index (PCDAI) before and after treatment were conducted with paired sample t-tests (parametric data) or Wilcoxon paired t-tests (non-parametric data) depending on the normal distribution (tested with Shapiro–Wilks test). Paired comparisons between cytokines before and after treatment were conducted with Wilcoxon paired t-tests while the comparisons between groups were conducted with Mann–Whitney U test after control of normality with Shapiro–Wilks test. All analyses were performed with the IBM SPSS Statistics Data Editor, version 23® (Armonk, NY, USA). Statistical significance was set at $p < 0.05$.

3. Results

Thirteen children were included with a CD diagnosis according to the ECCO/ESPGHAN guidelines. One CD patient left the study after the first colonoscopy due to social circumstances. Out of 12 patients who completed EEN treatment, two patients were re-diagnosed with UC and one with IBD-unclassified (IBD-U) at the time of histopathological review after study completion (Table 1 for Paris classification at inclusion).

3.1. EEN Treatment

Eleven children completed six weeks of EEN and one CD patient completed only four weeks of EEN due to a lack of motivation, but fulfilled participation in all other aspects of the study. All patients accepted the prescribed EEN by oral intake without the use of nasogastric tube.

3.2. Clinical Activity Scoring

Clinical scoring of the children diagnosed with CD was measured by PCDAI, which was also used for the children who had their diagnoses changed to UC ($n = 2$) or IBD-U ($n = 1$). At inclusion, six children were considered to have mild disease (PCDAI 10–27.5) and seven patients showed moderate to severe disease (PCDAI > 27.5). There was a significant decrease in PCDAI at CC ($p = 0.02$).

The median PCDAI was 26.5 (IQR 20.0–36.6, range 20–40) at inclusion and 5 (IQR 0-5, range 0–15) after EEN treatment. Ten of twelve patients (83%) showed clinical remission (PCDAI < 10) after EEN induction treatment.

3.3. Laboratory Values

ESR, CRP, hemoglobin, plasma-albumin and F-calprotectin were monitored in all patients. There were significant decreases in ESR (p = 0.005), CRP (p = 0.016) and f-calprotectin (p = 0.033) and significant increases in hemoglobin (p = 0.001) and p-albumin (p = 0.003) after EEN treatment (Table 2).

Table 2. Laboratory values and weight in 12 patients at inclusion and at control colonoscopy.

Value	At Inclusion Median (IQR) Range	After EEN Treatment Median (IQR) Range
Weight (kg)	37.9 (31.5–52.6) 27.5–59.7	40.5 (32.8–55.4) 29.8–59.1
ESR (mm/h)	28 (17.3–27.5) 8–53	9 (8–11) 2–21
CRP (mg/L)	14 (2–49.3) 1–86	2.5 (1–8.3) 1–20
Albumin (g/L)	33 (25–36) 24–41	36.3 (33.5–40.5) 31–44
Hemoglobin (g/L)	113 (101–119.5) 83–142	129 (121–135) 116–144
F-calprotectin (mg/kg)	2640 (1191–3169) 580–6360	620 (198–1556) 5–2256

3.4. Anthropometric Data

There was a significant gain in weight (p = 0.003) after EEN treatment (Table 2).

3.5. Endoscopic Healing

All patients were examined with a control upper and lower endoscopy at a median of 13 days (range 1–45 days) after completion of EEN. A significant decrease (p = 0.008) was seen in SES-CD after EEN (median SES-CD 9.5, IQR 4.5–14.3, range 4–28 at inclusion compared to median 3.5, IQR 1–10, range 0–16 at CC).

3.6. Clinical Outcome of the Two UC Patients

One UC patient showed a reduction in PCDAI (23 to 5 points) and ESR (28 to 11 mm/h) and an increased hemoglobin value (110 to 116 g/L). However, no considerable effect was seen in SES-CD, CRP and F-calprotectin. The other UC patient showed a decrease in PCDAI (40 to 15 points), ESR (53 to 2 mm/h), CRP (47 to 11 mg/L), F-calprotectin (3169 to 1430 mg/kg) and SES-CD (21 to 16 points) and a raise in albumin (28 to 31 g/L) and Hb (83 to 128 g/L).

3.7. Mucosal Healing

The histopathological scoring using the Geboes score showed an improvement in ten patients, worsening in one patient and resolution of inflammation in one patient after EEN treatment (Tables A1 and A2).

3.8. Adverse Events

Two patients reported initial mild abdominal pain related to the intake of nutritional drinks. The treatment was tolerated without any additional side effects in all 12 patients.

3.9. Mucosal Cytokine Profile

In six of twelve EEN-treated children, the cytokine profile in biopsies were analyzed both at diagnosis and at CC. In the remaining seven patients, mucosal cytokines in biopsies were analyzed either at diagnosis or at CC, but could not be analyzed both at diagnosis and CC due to technical circumstances.

3.9.1. Cytokine Profiles in Six Patients Pre- and Post EEN

No significant differences were found in any cytokine profile in six patients (five with CD and one with IBD-U) who completed six weeks of EEN. Furthermore, there were no associations in the cytokine profile in relation to gender, age or disease extension. In individual patients, both reductions and increases in the cytokine expression were seen. With regards to the key proinflammatory cytokine IL-12β, only one patient demonstrated a decrease while four patients showed an increase after EEN (one sample missing). In addition, the antiinflammatory IL-10 decreased in three patients and increased in three patients, while two patients had a reduction of the regulatory TGF-β1, one patient had no change and three patients showed increased expression after EEN treatment. The regulatory cytokine CSF-2 was downregulated in four out of five patients after EEN treatment (Table 3 and Figure 1). Table A3 for real-time PCR values per patient pre- and post-EEN.

Table 3. MCP in biopsies from six children at IBD onset and after treatment harvested from colon (in some patients, it was not possible to analyze all MCPs).

CYTOKINE	Decreased	Unchanged	Increased
CSF-2	4		1
IFN-γ	3		2
TNF-α	4		2
IL-1β	4		2
IL-4	3		
IL-6	2	2	2
IL-10	3		3
IL-12β	1		4
IL-22	2		
IL-23α	5		1
IL-36γ	4		1
TGF-β1	2	1	3

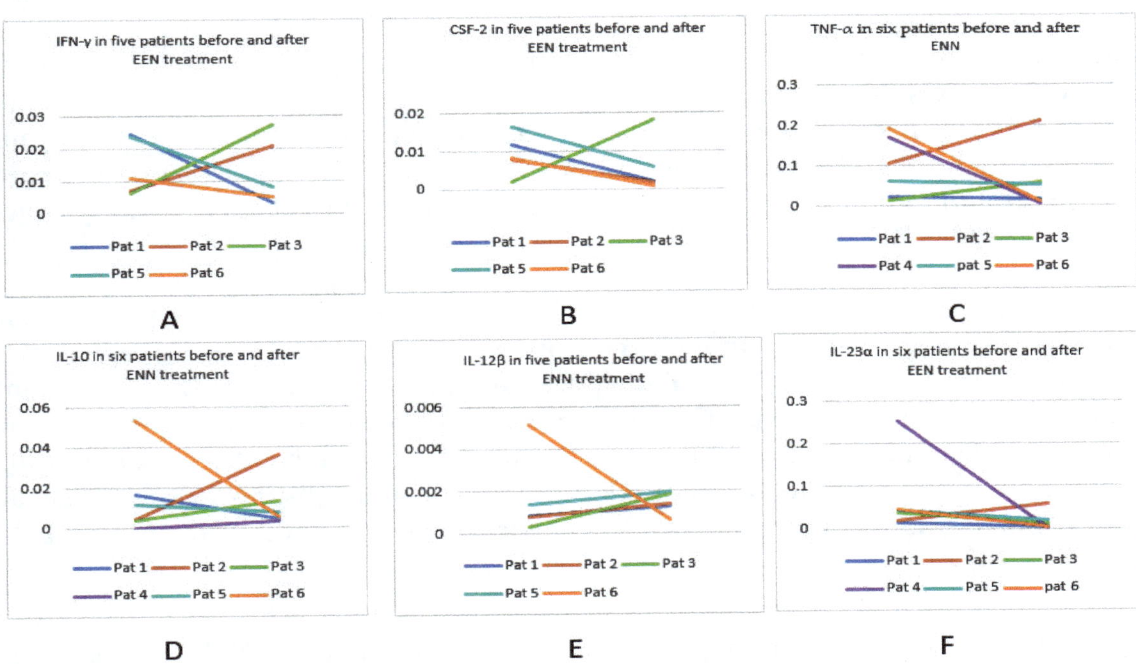

Figure 1. Six cytokine profiles in mucosal biopsies according to mRNA levels measured by q-PCR at disease onset and after EEN treatment. (**A**). IFN-γ at onset and after EEN treatment. (**B**). CSF-2 at onset and after EEN treatment. (**C**). TNF-α at onset and after EEN treatment. (**D**). IL-10 at onset and after EEN treatment. (**E**). IL-12β at onset and after EEN treatment. (**F**). IL-23α at onset and after EEN treatment.

3.9.2. Cytokine Comparison between IBD Patients and Non-IBD Controls

When 12 MCPs in eight IBD-patients were compared to six non-IBD patients at inclusion, significantly higher values of IL-12β ($p = 0.007$) and IL-23α ($p = 0.025$) were measured in the IBD patients compared to non-IBD controls.

4. Discussion

In the present study, we aimed to investigate the effect of EEN treatment on symptoms, biochemistry, endoscopy, histopathology and mucosal cytokine profile in children with new onset IBD.

We found a significant reduction of PCDAI, CRP, ESR and F-calprotectin; a significant increase in hemoglobin and albumin levels; and a significant gain in weight between the baseline and after completion of the EEN treatment. Mucosal healing (MH), measured by SES-CD, was seen in the majority of the patients at CC compared to diagnosis. Our results are consistent with other reports, which have showed that EEN is effective for clinical and biochemical remission in up to 80% in children with newly diagnosed CD [19,20].

Interestingly, in the two patients with a subsequent change of diagnosis from CD to UC, EEN also had an antiinflammatory effect. To the best of our knowledge, the literature on the evaluation of EEN in UC is limited [21,22].

MCP

In this pilot study, no significant differences in MCP were found after EEN treatment in children with IBD. However, we found significant higher levels of baseline IL-12β and IL-23α in the IBD-patients compared to non-IBD controls. These cytokines are known to play an important role in the pathogenesis of CD [23].

Our intention was to investigate the effects of EEN on the mucosal cytokine profile in addition to its clinical effects. It is likely that MCP mirrors the inflammatory activity more adequately than cytokines analyzed in peripheral blood [24]. Even though the reduced expression of proinflammatory cytokines was seen after EEN treatment, no consistent effect of EEN variations was identified. This is probably due to individual variations and a limited number of patients, which is an important limitation of the study.

The expression of TGF-β1, CSF-2 and IL-10, which are known as regulatory cytokines, demonstrated conflicting changes in the patient group after treatment. There are only a few reports published on mucosal cytokines after EEN. Yamamoto et al. investigated IL-1β, IL-1 receptor antagonist (IL-1ra), IL-6, IL-8 and TNF-α with enzyme-linked immunosorbent assay (ELISA) before and after four weeks of elemental diet in 28 adult patients. After treatment, a reduction in the mucosal expression of IL-1β, IL-1ra, IL-6, IL-8 and TNF-α was noticed. Furthermore, when they compared IBD patients to healthy controls, significantly higher levels of all cytokines were observed in the IBD patients [12].

Fell et al. investigated clinical efficacy and mucosal healing after eight weeks of CT3211 (a polymeric nutritional diet) in 29 children with active CD. In addition, IL-1β, IL-8, IL-10, TGF-β1 and IFN-γ were analyzed with PCR in ileal- and colonic biopsies from 18 children [11]. Complete clinical remission was seen in 79% of the patients. Furthermore, macroscopic and histological healing was associated with a significant downregulation of mucosal proinflammatory cytokines in ileum or/and colon. Elevated mucosal cytokines were observed in CD patients before EEN treatment compared to non-IBD controls and ileal TGF-β1 increased during treatment.

Thus, the reports on MCP and EEN show contradictory results and one explanation may be the diversity in methodology, but also in the types and length of EEN treatment. The individual expression of the mucosal cytokines may also reflect the diversity in patients and their immunological status since CD probably comprises several pathogenic mechanisms that differ between patients [25,26]. Nevertheless, earlier reports show aberrant gene expression in patients with CD, which involves cytokine expression. In 2006, Carr et al. found a strong association between an aberrant gene-expression of the proinflammatory cytokine IL23R and CD while Waschke et al. connected various single nucleotide polymorphisms in the TNF receptors to different CD phenotypes [27–29]. In our report, the expression of regulatory IL-10, TGF-β1 and CSF-2 was shown to decrease and increase in individual patients after EEN treatment. This may reflect the temporal aspect, i.e., the same cytokine may be protective during acute inflammation but harmful and perpetuate the chronic inflammation [30]. Thus, cytokines may exert variable functions during different immunological conditions [31–33].

5. Conclusions

Complete remission after 6 weeks of EEN was achieved in a majority of children with new onset IBD. We found a higher level of expression of IL-12β and IL-23α in these children compared to controls at inclusion. There were individual changes in the mucosal cytokine profiles after EEN-treatment but there were no consistent trends. Further understanding of the role of both antiinflammatory and regulatory cytokines as well as the aspects of temporal changes in the cytokine expression from diagnosis to remission requires larger studies.

Author Contributions: Conceptulization and methodology: H.R., Y.F., M.E. and U.L.F. Software and formal analysis: H.R. Validation: H.R., Y.F., M.E. and U.L.F. Investigation: H.R., Y.F. and K.J.-V. Supervision: Y.F., M.E. and U.L.F. Writing—Original Draft preparation H.R. Writing—Review and Editing: H.R., Y.F., M.E., U.L.F. and K.J.-V. Project administration: H.R.

Appendix A

Table A1. Geboes scoring: Grades < 3 were regarded as absence of IBD inflammation, while grades $\geq$ 3 were regarded as presence of IBD inflammation of varying degree (3:1–3:7) with the following subgroups: a = basal plasmacytosis, b = lymphoid nodules, c = Paneth cell hyperplasia, d = eosinophils in the lamina propria, e = histiocytic cell proliferation, f = giant cells, g = granuloma, h = vasculitis and i = dysplasia. The table shows 11 segments (segment 1 = ileum, segment 11 = rectum) before and after EEN treatment.

	Segm. 1	Segm. 2	Segm. 3	Segm. 4	Segm. 5	Segm. 6	Segm. 7	Segm. 8	Segm. 9	Segm. 10	Segm. 11
Patient Endoscopy1 | Endoscopy2											
Pat 1 CD	mult.g | g	<3 | <3	<3 | <3	<3 | <3	<3 | <3	<3 | <3	<3 | <3	<3 | <3	<3 | <3	<3 | <3	<3 | <3
Pat 2 UC	<3 | 3:3	5 | 3:7	3:7 | 3:7	3:3 | 3:3	3:3 | 3:7	5 | 3:7	5 | 3:3	4 | 3:7	3:7 | 3:7		<3 | 3:7
Pat 3 CD	<3 | <3	<3+g | <3	5+b | <3+e	<3 | mult.g	<3 | <3+e	<3 | <3+e	<3 | <3	<3 | <3+g	<3 | <3	<3 | <3	<3 | <3
Pat 4 CD	3:3+b+g | 3:1	3:3+b+g | 3:1	3:3+b+g | 3:1	<3 | <3	<3 | <3	<3 | <3	<3 | <3	3:3 | <3	<3 | <3	<3 | <3	<3 | <3
Pat 5 CD	<3 | <3	<3 | <3	<3 | <3	<3 | <3	<3 | <3	<3 | <3	<3 | <3	<3 | <3	<3 | <3	<3 | <3	<3 | <3
Pat 6 CD	3:3+e | <3	<3 | <3	<3 | <3	<3 | <3	<3 | <3	<3 | <3	<3 | <3	<3 | <3	<3 | <3	<3 | <3	4+g | <3
Pat 7 UC	<3 | <3	3:7 | 3:3	3:7+e | 3:3	3:7 | 3:3	3:7 | 3:3	3:3 | 3:3	3:7 | 3:7	3:7 | 3:3	4+e | 3:7	3:7+c | 3:3	3:7 | 3:3
Pat 8 CD	infl.polyp | 3:7	<3 | <3+g	<3+g | <3	<3+e | 3:3	<3+g | 3:3	3:2 | <3	3:2+g | 3:1	<3 | <3	<3+g | <3	<3+g | <3	<3+g | <3
Pat 9 I-BDU	<3 | <3	<3 | <3	<3 | <3	3:2 | <3	<3 | <3	<3 | <3	3:1 | <3	3:1 | <3	3:1 | <3	<3 | <3	<3 | <3
Pat 10 CD	<3+g | <3+g	<3+g | <3+g	<3 | <3+g	<3 | <3	<3+g | <3	<3 | <3	<3 | <3+g	<3+g | <3	<3 | <3	<3+g | <3	<3+g | <3
Pat 11	<3 | <3	<3 | <3	3:4 | <3	3:7+e | <3	3:7+e | <3	4+e | <3	4 | <3:4	4 | <3	4 | 3:4	3:7+e | <3	4 | <3
Pat 12	5+e | 3:2	3:3 | 3:2	3:3 | 3:2	<3 | <3	<3 | 3:7	<3 | 3:7	<3 | <3	<3 | <3	<3 | <3	<3 | <3	3:7 | <3

Table A2. Geboes results summarized (every patient, 11 segments) as improvement, no change, aggravated inflammation or no inflammation after EEN.

Patient	Improvement	No Change	Aggravated Inflammation	No Inflammation
1	1			10
2	4	4	3	
3	2		4	5
4	4			7
5				11
6	2	1		8
7	8		3	
8	7	2	1	1
9	4			7
10	4	5	2	
11	9			2
12	4		2	5

Table A3. Real-time PCR values per patient pre- and post-EEN and mean values and SD for group per cytokine.

Patient	CSF-2 RQ pre-post EEN	IFN-γ RQ pre-post EEN	TNF-α RQ pre-post EEN	IL1-β:1 RQ pre-post EEN	IL-4:1 RQ pre-post EEN	IL-6:1 RQ pre-post EEN
1	0.011651–0.001997	0.024588–0.003389	0.024577–0.016915	0.573893–0.020431	0.000275–4.72×10^{-5}	0.001001–0.001825
2	0.007851–0.001629	0.007228–0.020651	0.106451–0.21017	0.051899–0.924653	0.001325–########	0.020791–0.172768
3	0.001862–0.018126	0.00664–0.02729	0.014612–0.059869	0.218129–0.408354	0.000282–8.68×10^{-5}	0.008237–0.029142
4	########–########	########–0.00048	0.168562–0.007131	1.021516–0.010524	########–########	########–0.003238
5	0.016589–0.005784	0.023729–0.008329	0.06296–0.054617	2.175898–0.061581	0.000737–0.000148	0.042764–0.022326
6	0.008264–0.000895	0.010918–0.00516	0.190799–0.012544	3.225579–0.108797	########–########	0.32355–0.00282
Mean for group pre-post EEN	0.0092434–0.005686	0.014621–0.010883	0.09466–0.060208	1.211152–0.255723	0.0006548–9.39959×10^{-5}	0.158537–0.038687
SD for group pre-post EEN	0.0048404–0.006446	0.007929–0.009732	0.09466–0.060208	1.137297–0.328006	0.0004296–4.14339×10^{-5}	0.122961–0.06088

Patient	IL-10:1 RQ pre-post EEN	IL-12β:1 RQ pre-post EEN	IL-22:1 RQ pre-post EEN	IL-23α:1 RQ pre-post EEN	IL-36γ:1 RQ pre-post EEN	TGFβ1:1 RQ pre-post EEN
1	0.016987–0.004407	0.000851–0.001291	#######–0.002077	0.015346–0.005568	0.000435–0.000911	0.653298–0.657096
2	0.004295–0.03603	0.000767–0.001354	########–0.016029	0.020307–0.060188	0.002836–0.002475	1.013262–4.188852
3	0.003799–0.013653	0.000296–0.001842	0.000458–0.004207	0.037239–0.012223	0.002853–0.002125	0.425452–0.726292
4	########–0.003523	########–########	########–#######	0.254504–0.003021	########–########	1.497149–0.271375
5	0.01185–0.007582	0.001391–0.001984	0.014448–0.008729	0.044249–0.019889	0.00407–0.000911	0.988215–1.261974
6	0.053329–0.005778	0.005143–0.000639	0.008147–8.46×10^{-5}	0.046621–0.004837	0.001272–0.000563	0.83872–0.52586
Mean for group pre-post EEN	0.018052–0.011829	0.00169–0.001422	0.007684–0.006225	0.069711–0.017621	0.002293–0.001397	0.902683–1.271908
SD for group pre-post EEN	0.018311–0.011312	0.001761–0.000475	0.005721–0.005681	0.083447–0.019867	0.001285–0.000756	0.333408–1.338034

References

1. Van Limbergen, J.; Russell, R.K.; Drummond, H.E.; Aldhous, M.C.; Round, N.K.; Nimmo, E.R.; Smith, L.; Gillett, P.M.; McGrogan, P.; Weaver, L.T.; et al. Definition of phenotypic characteristics of childhood-onset inflammatory bowel disease. *Gastroenterology* **2008**, *135*, 1114–1122. [CrossRef] [PubMed]
2. Baumgart, D.C.; Sandborn, W.J. Crohn's disease. *Lancet* **2012**, *380*, 1590–1605. [CrossRef]

3. Ruemmele, F.M.; Veres, G.; Kolho, K.L.; Griffiths, A.; Levine, A.; Escher, J.C.; Amil Dias, J.; Barabino, A.; Braegger, C.P.; Bronsky, J.; et al. Consensus guidelines of ECCO/ESPGHAN on the medical management of pediatric Crohn's disease. *J. Crohns Colitis* **2014**, *8*, 1179–1207. [CrossRef] [PubMed]
4. Zachos, M.; Tondeur, M.; Griffiths, A.M. Enteral nutritional therapy for induction of remission in Crohn's disease. *Cochrane Database Syst. Rev.* **2008**, *4*, Cd000542.
5. Dziechciarz, P.; Horvath, A.; Shamir, R.; Szajewska, H. Meta-analysis: Enteral nutrition in active Crohn's disease in children. *Aliment. Pharmacol. Ther.* **2007**, *26*, 795–806. [CrossRef] [PubMed]
6. Day, A.S.; Whitten, K.E.; Lemberg, D.A.; Clarkson, C.; Vitug-Sales, M.; Jackson, R.; Bohane, T.D. Exclusive enteral feeding as primary therapy for Crohn's disease in Australian children and adolescents: A feasible and effective approach. *J. Gastroenterol. Hepatol.* **2006**, *21*, 1609–1614. [CrossRef] [PubMed]
7. Cuiv, P.O.; Begun, J.; Keely, S.; Lewindon, P.J.; Morrison, M. Towards an integrated understanding of the therapeutic utility of exclusive enteral nutrition in the treatment of Crohn's disease. *Food Funct.* **2016**, *7*, 1741–1751. [CrossRef] [PubMed]
8. Furness, J.B.; Kunze, W.A.; Clerc, N. Nutrient tasting and signaling mechanisms in the gut. II. The intestine as a sensory organ: Neural, endocrine and immune responses. *Am. J. Physiol.* **1999**, *277 Pt 1*, G922–G928. [PubMed]
9. Korzenik, J.R.; Dieckgraefe, B.K. Is Crohn's disease an immunodeficiency? A hypothesis suggesting possible early events in the pathogenesis of Crohn's disease. *Dig. Dis. Sci.* **2000**, *45*, 1121–1129. [CrossRef]
10. Neurath, M.F. Cytokines in inflammatory bowel disease. *Nat. Rev. Immunol.* **2014**, *14*, 329–342. [CrossRef]
11. Fell, J.M.; Paintin, M.; Arnaud-Battandier, F.; Beattie, R.M.; Hollis, A.; Kitching, P.; Donnet-Hughes, A.; MacDonald, T.T.; Walker-Smith, J.A. Mucosal healing and a fall in mucosal proinflammatory cytokine mRNA induced by a specific oral polymeric diet in paediatric Crohn's disease. *Aliment. Pharmacol. Ther.* **2000**, *14*, 281–289. [CrossRef] [PubMed]
12. Yamamoto, T.; Nakahigashi, M.; Umegae, S.; Kitagawa, T.; Matsumoto, K. Impact of elemental diet on mucosal inflammation in patients with active Crohn's disease: Cytokine production and endoscopic and histological findings. *Inflamm. Bowel Dis.* **2005**, *11*, 580–588. [CrossRef] [PubMed]
13. Schwerd, T.; Frivolt, K.; Clavel, T.; Lagkouvardos, I.; Katona, G.; Mayr, D.; Uhlig, H.H.; Haller, D.; Koletzko, S.; Bufler, P. Exclusive enteral nutrition in active pediatric Crohn disease: Effects on intestinal microbiota and immune regulation. *J. Allergy Clin. Immunol.* **2016**, *138*, 592–596. [CrossRef] [PubMed]
14. Levine, A.; Koletzko, S.; Turner, D.; Escher, J.C.; Cucchiara, S.; de Ridder, L.; Kolho, K.L.; Veres, G.; Russell, R.K.; Paerregaard, A.; et al. ESPGHAN revised porto criteria for the diagnosis of inflammatory bowel disease in children and adolescents. *J. Pediatr. Gastroenterol. Nutr.* **2014**, *58*, 795–806. [CrossRef] [PubMed]
15. Turner, D.; Griffiths, A.M.; Walters, T.D.; Seah, T.; Markowitz, J.; Pfefferkorn, M.; Keljo, D.; Waxman, J.; Otley, A.; LeLeiko, N.S.; et al. Mathematical weighting of the pediatric Crohn's disease activity index (PCDAI) and comparison with its other short versions. *Inflamm. Bowel Dis.* **2012**, *18*, 55–62. [CrossRef] [PubMed]
16. Levine, A.; Griffiths, A.; Markowitz, J.; Wilson, D.C.; Turner, D.; Russell, R.K.; Fell, J.; Ruemmele, F.M.; Walters, T.; Sherlock, M.; et al. Pediatric modification of the Montreal classification for inflammatory bowel disease: The Paris classification. *Inflamm. Bowel Dis.* **2011**, *17*, 1314–1321. [CrossRef]
17. Daperno, M.; D'Haens, G.; Van Assche, G.; Baert, F.; Bulois, P.; Maunoury, V.; Sostegni, R.; Rocca, R.; Pera, A.; Gevers, A.; et al. Development and validation of a new, simplified endoscopic activity score for Crohn's disease: The SES-CD. *Gastrointest. Endosc.* **2004**, *60*, 505–512. [CrossRef]
18. Geboes, K.; Riddell, R.; Ost, A.; Jensfelt, B.; Persson, T.; Lofberg, R. A reproducible grading scale for histological assessment of inflammation in ulcerative colitis. *Gut* **2000**, *47*, 404–409. [CrossRef]
19. Day, A.S.; Lopez, R.N. Exclusive enteral nutrition in children with Crohn's disease. *World J. Gastroenterol.* **2015**, *21*, 6809–6816. [CrossRef]
20. Bannerjee, K.; Camacho-Hubner, C.; Babinska, K.; Dryhurst, K.M.; Edwards, R.; Savage, M.O.; Sanderson, I.R.; Croft, N.M. Antiinflammatory and growth-stimulating effects precede nutritional restitution during enteral feeding in Crohn disease. *J. Pediatr. Gastroenterol. Nutr.* **2004**, *38*, 270–275. [CrossRef]
21. Gonzalez-Huix, F.; Fernandez-Banares, F.; Esteve-Comas, M.; Abad-Lacruz, A.; Cabre, E.; Acero, D.; Sanderson, I.R.; Croft, N.M. Enteral versus parenteral nutrition as adjunct therapy in acute ulcerative colitis. *Am. J. Gastroenterol.* **1993**, *88*, 227–232. [PubMed]

22. Shaoul, R.; Brown, S.; Day, A.S. Reasoning Beyond the Potential Use of Exclusive Enteral Nutrition and Other Specified Diets in Children with Ulcerative Colitis. *J. Pediatr. Gastroenterol. Nutr.* **2018**, *66*, 378–382. [CrossRef]
23. Guan, Q.; Zhang, J. Recent Advances: The Imbalance of Cytokines in the Pathogenesis of Inflammatory Bowel Disease. *Mediators Inflamm.* **2017**, *2017*, 4810258. [CrossRef] [PubMed]
24. Dock, J.; Ramirez, C.M.; Hultin, L.; Hausner, M.A.; Hultin, P.; Elliott, J.; Yang, O.O.; Anton, P.A.; Jamieson, B.D.; Effros, R.B. Distinct aging profiles of CD8+ T cells in blood versus gastrointestinal mucosal compartments. *PLoS ONE* **2017**, *12*, e0182498. [CrossRef]
25. Roggenbuck, D.; Reinhold, D.; Baumgart, D.C.; Schierack, P.; Conrad, K.; Laass, M.W. Autoimmunity in Crohn's Disease-A Putative Stratification Factor of the Clinical Phenotype. *Adv. Clin. Chem.* **2016**, *77*, 77–101. [PubMed]
26. Cleynen, I.; Boucher, G.; Jostins, L.; Schumm, L.P.; Zeissig, S.; Ahmad, T.; Andersen, V.; Andrews, J.M.; Annese, V.; Brand, S.; et al. Inherited determinants of Crohn's disease and ulcerative colitis phenotypes: A genetic association study. *Lancet* **2016**, *387*, 156–167. [CrossRef]
27. Ek, W.E.; D'Amato, M.; Halfvarson, J. The history of genetics in inflammatory bowel disease. *Ann. Gastroenterol.* **2014**, *27*, 294–303. [PubMed]
28. Duerr, R.H.; Taylor, K.D.; Brant, S.R.; Rioux, J.D.; Silverberg, M.S.; Daly, M.J.; Steinhart, A.H.; Abraham, C.; Regueiro, M.; Griffiths, A.; et al. A genome-wide association study identifies IL23R as an inflammatory bowel disease gene. *Science* **2006**, *314*, 1461–1463. [CrossRef]
29. Waschke, K.A.; Villani, A.C.; Vermeire, S.; Dufresne, L.; Chen, T.C.; Bitton, A.; Cohen, A.; Thomson, A.B.; Wild, G.E. Tumor necrosis factor receptor gene polymorphisms in Crohn's disease: Association with clinical phenotypes. *Am. J. Gastroenterol.* **2005**, *100*, 1126–1133. [CrossRef]
30. Bamias, G.; Cominelli, F. Cytokines and intestinal inflammation. *Curr. Opin. Gastroenterol.* **2016**, *32*, 437–442. [CrossRef]
31. Sanjabi, S.; Zenewicz, L.A.; Kamanaka, M.; Flavell, R.A. Antiinflammatory and proinflammatory roles of TGF-beta, IL-10 and IL-22 in immunity and autoimmunity. *Curr. Opin. Pharmacol.* **2009**, *9*, 447–453. [CrossRef] [PubMed]
32. Egea, L.; Hirata, Y.; Kagnoff, M.F. GM-CSF: A role in immune and inflammatory reactions in the intestine. *Expert Rev. Gastroenterol. Hepatol.* **2010**, *4*, 723–731. [CrossRef] [PubMed]
33. Dabritz, J. Granulocyte macrophage colony-stimulating factor and the intestinal innate immune cell homeostasis in Crohn's disease. *Am. J. Physiol. Gastrointest. Liver Physiol.* **2014**, *306*, G455–G465. [CrossRef] [PubMed]

15

Micronutrient Absorption and Related Outcomes in People with Inflammatory Bowel Disease

Kyle Kilby [1], Holly Mathias [2], Lindsay Boisvenue [3], Courtney Heisler [4] and Jennifer L. Jones [4,*]

1 Faculty of Medicine, Dalhousie University, 1459 Oxford Street, Halifax, NS B3J 4R2, Canada; Kyle.Kilby@dal.ca
2 School of Health and Human Performance, Dalhousie University, 6230 South Street, Halifax, NS B3H 1T8, Canada; Holly.Mathias@dal.ca
3 Seaway Valley Community Health Care, 353 Pitt Street, Cornwall, ON K6J 3R1, Canada; BoisvenueL@seawayvalleychc.ca
4 Nova Scotia Collaborative Inflammatory Bowel Disease Program, Division of Digestive Care and Endoscopy, QEII Health Science Centre, Room 932, Victoria Building, 1276 South Park Street, Halifax, NS B3H 2Y9, Canada; courtney.heisler@nshealth.ca
* Correspondence: jljones@dal.ca

Abstract: Inflammatory Bowel Disease (IBD) is a chronic disorder associated with immune dysregulation and chronic inflammation of the digestive tract. While it is poorly understood, the role of nutrition and nutrient status in the etiology of IBD and its associated outcomes has led to increased research relating to micronutrient deficiency. This review offers an overview of recent literature related to micronutrient absorption and outcomes in adults with IBD. Although the absorption and IBD-related outcomes of some micronutrients (e.g., vitamin D and iron) are well understood, other micronutrients (e.g., vitamin A) require further research. Increased research and clinician knowledge of the relationship between micronutrients and IBD may manifest in improved nutrient screening, monitoring, treatment, and outcomes for people living with IBD.

Keywords: Inflammatory Bowel Disease; micronutrients; vitamin; mineral; deficiency

---

1. Introduction

Inflammatory Bowel Diseases (IBD) (including Crohn's Disease (CD) and Ulcerative Colitis (UC)) are complex disorders involving immune dysregulation, leading to infiltration and destruction of the gastrointestinal tract. At its core, IBD results from an imbalance between pro-inflammatory and anti-inflammatory signaling, however the etiology of this imbalance, and of IBD itself, remains poorly understood [1]. An expanding body of literature implicates a shared role of genetics and the environment in the development of disease. The contributing role of environmental factors in the pathogenesis of IBD is further substantiated by observed rising IBD incidence rates in populations that have immigrated from geographic regions of low disease prevalence to regions where the disease is more prevalent [2]. Population-based studies highlight an association between increased intake of total fat, processed meat, and protein (common components of 'Western' diets), and the incidence of IBD [3,4].

In turn, IBD itself affects nutrition intrinsically by disrupting the absorption of nutrients in the gut, and extrinsically through reduced total food intake due to pain and fatigue, as well as the avoidance of food groups that exacerbate their symptoms [5–11]. Given differences in disease location between CD (commonly involving the ileocecal junction but can affect any part of the gastrointestinal tract) and UC (localized to the rectum and colon), and the distribution of nutrient absorption sites within the gut, the spectrum of the association between IBD and nutrient status varies in both magnitude and selectivity [12,13]. Micronutrient status is further impacted by increased gastrointestinal losses and the surgical treatment of IBD itself, which decreases the amount of mucosal surface area available for absorption [14]. The effect of selected micronutrient deficiencies on patient outcomes has been difficult to characterize. The severity of deficiency often moves lockstep with disease severity, making it difficult to draw conclusions about the specific impact of micronutrient levels on patient outcomes without experimental interventional studies to eliminate known or residual confounding effect. This review seeks to highlight many of the common micronutrient deficiencies associated with IBD and examine the reciprocal relationship between micronutrients and IBD with respect to absorption and outcomes. Furthermore, this review aims to examine current recommendations for micronutrient supplementation and screening for patients with IBD.

2. Literature Review

2.1. Materials & Methods

An initial literature search was performed in order to develop a set of well-studied and clinically relevant micronutrients. Medline, Pubmed, Embase and CINAHL databases were searched for English language peer-reviewed articles published during 2009–2019 using the keywords 'inflammatory bowel disease' and, 'micronutrients' alongside, 'deficiency', 'outcomes', 'screening', and/or 'treatment'. This search strategy resulted in 1334 articles. Articles were excluded if they did not focus on the adult IBD patients or patient outcomes. From this, a subset of 160 papers were used to determine which micronutrient deficiencies warranted further investigation.

Individual literature searches for each micronutrient were performed, with no exclusion criteria. Each search followed the same formula of keywords, with 'inflammatory bowel disease' and the vitamin in question, as well as the modifiers, 'outcomes', 'deficiency', 'supplementation', or 'therapy'. From these subsearches, all relevant results were included. Finally, snowballing was used to find additional sources that were not returned by the search.

2.2. Micronutrients

Micronutrients are categorized as having four main roles in supporting major body function: cofactors in metabolism, coenzymes in metabolism, genetic controls, and antioxidants [15]. Therefore, deficiency of essential micronutrients leads to deleterious downstream effects involving metabolism, gene expression and oxidative stress [15]. In the context of IBD, the role of micronutrients in genetic control and antioxidation are of particular importance [16]. Vitamin A, B, and E have been implicated in regulating immune responses and homeostasis within the gut, inhibiting the release of inflammatory cytokines and favoring the differentiation of regulatory (T_{REG}) lymphocytes over proinflammatory T_H17 lymphocytes [16]. In healthy patients, production of reactive oxygen species (ROS) is balanced by the activity of antioxidative micronutrients such as vitamins A and E, as well as enzymes requiring trace metals (zinc and selenium as examples) as cofactors [16]. In IBD, immune dysregulation and inflammation result in the increased production of ROS, further underlying the importance of antioxidative micronutrients in mitigating IBD pathogenesis [17]. This relationship creates a chicken and the egg situation: Is increasing disease severity responsible for micronutrient deficiencies by impairing absorption? Or are dwindling levels of micronutrients, which act as antioxidants and immune regulators, responsible for progression of disease?

2.3. Vitamins

2.3.1. Vitamin A

Vitamin A, and its active metabolite retinoic acid, have widespread effects through the body. In the context of the immune response, retinoic acid signaling results in expression of Foxp3, a transcription factor that leads to the differentiation of naïve T cells to T_{REG} cells [18–21]. These T_{REG} cells attenuate the immune response through the release of anti-inflammatory cytokines [22,23]. Conversely, retinoic acid inhibits the expression of IL-6 receptors, preventing the differentiation of naïve cells into proinflammatory T_H17 cells [20]. Furthermore, retinoic acid induces the expression of $\alpha 4\beta 7$ and CCR9 on T cells [24]. The expression of these molecules causes T cells to preferentially migrate into the gut wall following exposure to antigen [25].

Vitamin A absorption chiefly occurs in the proximal intestine and can be directly converted into retinoic acid in the gut by enterocytes [26]. Given that vitamin A stores in the liver buffer decreasing levels in the blood, measuring serum vitamin A does not accurately assess the total amount present in the body [27]. Soares-Mota et al., 2015 used relative dose response testing to indirectly assess liver stores of vitamin A in 38 Brazilian patients with CD and 34 healthy subjects. They found that deficiencies in vitamin A stores were significantly more common in those suffering from CD (37% vs. 12%, $p < 0.005$). Interestingly, they did not find any association between vitamin A deficiency, disease location, or disease activity [27].

Provitamins of vitamin A have also been examined in the context of IBD. One such provitamin, β-carotene, has been well studied [28]. Compared to controls, β-carotene levels in IBD patients have been shown to be significantly decreased, with further decrease in those with active disease [29]. As well, supplementation with β-carotene lead to disease amelioration in a dextran sodium sulfate (DSS) murine model of colitis [30]. Conclusions are much harder to draw from results of human trials. Firstly, in the articles reviewed by Rezaie et al., 2007, each study uses β-carotene alongside other antioxidative micronutrients, making it difficult to judge its effect [31]. Furthermore, the review notes that the studies used small doses of β-carotene and did not see normalization of β-carotene serum levels. The one study reviewed that used high dose antioxidants, including β-carotene, saw decreases in the required corticosteroid dose, while all other studies were negative [31,32]. Again, without elucidating the effect of β-carotene supplementation in isolation, it is impossible to determine its clinical utility. It is also difficult to distinguish whether any effects are due to its conversion to vitamin A or its own antioxidative ability.

The role of non-provitamin A carotenoids in IBD will only be described briefly, as their role in the context of IBD requires further elucidation. Presently, deficiencies of these carotenoids, namely lycopene and lutein, have been described in IBD patients [30,33]. However, the clinical significance of these deficiencies in IBD is unclear. While the effect of dietary supplementation has not been determined, a single retrospective study using the self-reported dietary records of 56 UC patients in remission associated higher lycopene and lutein intake with decreased fecal blood and mucus, with no change in abdominal pain [34]. Lutein was also able to attenuate ulceration of the GI tract in DSS murine models [35]. Given the exceeding rarity of clinical serum testing for these compounds, and the lack of data surrounding their supplementation, significant further research is required before any recommendation can be made.

Given the ability of vitamin A to attenuate intestinal inflammation in murine models and the prevalence of deficiency in the Brazilian CD population, further research into the role of vitamin A in IBD is warranted [27,36]. At this point, research regarding vitamin A supplementation in IBD is limited to two small studies published in 1985, (Wright et al., 1985: $n = 86$; Norrby et al., 1985, $n = 8$) [37,38]. Neither of these papers found a significant benefit of supplementation. However, drastic changes in the management and treatment of IBD over the past 30 years, combined with small sample sizes in both studies make this an attractive topic to revisit using well-designed clinical trials [39].

2.3.2. Folate

While folate (also known as vitamin B9) deficiency has classically been associated with anemia in IBD patients, it's role in IBD is likely more complex than previously thought. Not only is folate essential in the synthesis of nucleotides, but it is implicated in the regulation of T_{REG} cells [40]. In vitro, folate acts as a pro-survival signal for T_{REG} cells [41,42]. Similarly, in murine models, deficiency in folate leads to the reduction of T_{REG} cells in the intestine [40]. Murine models have also demonstrated a predisposition towards intestinal inflammation in mice being fed diets deficient in folate [42,43]. Furthermore, folate deficiency (as well as B12 deficiency) inhibits the conversion of homocysteine to methionine, which results in increased levels of homocysteine in the blood and intestinal mucosa of a significant portion of IBD patients [44]. Homocysteine acts as a pro-oxidant amino acid, increasing oxidative stress in the body [45]. Homocysteine also promotes the secretion of pro-inflammatory chemokines, and the differentiation of naïve CD4+ T cells into pro-inflammatory T_H17 cells [46]. Homocysteine levels are correlated with thrombotic events, and interestingly, IBD patients have an increased prevalence of thrombosis compared to those without IBD (5-year prevalence, 7.5% vs. 4.5%, $p < 0.001$) [47]. Furthermore, the patients are at increased risk of mesenteric ischemia (HR 11.2), and female IBD patients have significantly higher risk of MI (HR 1.6) and stroke (HR 2.1) [48].

Folate is absorbed in the jejunum following its conversion from folate polyglutamate to monoglutamate in the gut [49]. Further conversion in the liver results in the production of the metabolically active tetrahydrofolate (THF) [49]. Folate levels are significantly lower in patients with both CD and UC, with one prospective study of 180 IBD patients suggesting that 22.2% of CD patients and 4.3% of UC patients are deficient [50]. While the mechanism behind folate deficiency has not been well categorized, jejunal dysfunction and reduced intake of folate-containing foods are likely contributors. Furthermore, the use of methotrexate or sulfasalazine in IBD treatment leads to errors of folate metabolism and absorption [51,52].

While anemia is common in IBD patients, the authors were unable to find a study that assessed the proportion of patients with megaloblastic anemias in the setting of folate deficiency. Furthermore, folate supplementation remains a relatively unexplored topic. At this point, only the effect of supplementation on colorectal cancer has been described. A meta-analysis of 10 such articles determined that folate supplementation significantly lowers the risk of colorectal cancer in IBD patients (HR 0.58; 95% CI: 0.36–0.66) [53]. However, the studies analyzed used varying doses of folate, making recommendations difficult. The effect of folate supplementation on homocysteine levels in the intestinal mucosa, and the risk of thrombotic event, are logical targets of future research.

2.3.3. Vitamin B12

Unlike the micronutrients discussed above, no direct connection between vitamin B12 (cobalamin) and immune regulation has been described. Vitamin B12 has been included in this review due to the clinical consequences of its deficiency, as well as the impact of CD on the site of its intestinal absorption. Vitamin B12 is essential in the metabolism of macronutrients, synthesis of DNA, and nerve function [54]. Deficiency is associated with macrocytic anemia via impaired folate metabolism, neurologic damage, and hyperhomocysteinemia [54]. While serious, these complications are uncommonly reported in IBD patients. In order to be absorbed, vitamin B12 requires activation by intrinsic factor produced in the stomach. Following activation, vitamin B12 is only absorbed via specific receptors present in the terminal ileum [55]. This location makes its deficiency a particular concern in CD, as a significant proportion of CD patients develop ileal disease [56].

Numerous studies exist that assess B12 status in IBD patients and the results vary [50,57–60]. In recent years, both a systemic review and meta-analysis of the literature have concluded that IBD is not associated with significantly lower serum B12 levels [61]. However, surgical resection of the ileum is associated with B12 deficiency [61]. Meta-analysis by Pan et al., 2017 suggests that patients with ileal resections were disproportionately underrepresented in the literature surrounding B12 deficiency [61]. Considering that ileal disease is common in CD, and upwards of 50% of CD patients require surgery within 10 years of diagnosis, patients with ileal resection, and therefore B12 deficiency, likely represent a larger group than described [62].

2.3.4. Vitamin D

The relationship of IBD and vitamin D is likely the most complicated of the IBD-micronutrient relationships. While normally associated with calcium metabolism and bone health, the role of vitamin D in the regulation of the immune response has been the topic of much research in recent years [16]. In the gut, vitamin D's active form 1α,25-dihydroxyvitamin D3 (calcitriol) alters the T cell response, favoring T_{REG} cells and inhibiting production of proinflammatory cytokines [63]. Calcitriol also impairs the function of interstitial dendritic cells, limiting their ability to activate T cells within the gut [63]. Furthermore, direct signaling via vitamin D receptors on T cells leads to upregulation of programmed death receptors and the downregulation of the activating receptor CD69 [64]. These properties provide a rational physiological means by which vitamin D deficiency affects IBD pathogenesis. This is further substantiated by murine models of IBD in which vitamin D supplementation improves symptoms, and deficiency increases symptoms [65,66].

Vitamin D is acquired through the diet, however the majority of vitamin D is synthesized endogenously in the skin [67]. Once acquired, vitamin D must then be metabolized step-wise in the liver and kidney into its active form 1α,25-dihydroxyvitamin D3 [67]. Vitamin D deficiency is common in IBD patients, with a meta-analysis identifying deficient vitamin D levels in 57.7% of CD patients [68]. The exact reason for vitamin D deficiency in IBD is not well understood. Considering that few foods naturally contain vitamin D, deficiency is likely a combination of reduced intake to diet restrictions and aversions, as well as impairment of the absorption of fat-soluble vitamins [69].

Literature correlating vitamin D deficiency with IBD disease activity is abundant and relatively homogenous [70–75]. However, there exists a limited amount of data in patients whose vitamin D levels have been restored through supplementation. Broadly, vitamin D levels are inversely associated with inflammatory markers, while positively associated with bone mineral density (BMD), anti-inflammatory cytokine production, and response to anti-tumor necrosis factor (TNF) therapy [70,76–80]. In both CD and UC, vitamin D deficiency is also associated with more frequent relapses of disease, disease severity, risk of colorectal cancer [81–83]. Similarly, a landmark longitudinal study of 965 American IBD patients saw a significant association between low vitamin D concentration and increased utilization of healthcare, increased pain, and decreased quality of life [84]. This study also found that vitamin D normalization significantly reduced healthcare utilization in the same population [84]. Ananthakrishnan et al., 2013 have corroborated this finding, showing that normalization of vitamin D levels reduces risk of surgery in CD patients [85]. In terms of BMD, concurrent supplementation with calcium and vitamin D led to significantly increased BMD in the hip and lumbar spine [86,87].

Dosing of vitamin D for effect in IBD is not well-established [88]. Doses of vitamin D3 at 4000 IU/day are adequate in correcting deficiency but given the conflicting evidence around the effect of supplementation on disease course in the first place, the most appropriate therapeutic dose has not been determined [88,89].

2.3.5. Calcium

Calcium homeostasis is a complex, multifaceted phenomenon. Bone, which is 60% comprised of calcium hydroxyapatite ($Ca_{10}(PO_4)_6(OH)_2$, undergoes constant remodeling throughout life. Therefore, the pathways responsible for the control of calcium homeostasis are critically important. The supply of calcium involves paracellular and transcellular intestinal and renal absorption and reabsorption [90]. Chronic intestinal inflammation of IBD, as well as dietary and lifestyle alterations and medications used to treat IBD, impact these physiologic homeostatic pathways [7,9,87,90,91]. Intestinal malabsorption, as a result of decreased dairy product intake, leads to low luminal ionic calcium (Ca^{2+}) concentrations resulting in increased transcellular active transport (versus more non-active paracellular transport when luminal Ca^{2+} concentrations are high via decreased duodenal transit time and down regulation of protein responsible for transcellular Ca^{2+} transport proteins). Ca^{2+} is absorbed through facilitated diffusion mediated by transient receptor potential villanoid channels (TRPV6 and 5), which are regulated by vitamin D3, parathyroid hormone, estrogens, pH- and Ca^{2+} dependent regulatory mechanisms, and bidirectional Na+/Ca^{2+} exchange [90].

Beyond the known negative influence of vitamin D insufficiency and malnutrition, there is a relative paucity of knowledge relating to the impact of acute and chronic intestinal inflammation itself on Ca^{2+} homeostasis in the kidneys and intestine. A study by Huybers et al. demonstrated in a TNF-α overexpressing mouse model of Crohn's ileitis that multiple epithelial proteins involved in Ca^{2+} absorption and transport, including TRPV6, were down regulated [92]. As a result of changes in the expression of Ca^{2+} transport genes, bone resorption increased. When these same mice were treated with methylprednisone, similar inhibitory effects were seen in TRPV6 and calbindin D9K mRNA and protein. Although limited data exists in IBD, a very small (n = 4) study of CD patients in remission revealed intestinal absorption of Ca^{2+}, as well as response to $1{,}25(OH)_2D_3$, to be similar to that of controls [92].

In addition to calcium, phosphate (P_i) homeostasis is important in the maintenance of BMD. Prolonged phosphate deficiency may lead to bone demineralization (osteomalacia and rickets). Although little is known about the impact of intestinal inflammation on P_i absorption, as with serum Ca^{2+} it is known that serum levels of P_i do not reflect minor alterations in active mineral transport. Therefore, it is very uncommon to observe changes in serum Ca^{2+} or P_i in IBD patients. The *Klotho* gene, a multifunctional protein, has been implicated in the regulation of both Ca^{2+} and P_i metabolism through its influence on transepithelial Ca^{2+} transport via promotion of transport channel recruitment and retention. Thurston et al., have demonstrated renal Klotho to be significantly down-regulated in various murine models of colitis via TNF and IFN-gamma [93].

Through complex absorptive, transport, and hydroxylation mechanisms, vitamin D3 is converted to the hormonally active form of vitamin D, $1{,}25(OH)_2D_3$, which is responsible for most, if not all, of the biological effects of vitamin D. $1{,}25(OH)_2D_3$ has a pleiotropic role and is a key regulator of bone turn-over, with the potential to facilitate both osteoclastic and osteoblastic pathways. Numerous studies have demonstrated the association between vitamin D deficiency or insufficiency and IBD when compared with control or healthy individuals [94,95]. The mechanisms for this observed associations in IBD may include intestinal malabsorption, decreased dietary intake, disrupted enterohepatic circulation, renal insufficiency and inadequate sunshine exposure. Given the association between IBD and decreased vitamin D status, numerous interventional studies have been conducted in an attempt to determine the impact of vitamin D supplementation on IBD-related clinical outcomes. The data related to BMD loss or accrual have been mixed [90,96,97]. In fact, there have been several studies that suggest, in the setting of active inflammation, that high concentrations of $1{,}25(OH)_2D_3$ may promote the development of osteoporosis in CD [98]. Likewise, the outcomes of studies relating to bone formation and resorption in IBD patients have been conflicting, likely due to flaws in study design, power, confounding factors, IBD complexity, and challenges related to understanding and measuring bone turn-over rates in both adults and children with IBD. More well designed and adequately powered clinical studies are required to definitely answer these questions relating to bone formation and resorption in IBD [90].

The presumption that the BMD effects observed in IBD are simply as a result of vitamin D3 and calcium deficiency has more recently been recognized to be overly simplistic. The complex interplay between the inflammatory disease process itself and the mediators of mineral homeostasis and bone (re)absorption complicates efforts to clearly elucidate the role that these nutrients and hormones play in the pathogenesis of metabolic bone disease in patients with IBD, as well as the role that acute and chronic inflammation may play in alterations of mineral and hormonal homeostasis.

2.3.6. Vitamin K

The mechanism of vitamin K absorption is two-fold. Vitamin K is both directly absorbed from the diet and produced in the gut by commensal GI flora. As a cofactor, vitamin K is crucial to the production of coagulation factors and in the maintenance of bone [99]. As well, much like many of the other micronutrients discussed, vitamin K is implicated in immune signaling and inflammation [16]. Poor vitamin K levels are associated with increasing levels of IL-6 in the blood, a pro-inflammatory cytokine that is implicated in IBD pathology [100,101]. Similarly, in murine models, vitamin K supplementation reduced intestinal inflammation in the presence of the bacterial antigen lipopolysaccharide (LPS), while deficiency aggravated disease in DSS models of colitis in mice [102,103]. This provides a dual rationale for vitamin K supplementation in IBD: avoid complications such as bleeding and bone loss, while hopefully pushing the body away from pro-inflammatory immune pathways.

Vitamin K deficiency is found in 31% of IBD patients, with dysregulation of the gut biota and bile salt malabsorption proposed as mechanisms [69]. In these patients, low levels of vitamin K are associated with low BMD, as well as clinical activity and duration of disease [104–106]. In long-standing IBD, the prevalence of osteoporosis can be as high as 41% [107]. Considering this, and the adverse outcomes associated with fractures, BMD is of critical importance in IBD management. Daily supplementation of vitamin K over 12 months was unable to alter the indices of bone health in IBD patients with vitamin K deficiencies [108]. Furthermore, in rheumatoid arthritis, which shares some common inflammatory pathophysiology with IBD, vitamin K supplementation did not significantly alter the level of IL-6 or the clinical activity of disease in patients [109]. Given the link of vitamin K deficiency to low BMD and high IL-6, these results are disappointing.

2.4. *Metals*

2.4.1. Iron

Aside from vitamin D, iron is likely the micronutrient that has been most heavily studied in the context of IBD. Iron has attracted attention due to the high portion of IBD patients who suffer from anemia [110]. The mean prevalence of anemia calculated by meta-analysis is 16% in outpatients, increasing to 68% in inpatients [99]. As well, the overall portion of IBD patients with iron deficiency is 45% [111]. The physiological means by which IBD causes iron-deficiency is straight forward. Mucosal bleeding leads to iron loss in the stool, meanwhile inflammatory changes altering hepcidin and iron metabolism impact iron absorption [112].

Anemia, and the associated fatigue, can be one of the most crippling symptoms of IBD, with quality of life scores mirroring hemoglobin (Hb) levels [113]. On this basis alone, the treatment of iron-deficiency anemia in IBD is paramount. Current recommendations suggest the end goal of iron supplementation is the normalization of iron store levels, as well as Hb [114]. Oral and intravenous iron products are available for use in IBD. Clinically, and in meta-analysis, intravenous iron supplementation is associated with significantly fewer GI side effects, as well as slightly greater increases in Hb [115]. However, the patient's quality of life did not significantly differ between intravenous and oral iron [116]. Importantly, anemia reoccurs rapidly in IBD, further necessitating the use of iron maintenance therapies [117]. In line with this, European Crohn's and Colitis Organization (ECCO) guidelines suggest that patients who have been treated for iron-deficiency anemia be monitored every 3 months for the first year, and every 6–12 months for the recurrence of anemia [114].

2.4.2. Zinc

As a cofactor, zinc is intimately involved in the regulation of both the innate and adaptive arms of the immune system [118]. Importantly, zinc downregulates NF-κB signaling through the zinc-finger protein A20, leading to decreased expression of its downstream products (namely IL-6 and TNF-α) [119–121]. It is worth noting that certain mutations in the gene that encodes A20 (*TNFAIP3*) are positively associated with the risk of developing numerous inflammatory conditions, including IBD [121]. As well, deletion of *TNFAIP3* in mice intestinal cells leads to sensitivity to DSS-induced colitis. Conversely, zinc deficiency results in increased production of pro-inflammatory molecules in murine models [122]. Finally, zinc also exerts an anti-oxidative effect through its inhibition of NADPH oxidase, and its role as a cofactor for superoxide dismutase [123,124]. The relationship between zinc and IBD on both a theoretical and genetic level, make it a micronutrient of interest to explore further.

Zinc deficiency is present in a significant portion of IBD patients (15.2–65%) [8,125]. Zinc levels are balanced through absorption in the proximal small intestine, and excretion in intestinal and pancreatic secretions [126]. Losses are increased in association with chronic diarrhea, high output ostomies, and high output fistulas, which often pose a problem for IBD patients. These increased losses combined with the malabsorptive state of intestinal inflammation are likely responsible for zinc deficiency in IBD patients.

Clinically, an association has also been observed between zinc deficiency and IBD. A prospective study of 170,756 women over 26 years found that increasing zinc intake was inversely corelated with CD risk [127]. Furthermore, an American cohort study of 773 CD and 233 UC patients highlighted the relationship between zinc deficiency and adverse patient outcomes. They found that zinc deficiency was associated with a significant increase in hospitalizations (CD: OR 1.44. 95% CI [1.02–2.04]; UC: OR 2.14, 95% CI [1.07–4.29]), surgery (CD: OR 2.05, 95% CI [1.38–3.05]; UC: OR 1.64, 95% CI [0.59–4.52]), and complications (CD: OR 1.50, 95% CI [1.04–2.15]; UC: OR 1.97, 95% CI [0.94–4.11]) [128]. In patients who were able to achieve normal zinc levels within 12 months, the risk of adverse outcomes returned to baseline [128]. Although zinc deficiency is associated with disease activity and worse outcomes, a single small cross-over trial (n = 14) that explored the effect of daily zinc supplementation did not show changes in the level of pro-inflammatory cytokines, or disease activity [129]. Given the positive results seen by Siva et al., 2017, larger trials following zinc supplementation may be a reasonable step forward [128].

2.4.3. Selenium

Much like zinc, selenium is integral to the immune function. Selenoproteins, through which selenium exerts its effect, encompass a group of proteins with diverse pro- and anti-inflammatory effects that are beyond the scope of this review. Relevant to IBD, glutathione peroxidases (GPx) utilize selenium to mitigate the effect of ROS [130]. Whereas loss of the genes encoding GPx proteins results in increased severity of disease in DSS murine models [131–133].

Selenium deficiency is common in IBD patients with a recent study reporting 30.9% of patients as deficient, and numerous others observing levels that were significantly decreased compared to control [134–139]. In DSS-treated mice, selenium deficiency leads to increased severity of disease and upregulation of pro-inflammatory TH1 cytokines [140,141]. In humans, selenium deficiency has been investigated for its possible role in cardiovascular disease, however a recent review by Benstoem et al., 2015 describes the literature as "inconclusive" [142].

Selenium supplementation in the context of IBD has not been documented in the literature outside of murine models. In these models, supplementation ameliorated cox-dependent inflammation by altering the PGE2 pathway [143,144]. Given the abundance of animal data, and the strong physiological link between selenium and immune function, the study of selenium therapy should be a future focus. Table 1 presents the immune implications of micronutrient deficiencies, including selenium, in adult IBD patients.

Table 1. Immune implications of micronutrient deficiencies in IBD.

Micronutrient	Level in IBD	Purported Pathogenic Role of Deficiency
Vitamin A	↓ [27]	↓ T_{REG} cell differentiation [18–21] ↑ T_{H17} cell differentiation [20] ↓ T cell migration into the gut [25]
Folate	↓ [43]	↓ T_{REG} cell survival [31,32] ↑ Proinflammatory signaling [37,39] ↑ Oxidative stress [37,38]
Vitamin B12	=↓ in patients with ileal resection [54]	–
Vitamin D	↓ [61]	↑ T cell activation [56] ↑ Proinflammatory signaling [56] ↓ Decreased T cell turnover [57]
Calcium	↓ [87,90,91]	–
Vitamin K	↓ [62]	↑ Proinflammatory signaling [84,85]
Iron	↓ [104]	–
Zinc	↓ [8,118]	↑ Proinflammatory signaling [114] ↑ Oxidative stress [116,117]
Selenium	↓ [134–139]	↑ Proinflammatory signaling [141] ↑ Oxidative stress [130]

This table presents the immune implications of micronutrient deficiencies in adult IBD patients. The arrows describe the effect of IBD on the level of micronutrient present in the individual, as well as the effect on the purported pathogenic role related to that micronutrient. For example, ↑ indicates an increase, ↓ indicates a decrease, and =↓indicates about the same or less.

3. Recommendations and Conclusions

The understanding of the role of micronutrients in immune system function has changed greatly in recent years, as has our understanding of the pathophysiologic mechanism(s) of Inflammatory Bowel Disease (IBD). However, the etiology of IBD and the role that micronutrients play in the development of IBD is still unclear. There are clear physiologic links between immune-regulating micronutrients and the balance of pro- and anti-inflammatory processes in the gut (see Table 1) [16]. However, experimental models often oversimplify what is experienced clinically (see Table 2). The same is true of micronutrients with anti-oxidative effects [16,17]. In addition, the bidirectional relationship of deficiency and disease makes the exact role of each micronutrient difficult to characterize, as IBD impacts nutritional status through both decreased intake (impaired absorption, avoidance of trigger foods, decreased appetite, decreased surface area secondary to resection, etc.), and increased gastric losses (chronic diarrhea, intestinal blood loss, mucus losses, etc.). The effect of micronutrients on outcomes is most easily understood in the context of iron, in which IBD leads to iron deficiency, and deficiency leads to anemia. However, for the other micronutrients, the relationship between IBD, deficiency, and clinical outcomes is much less clear. Table 2 presents the clinical outcomes associated with level of micronutrients discussed in this paper, in adult IBD patients.

Table 2. Clinical outcomes associated with micronutrient levels in IBD.

Micronutrient	Effect of Deficiency	Effect of Supplementation
Vitamin A	–	–
Folate	Macrocytic anemia ↑ Homocysteinemia [44]	↓ Risk of colorectal cancer [53]
Vitamin B12	Macrocytic anemia ↑ Homocysteinemia Neurologic damage [54]	–
Vitamin D	↑ Inflammatory markers [70,77] ↑ Healthcare utilization [84] ↑ Disease activity [70–75] ↑ Risk of colorectal cancer [83] ↓Quality of life [72,85]	↑ Bone mineral density ↓ Risk of surgery
Vitamin K	↓ Bone mineral density [104–106] ↑ Bleeding risk [99]	↔ Disease activity ↔ Bone mineral density
Iron	Iron-deficiency anemia	Resolution of anemia ↑ Quality of life [113]
Zinc	↑ CD risk [127] ↑ Hospitalizations ↑ Surgery ↑ Complications [126]	↔Disease activity
Selenium	? Cardiovascular disease [142]	–

This table presents the clinical outcomes associated with micronutrient levels in IBD. The arrows describe the effect of IBD on the level of micronutrient present in the individual, as well as the effect on the purported pathogenic role related to that micronutrient. For example, ↑ indicates an increase, ↓ indicates a decrease, ↔ indicates a potential increase or decrease, and ? indicates that the outcome is unknown.

hile association studies suggest the benefit of treating deficiency of iron, zinc and vitamin D, similar studies have not been performed for other micronutrients. Similarly, literature regarding the use of supplementation as therapy is limited to a few, small scale studies that only targeted specific subgroups of patients [37,38,129]. These factors make specific recommendations on dosage for supplementation difficult. At this point, current European Society for Clinical Nutrition and Metabolism (ESPEN) recommendations suggest that micronutrient levels be assessed annually in IBD patients, with the correction of any deficit with supplementation [145]. Guidelines for iron supplementation are more specific, suggesting iron repletion therapy in all IBD patients with iron-deficiency anemia, with the end goal of therapy being the normalization of both hemoglobin and iron stores [114]. Intravenous iron should be considered in patients with clinically active disease and those who are intolerant of oral iron, while oral iron should be considered in those with inactive disease or milder anemia [114]. The dose of iron is dependent on the route and formulation chosen, however a response of 2 g/dL within 4 weeks is appropriate [114]. As for zinc, a 3-month course of daily supplementation with 200 mg of $ZnSO_4$ normalizes zinc serum concentrations in deficient IBD patients [146]. Given that zinc citrate has similar bioavailability and is more palatable to patients its use may be preferred [147]. In addition, one author suggests increasing zinc supplementation in patients with diarrhea in order to offset increased GI loses at a rate of 30–40 mg elemental zinc for every liter of stool output [148].

For the other nutrients discussed in this paper, evidence-based recommendations for supplementation in the context of IBD do not exist. Rather, clinicians should focus on the correction of any micronutrient deficiencies that are found using appropriate oral therapy. Previous authors have posited varying suggestions on dosage with regards to reversing deficit, with high dose oral therapy as the common theme among them. A 2003 review by Eiden highlights such suggestions in IBD patients and is a valuable reference for clinicians with deficient IBD patients [149].

The development of specific recommendations for supplementation and micronutrient levels to targets is a priority. In order to do so, large, well-designed, controlled studies focused on supplementation are required. Given the consistency of the observed association between zinc and vitamin D and IBD clinical disease activity and inflammation, further study of supplementation of vitamin D and zinc as an adjunct to therapy is appropriate [16,36]. Given their link to immunity and oxidation, further characterization of the role of vitamin A, B9, and K in IBD pathogenesis is also warranted.

Author Contributions: Conceptualization, J.L.J. and L.B.; Methodology, J.L.J. and H.M.; Formal Analysis, K.K.; Data Curation, H.M.; Writing-Original Draft Preparation, K.K.; Writing-Review & Editing, K.K., L.B., H.M., C.C., J.L.J.; Supervision, J.L.J.; Project Administration, H.M.

References

1. Lee, S.H.; Kwon, J.e.; Cho, M.-L. Immunological pathogenesis of inflammatory bowel disease. *Intest. Res.* **2018**, *16*, 26–42. [CrossRef] [PubMed]
2. Benchimol, E.I.; Mack, D.R.; Guttmann, A.; Nguyen, G.C.; To, T.; Mojaverian, N.; Quach, P.; Manuel, D.G. Inflammatory bowel disease in immigrants to Canada and their children: A population-based cohort study. *Am. J. Gastroenterol.* **2015**, *110*, 553–563. [CrossRef] [PubMed]
3. Hou, J.K.; Abraham, B.; El-Serag, H. Dietary intake and risk of developing inflammatory bowel disease: A systematic review of the literature. *Am. J. Gastroenterol.* **2011**, *106*, 563–573. [CrossRef] [PubMed]
4. Racine, A.; Carbonnel, F.; Chan, S.S.M.; Hart, A.R.; Bueno-De-Mesquita, H.B.; Oldenburg, B.; Van Schaik, F.D.M.; Tjønneland, A.; Olsen, A.; Dahm, C.C.; et al. Dietary patterns and risk of inflammatory bowel disease in Europe: Results from the EPIC study. *Inflamm. Bowel Dis.* **2016**, *22*, 345–354. [CrossRef] [PubMed]
5. Limdi, J.K. Dietary practices and inflammatory bowel disease. *Indian J. Gastroenterol.* **2018**, *37*, 284–292. [CrossRef] [PubMed]
6. Taylor, L.; Almutairdi, A.; Shommu, N.; Fedorak, R.; Ghosh, S.; Reimer, R.A.; Panaccione, R.; Raman, M. Cross-sectional analysis of overall dietary intake and mediterranean dietary pattern in patients with Crohn's disease. *Nutrients* **2018**, *10*, 1761. [CrossRef] [PubMed]
7. Urbano, A.P.S.; Sassaki, L.Y.; Dorna, M.S.; de Barros Leite Carvalhaes, M.A.; Martini, L.A.; Ferreira, A.L.A. Nutritional intake according to injury extent in ulcerative colitis patients. *J. Hum. Nutr. Diet.* **2013**, *26*, 445–451. [CrossRef] [PubMed]
8. Vagianos, K.; Clara, I.; Carr, R.; Graff, L.A.; Walker, J.R.; Targownik, L.E.; Lix, L.M.; Rogala, L.; Miller, N.; Bernstein, C.N. What are adults with inflammatory bowel disease (IBD) eating? A closer look at the dietary habits of a population-based Canadian IBD cohort. *J. Parenter. Enter. Nutr.* **2016**, *40*, 405–411. [CrossRef]
9. Vidarsdottir, J.B.; Johannsdottir, S.E.; Thorsdottir, I.; Bjornsson, E.; Ramel, A. A cross-sectional study on nutrient intake and -status in inflammatory bowel disease patients. *Nutr. J.* **2016**, *15*, 61. [CrossRef] [PubMed]
10. Zallot, C.; Quilliot, D.; Chevaux, J.B.; Peyrin-Biroulet, C.; Guéant-Rodriguez, R.M.; Freling, E.; Collet-Fenetrier, B.; Williet, N.; Ziegler, O.; Bigard, M.A.; et al. Dietary beliefs and behavior among inflammatory bowel disease patients. *Inflamm. Bowel Dis.* **2013**, *19*, 66–72. [CrossRef]
11. Walton, M.; Alaunyte, I. Do patients living with ulcerative colitis adhere to healthy eating guidelines? A cross-sectional study. *Br. J. Nutr.* **2014**, *112*, 1628–1635. [CrossRef] [PubMed]
12. Tontini, G.E.; Vecchi, M.; Pastorelli, L.; Neurath, M.F.; Neumann, H. Differential diagnosis in inflammatory bowel disease colitis: State of the art and future perspectives. *World J. Gastroenterol.* **2015**, *21*, 21–46. [CrossRef] [PubMed]
13. Basu, T.K.; Donaldson, D. Intestinal absorption in health and disease: Micronutrients. *Best Pract. Res. Clin. Gastroenterol.* **2003**, *17*, 957–979. [CrossRef]
14. Lucendo, A.J.; De Rezende, L.C. Importance of nutrition in inflammatory bowel disease. *World J. Gastroenterol.* **2009**, *15*, 2081–2088. [CrossRef] [PubMed]
15. Shenkin, A. Micronutrients in health and disease. *Postgrad. Med. J.* **2006**, *82*, 559–567. [CrossRef] [PubMed]
16. Hosomi, K.; Kunisawa, J. The specific roles of vitamins in the regulation of immunosurveillance and maintenance of immunologic homeostasis in the gut. *Immune Netw.* **2017**, *17*, 13–19. [CrossRef] [PubMed]
17. Tian, T.; Wang, Z.; Zhang, J. Pathomechanisms of oxidative stress in inflammatory bowel disease and potential antioxidant therapies. *Oxid. Med. Cell. Longev.* **2017**, *2017*, 4535194. [CrossRef]

18. Elias, K.M.; Laurence, A.; Davidson, T.S.; Stephens, G.; Kanno, Y.; Shevach, E.M.; O'Shea, J.J. Retinoic acid inhibits TH17 polarization and enhances FoxP3 expression through a Stat-3/Stat-5 independent signaling pathway. *Blood* **2008**, *111*, 1013–1020. [CrossRef]
19. Hill, J.A.; Hall, J.A.; Sun, C.M.; Cai, Q.; Ghyselinck, N.; Chambon, P.; Belkaid, Y.; Mathis, D.; Benoist, C. Retinoic acid enhances Foxp3 induction indirectly by relieving inhibition from $CD4^+$CD44hi cells. *Immunity* **2008**, *29*, 758–770. [CrossRef]
20. Mucida, D.; Park, Y.; Kim, G.; Turovskaya, O.; Scott, I.; Cheroutre, H. Reciprocal TH17 and regulatory T Cell differentiation mediated by retinoic acid. *Science* **2007**, *317*, 256–260. [CrossRef]
21. Sun, C.-M.; Hall, J.A.; Blank, R.B.; Bouladoux, N.; Oukka, M.; Mora, J.R.; Belkaid, Y. Small intestine lamina propria dendritic cells promote de novo generation of Foxp3 T REG cells via retinoic acid. *J. Exp. Med.* **2007**, *204*, 1775–1785. [CrossRef] [PubMed]
22. Lewkowicz, N.; Klink, M.; Mycko, M.P.; Lewkowicz, P. Neutrophil—$CD4^+CD25^+$ T regulatory cell interactions: A possible new mechanism of infectious tolerance. *Immunobiology* **2013**, *218*, 455–464. [CrossRef] [PubMed]
23. Owczarczyk-Saczonek, A.; Czerwińska, J.; Placek, W. The role of regulatory T cells and anti-inflammatory cytokines in psoriasis. *Acta Dermatovenerol. Alp. Pannonica Adriat.* **2018**, *27*, 17–23. [CrossRef] [PubMed]
24. Iwata, M.; Hirakiyama, A.; Eshima, Y.; Kagechika, H.; Kato, C.; Song, S.Y. Retinoic acid imprints gut-homing specificity on T cells. *Immunity* **2004**, *21*, 527–538. [CrossRef] [PubMed]
25. Iwata, M. Retinoic acid production by intestinal dendritic cells and its role in T-cell trafficking. *Semin. Immunol.* **2009**, *21*, 8–13. [CrossRef] [PubMed]
26. Reboul, E. Absorption of vitamin A and carotenoids by the enterocyte: Focus on transport proteins. *Nutrients* **2013**, *5*, 3563–3581. [CrossRef] [PubMed]
27. Soares-Mota, M.; Silva, T.A.; Gomes, L.M.; Pinto, M.A.S.; Mendonça, L.M.C.; Farias, M.L.F.; Nunes, T.; Ramalho, A.; Zaltman, C. High prevalence of vitamin A deficiency in Crohn's disease patients according to serum retinol levels and the relative dose-response test. *World J. Gastroenterol.* **2015**, *21*, 1614–1620. [CrossRef] [PubMed]
28. Biasi, F.; Leonarduzzi, G.; Oteiza, P.I.; Giuseppe, P. Inflammatory bowel disease: Mechanisms, redox considerations, and therapeutic targets. *Antioxid. Redox Signal.* **2013**, *19*, 1711–1747. [CrossRef]
29. Trivedi, P.P.; Jena, G.B. Mechanistic insight into beta-carotene-mediated protection against ulcerative colitis-associated local and systemic damage in mice. *Eur. J. Nutr.* **2015**, *54*, 639–652. [CrossRef] [PubMed]
30. Hengstermann, S.; Valentini, L.; Schaper, L.; Buning, C.; Koernicke, T.; Maritchnegg, M.; Buhner, S.; Tillinger, W.; Regano, N.; Guglielmi, F.; et al. Altered status of antioxidant vitamins and fatty acids in patients with inactive inflammatory bowel disease. *Clin. Nutr.* **2008**, *27*, 571–578. [CrossRef] [PubMed]
31. Rezaie, A.; Parker, R.D.; Abdollahi, M. Oxidative stress and pathogenesis of inflammatory bowel disease: An epiphenomenon or the cause? *Dig. Dis. Sci.* **2007**, *52*, 2015–2021. [CrossRef] [PubMed]
32. Seidner, D.L.; Lashner, B.A.; Brzezinski, A.; Banks, P.L.C.; Goldblum, J.; Fiocchi, C.; Katz, J.; Lichtenstein, G.R.; Anton, P.A.; Kam, L.Y.; et al. An oral supplement enriched with fish oil, soluble fiber, and antioxidants for corticosteroid sparing in ulcerative colitis: A randomized, controlled trial. *Clin. Gastroenterol. Hepatol.* **2005**, *3*, 358–369. [CrossRef]
33. Wendland, B.E.; Aghdassi, E.; Tam, C.; Carrier, J.; Steinhart, A.H.; Wolman, S.L.; Baron, D.; Allard, J.P. Lipid peroxidation and plasma antioxidant micronutrients in Crohn disease. *Am. J. Clin. Nutr.* **2001**, *74*, 259–264 [CrossRef] [PubMed]
34. Glabska, D.; Guzek, D.; Zakrzemska, P.; Wiodarek, D.; Lech, G. Lycopene, lutein and zeaxanthin may reduce faecal blood, mucus and pus but not abdominal pain in individuals with ulcerative colitis. *Nutrients* **2016**, *8*, 613 [CrossRef] [PubMed]
35. Liu, C.; Bronson, R.; Wang, X.-D. Effects of lutein supplementation on the prevention of colonic inflammation and neoplasia in mice. *FASED J.* **2015**, *29*. [CrossRef]
36. Kang, S.G.; Wang, C.; Matsumoto, S.; Kim, C.H. High and low vitamin A therapies induce distinct FoxP3+ T cell subsets and effectively control intestinal inflammation. *Gastroenterology* **2009**, *137*, 1391–1402. [CrossRef] [PubMed]
37. Wright, J.P.; Mee, A.S.; Parfitt, A.; Marks, I.N.; Burns, D.G.; Sherman, M.; Tigler-Wybrandi, N.; Isaacs, S. Vitamin A therapy in patients with Crohn's disease. *Gastroenterology* **1985**, *88*, 512–514. [CrossRef]
38. Norrby, S.; Sjödahl, R.; Tagesson, C. Ineffectiveness of vitamin A therapy in severe Crohn's disease. *Acta Chir Scand.* **1985** *151*, 465–468. [PubMed]

39. Ghishan, F.K.; Kiela, P.R. Vitamins and minerals in inflammatory bowel disease. *Gastroenterol. Clin. N. Am.* **2017**, *46*, 797–808. [CrossRef]
40. Yamaguchi, T.; Hirota, K.; Nagahama, K.; Ohkawa, K.; Takahashi, T.; Nomura, T.; Sakaguchi, S. Control of immune responses by antigen-specific regulatory T cells expressing the folate receptor. *Immunity* **2007**, *27*, 145–159. [CrossRef]
41. Kunisawa, J.; Hashimoto, E.; Ishikawa, I.; Kiyono, H. A pivotal role of vitamin B9 in the maintenance of regulatory T cells in vitro and in vivo. *PLoS ONE* **2012**, *7*, e32094. [CrossRef]
42. Kinoshita, M.; Kayama, H.; Kusu, T.; Yamaguchi, T.; Kunisawa, J.; Kiyono, H.; Sakaguchi, S.; Takeda, K. Dietary folic acid promotes survival of Foxp3+ regulatory T cells in the Colon. *J. Immunol.* **2012**, *189*, 2869–2878. [CrossRef] [PubMed]
43. Zhu, S.; Li, J.; Bing, Y.; Yan, W.; Zhu, Y.; Xia, B.; Chen, M. Diet-induced hyperhomocysteinaemia increases intestinal inflammation in an animal model of colitis. *J. Crohn's Colitis* **2015**, *9*, 708–719. [CrossRef] [PubMed]
44. Oussalah, A.; Guéant, J.L.; Peyrin-Biroulet, L. Meta-analysis: Hyperhomocysteinaemia in inflammatory bowel diseases. *Aliment. Pharmacol. Ther.* **2011**, *34*, 1173–1184. [CrossRef] [PubMed]
45. Tyagi, N.; Sedoris, K.C.; Steed, M.; Ovechkin, A.V.; Moshal, K.S.; Tyagi, S.C. Mechanisms of homocysteine-induced oxidative stress. *Am. J. Physiol. Heart Circ. Physiol.* **2005**, *289*, H2649–H2656. [CrossRef]
46. Gao, X.; Li, J.; Chen, M. Effect of homocysteine on the differentiation of CD4 + T cells into TH17 cells. *Dig. Dis. Sci.* **2018**, *63*, 3339–3347. [CrossRef]
47. Cohen, J.; Ragni, M.V.; Comer, D.M.; Yabes, J.G. Inflammatory bowel disease and thrombosis: A national inpatient sample (NIS) study. *Blood* **2017**, *130*, 3372.
48. Ha, C.; Magowan, S.; Accortt, N.A.; Chen, J.; Stone, C.D. Risk of arterial thrombotic events in inflammatory bowel disease. *Am. J. Gastroenterol.* **2009**, *104*, 1445–1451. [CrossRef]
49. Milman, N. Intestinal absorption of folic acid—New physiologic & molecular aspects. *Indian J. Med. Res.* **2012**, *136*, 725–728.
50. Bermejo, F.; Algaba, A.; Guerra, I.; Chaparro, M.; De-La-Poza, G.; Valer, P.; Piqueras, B.; Bermejo, A.; García-Alonso, J.; Pérez, M.J.; et al. Should we monitor vitamin B12 and folate levels in Crohn's disease patients? *Scand. J. Gastroenterol.* **2013**, *48*, 1272–1277. [CrossRef]
51. Herfarth, H.H.; Kappelman, M.D.; Long, M.D.; Isaacs, K.L. Use of methotrexate in the treatment of inflammatory bowel diseases (IBD). *Inflamm. Bowel Dis.* **2016**, *22*, 224–233. [CrossRef] [PubMed]
52. Halstead, C.; Gandhi, G.; Tamura, T. Sulfasalazine inhibits the absorption of folates in ulcerative colitis. *N. Engl. J. Med.* **1981**, *305*, 1513–1517. [CrossRef] [PubMed]
53. Burr, N.E.; Hull, M.A.; Subramanian, V. Folic acid supplementation may reduce colorectal cancer risk in patients with inflammatory bowel disease: A systematic review and meta-analysis. *J. Clin. Gastroenterol.* **2017**, *51*, 247–253. [CrossRef] [PubMed]
54. O'Leary, F.; Samman, S. Vitamin B12 in health and disease. *Nutrients* **2010**, *2*, 299–316. [CrossRef] [PubMed]
55. Herbert, Y. Progress in gastroenterology: Absorption of vitamin B12 and folic acid. *Gastroenterology* **1968**, *54*, 110–115. [CrossRef]
56. Gasche, C.; Scholmerich, J.; Brynskov, J.; D'Haens, G.; Hanauer, S.B.; Irvine, E.J.; Jewell, D.P.; Rachmilewitz, D.; Sachar, D.B.; Sandborn, W.J.; et al. A simple classification of Crohn's disease: Report of the working party for the world congresses of gastroenterology, Vienna 1998. *Inflamm. Bowel Dis.* **2000**, *6*, 8–15. [CrossRef] [PubMed]
57. Battat, R.; Kopylov, U.; Szilagyi, A.; Saxena, A.; Rosenblatt, D.S.; Warner, M.; Bessissow, T.; Seidman, E.; Bitton, A. vitamin B12 deficiency in inflammatory bowel disease: Prevalence, risk factors, evaluation, and management. *Inflamm. Bowel Dis.* **2014**, *20*, 1120–1128. [CrossRef] [PubMed]
58. Battat, R.; Kopylov, U.; Byer, J.; Sewitch, M.J.; Rahme, E.; Nedjar, H.; Zelikovic, E.; Dionne, S.; Bessissow, T.; Afif, W.; et al. Vitamin B12 deficiency in inflammatory bowel disease: A prospective observational pilot study. *Eur. J. Gastroenterol. Hepatol.* **2017**, *29*, 1361–1367. [CrossRef]
59. Ward, M.G.; Kariyawasam, V.C.; Mogan, S.B.; Patel, K.V.; Pantelidou, M.; Sobczyńska-Malefora, A.; Porté, F.; Griffin, N.; Anderson, S.H.C.; Sanderson, J.D.; et al. Prevalence and risk factors for functional vitamin B12 deficiency in patients with Crohn's disease. *Inflamm. Bowel Dis.* **2015**, *21*, 2839–2847. [CrossRef]
60. Yakut, M.; Üstün, Y.; Kabaçam, G.; Soykan, I. Serum vitamin B12 and folate status in patients with inflammatory bowel diseases. *Eur. J. Int. Med.* **2010**, *21*, 320–323. [CrossRef]

61. Pan, Y.; Liu, Y.; Guo, H.; Jabir, M.S.; Liu, X.; Cui, W.; Li, D. Associations between folate and vitamin B12 levels and inflammatory bowel disease: A meta-analysis. *Nutrients* **2017**, *9*, 382. [CrossRef] [PubMed]
62. Frolkis, A.D.; Dykeman, J.; Negrón, M.E.; Debruyn, J.; Jette, N.; Fiest, K.M.; Frolkis, T.; Barkema, H.W.; Rioux, K.P.; Panaccione, R.; et al. Risk of surgery for inflammatory bowel diseases has decreased over time: A systematic review and meta-analysis of population-based studies. *Gastroenterology* **2013**, *145*, 996–1006. [CrossRef] [PubMed]
63. Jeffery, L.E.; Burke, F.; Mura, M.; Zheng, Y.; Qureshi, O.S.; Walker, L.S.K.; Lammas, D.A.; Raza, K.; Sansom, D.M. 1,25-dihydroxyvitamin D3 and interleukin-2 combine to inhibit T cell production of inflammatory cytokines and promote development of regulatory T cells expressing CTLA-4 and FoxP3. *J. Immunol.* **2009**, *183*, 5458–5467. [CrossRef] [PubMed]
64. Bendix, M.; Greisen, S.; Dige, A.; Hvas, C.L.; Bak, N.; Jørgensen, S.P.; Dahlerup, J.F.; Deleuran, B.; Agnholt, J. Vitamin D increases programmed death receptor-1 expression in Crohn's disease. *Oncotarget* **2017**, *8*, 24177–24186. [CrossRef] [PubMed]
65. Cantorna, M.T.; Munsick, C.; Bemiss, C.; Mahon, B.D. 1,25-dihydroxycholecalciferol prevents and ameliorates symptoms of experimental murine inflammatory bowel disease. *J. Nutr.* **2018**, *130*, 2648–2652. [CrossRef] [PubMed]
66. Lagishetty, V.; Misharin, A.V.; Liu, N.Q.; Lisse, T.S.; Chun, R.F.; Ouyang, Y.; McLachlan, S.M.; Adams, J.S.; Hewison, M. Vitamin D deficiency in mice impairs colonic antibacterial activity and predisposes to colitis. *Endocrinology* **2010**, *151*, 2423–2432. [CrossRef] [PubMed]
67. Jones, G.; Strugnell, S.A.; Deluca, H.F. Current understanding of the molecular actions of vitamin D. *Physiol. Rev.* **1998**, *78*, 1193–1231. [CrossRef]
68. Sadeghian, M.; Saneei, P.; Siassi, F.; Esmaillzadeh, A. Vitamin D status in relation to Crohn's disease: Meta-analysis of observational studies. *Nutrition* **2016**, *32*, 505–514. [CrossRef]
69. Fabisiak, N.; Fabisiak, A.; Watala, C.; Fichna, J. Fat-soluble vitamin deficiencies and inflammatory bowel disease: Systematic review and meta-analysis. *J. Clin. Gastroenterol.* **2017**, *51*, 878–889. [CrossRef]
70. Alrefai, D.; Jones, J.; El-Matary, W.; Whiting, S.J.; Aljebreen, A.; Mirhosseini, N.; Vatanparast, H. The association of vitamin d status with disease activity in a cohort of Crohn's disease patients in Canada. *Nutrients* **2017**, *9*, 1112. [CrossRef]
71. Blanck, S.; Aberra, F. Vitamin D deficiency is associated with ulcerative colitis disease activity. *Dig. Dis. Sci.* **2013**, *58*, 1698–1702. [CrossRef] [PubMed]
72. De Castro, F.D.; Magalhães, J.; Carvalho, P.B.; Moreira, M.J.; Mota, P.; Cotter, J. Lower levels of vitamin D correlate with clinical disease activity and quality of life in inflammatory bowel disease. *Arq. Gastroenterol.* **2016**, *52*, 260–265. [CrossRef] [PubMed]
73. Dolatshahi, S.; Pishgar, E.; Jamali, R. Does serum 25 hydroxy vitamin D level predict disease activity in ulcerative colitis patients? *Acta Clin. Belg. Int. J. Clin. Lab. Med.* **2016**, *71*, 46–50. [CrossRef] [PubMed]
74. Torki, M.; Gholamrezaei, A.; Mirbagher, L.; Danesh, M.; Kheiri, S.; Emami, M.H. Vitamin D deficiency associated with disease activity in patients with inflammatory bowel diseases. *Dig. Dis. Sci.* **2015**, *60*, 3085–3091. [CrossRef] [PubMed]
75. Ulitsky, A.; Ananthakrishnan, A.N.; Naik, A.; Skaros, S.; Zadvornova, Y.; Binion, D.G.; Issa, M. Vitamin D deficiency in patients with inflammatory bowel disease: Association with disease activity and quality of life. *J. Parenter. Enter. Nutr.* **2011**, *35*, 308–316. [CrossRef] [PubMed]
76. Abraham, B.P.; Prasad, P.; Malaty, H.M. Vitamin D deficiency and corticosteroid use are risk factors for low bone mineral density in inflammatory bowel disease patients. *Dig. Dis. Sci.* **2014**, *59*, 1878–1884. [CrossRef]
77. Garg, M.; Rosella, O.; Lubel, J.S.; Gibson, P.R. Association of circulating vitamin D concentrations with intestinal but not systemic inflammation in inflammatory bowel disease. *Inflamm. Bowel Dis.* **2013**, *19*, 2634–2643. [CrossRef] [PubMed]
78. Garg, M.; Hendy, P.; Ding, J.; Shaw, S.; Hold, G.; Hart, H. The effect of vitamin D on intestinal inflammation and faecal microbiota in patients with ulcerative colitis. *J. Crohn's Colitis* **2018**, *12*, 963–972. [CrossRef] [PubMed]
79. Gubatan, J.; Mitsuhashi, S.; Longhi, M.S.; Zenlea, T.; Rosenberg, L.; Robson, S.; Moss, A.C. Higher serum vitamin D levels are associated with protective serum cytokine profiles in patients with ulcerative colitis. *Cytokine* **2018**, *103*, 38–45. [CrossRef] [PubMed]

80. Winter, R.W.; Collins, E.; Cao, B.; Carrellas, M.; Crowell, A.M.; Korzenik, J.R. Higher 25-hydroxyvitamin D levels are associated with a greater odds of remission with anti-tumor necrosis factor-a medications among patients with inflammatory bowel disease. *Aliment. Pharmacol. Ther.* **2018**, *45*, 653–659. [CrossRef]
81. Ananthakrishnan, A.N.; CHeng, S.-C.; Cai, T.; Cagan, A.; Gainer, V.S.; Szolovits, P.; Shaw, S.Y.; Churchill, S.; Karlson, E.W.; Murphy, S.N.; et al. Association between reduced plasma 25-hydroxy vitamin D and increased risk of cancer in patients with inflammatory bowel diseases. *Clin. Gastroenterol. Hepatol.* **2014**, *13*, 821–827. [CrossRef]
82. Gubatan, J.; Mitsuhasi, S.; Zenlea, T.; Rosenberg, L.; Robson, S.; Moss, A.C. Low serum vitamin D during remission increases risk of clinical relapse in patients with ulcerative colitis. *Clin. Gastroenterol. Hepatol.* **2017**, *15*, 240–246. [CrossRef] [PubMed]
83. Meckel, K.; Li, Y.C.; Lim, J.; Kocherginsky, M.; Weber, C.; Almoghrabi, A.; Chen, X.; Kaboff, A.; Sadiq, F.; Hanauer, S.B.; et al. Serum 25-hydroxyvitamin D concentration is inversely associated with mucosal inflammation in patients with ulcerative colitis. *Am. J. Clin. Nutr.* **2016**, *104*, 113–120. [CrossRef] [PubMed]
84. Kabbani, T.A.; Koutroubakis, I.E.; Schoen, R.E.; Ramos-Rivers, C.; Shah, N.; Swoger, J.; Regueiro, M.; Barrie, A.; Schwartz, M.; Hashash, J.G.; et al. Association of vitamin D level with clinical status in inflammatory bowel disease: A 5-year longitudinal study. *Am. J. Gastroenterol.* **2016**, *111*, 712–719. [CrossRef]
85. Ananthakrishnan, A.N.; Cagan, A.; Gainer, V.S.; Cai, T.; Cheng, S.C.; Savova, G.; Chen, P.; Szolovits, P.; Xia, Z.; De Jager, P.L.; et al. Normalization of plasma 25-hydroxy vitamin D is associated with reduced risk of surgery in Crohn's disease. *Inflamm. Bowel Dis.* **2013**, *19*, 1921–1927. [CrossRef]
86. Bakker, S.F.; Dik, V.K.; Witte, B.I.; Lips, P.; Roos, J.C.; Van Bodegraven, A.A. Increase in bone mineral density in strictly treated Crohn's disease patients with concomitant calcium and vitamin D supplementation. *J. Crohn's Colitis* **2013**, *7*, 377–384. [CrossRef] [PubMed]
87. Casals-Seoane, F.; Chaparro, M.; Maté, J.; Gisbert, J.P. Clinical course of bone metabolism disorders in patients with inflammatory bowel disease: A 5-year prospective study. *Inflamm. Bowel Dis.* **2016**, *22*, 1929–1936. [CrossRef] [PubMed]
88. Mathur, J.; Naing, S.; Mills, P.; Limsui, D. A randomized clinical trial of vitamin D3 (Cholecalciferol) in ulcerative colitis patients with hypovitaminosis D3. *PeerJ* **2017**, *5*, e3654. [CrossRef] [PubMed]
89. Narula, N.; Cooray, M.; Anglin, R.; Muqtadir, Z.; Narula, A.; Marshall, J.K. Impact of high-dose vitamin D3 supplementation in patients with Crohn's disease in remission: A pilot randomized double-blind controlled study. *Dig. Dis. Sci.* **2017**, *62*, 448–455. [CrossRef] [PubMed]
90. Ghishan, F.; Kiela, P. Advances in the understanding of mineral and bone metabolism in inflammatory bowel diseases. *Am. J. Physiol. Gastrointest. Liver Physiol.* **2010**, *300*, G191–G201. [CrossRef]
91. Krela-Kazmierczak, I.; Szymczak, A.; Tomczak, M.; Lykowska-Szuber, L.; Linke, K.; Eder, P. Calcium and phosphate metabolism in patients with inflammatory bowel diseases. *Pol. Arch. Med. Wewn.* **2015**, *125*, 588–590. [CrossRef] [PubMed]
92. Huybers, S.; Apostolaki, M.; van der Eerden, B.C.; Kollias, G.; Naber, T.H.; Bindels, R.J.; Hoenderop, J.G. Murine $TNF^{\Delta ARE}$ Crohn's disease model displays diminished expression of intestinal Ca^{2+} transporters. *Inflamm. Bowel Dis.* **2008**, *14*, 803–811. [CrossRef] [PubMed]
93. Thurston, R.D.; Larmonier, C.B.; Majewski, P.M.; Ramalingam, R.; Mi-dura-Kiela, M.; Laubitz, D.; Vandewalle, A.; Besselsen, D.G.; Muhlbauer, M.; Jobin, C.; et al. Tumor necrosis factor and interferon-gamma down-regulate Klotho in mice with colitis. *Gastroenterology* **2010**, *138*, 1384–1394. [CrossRef] [PubMed]
94. El-Matary, W.; Sikora, S.; Spady, D. Bone mineral density, vitamin D, and disease activity in children newly diagnosed with inflammatory bowel disease. *Dig. Dis. Sci.* **2011**, *56*, 825–829. [CrossRef] [PubMed]
95. Leslie, W.D.; Miller, N.; Rogala, L.; Bernstein, C.N. Vitamin D status and bone density in recently diagnosed inflammatory bowel disease: The manitoba IBD cohort study. *Am. J. Gastroenterol.* **2008**, *103*, 1451–1459. [CrossRef] [PubMed]
96. Benchimol, E.I.; Ward, L.M.; Gallagher, J.C.; Rauch, F.; Barrowman, N.; Warren, J.; Beedle, S.; Mack, D.R. Effect of calcium and vitamin D supplementation on bone mineral density in children with inflammatory bowel disease. *J. Pediatr. Gastroenterol. Nutr.* **2007**, *45*, 538–545. [CrossRef] [PubMed]
97. Bernstein, C.N.; Sargent, M.; Leslie, W.D. Serum osteoprotegerin is in-creased in Crohn's disease: A population-based case control study. *Inflamm. Bowel Dis.* **2005**, *11*, 325–330. [CrossRef] [PubMed]
98. Abreu, M.T.; Kantorovich, V.; Vasiliauskas, E.A.; Gruntmanis, U.; Matuk, R.; Daigle, K.; Chen, S.; Zehnder, D.; Lin, Y.C.; Yang, H.; et al. Measurement of vitamin D levels in inflammatory bowel disease patients reveals a

subset of Crohn's disease patients with elevated 1,25-dihydroxyvitamin D and low bone mineral density. *Gut* **2004**, *53*, 1129–1136. [CrossRef]

99. Grober, U.; Reichrath, J.; Holick, M.; Kisters, K. Vitamin K: An old vitamin in a new. *Dermato-Endocrinology* **2014**, *6*, e968490. [CrossRef]
100. Shea, M.K.; Dallal, G.E.; Dawson-Hughes, B.; Ordovas, J.M.; O'Donnell, C.J.; Gundberg, C.M.; Peterson, J.W.; Booth, S.L. Vitamin K, circulating cytokines, and bone mineral density in older men and women. *Am. J. Clin. Nutr.* **2008**, *46*, 220–231. [CrossRef]
101. Yen, D.; Cheung, J.; Scheerens, H.; Poulet, F.; McClanahan, T.; Mckenzie, B.; Kleinschek, M.A.; Owyang, A.; Mattson, J.; Blumenschein, W.; et al. IL-23 is essential for T cell–mediated colitis and promotes inflammation via Il-17 and IL-6. *J. Clin. Investig.* **2006**, *116*, 1310–1316. [CrossRef] [PubMed]
102. Ohsaki, Y.; Shirakawa, H.; Hiwatashi, K.; Furukawa, Y.; Mizutani, T.; Komai, M. Vitamin K suppresses lipopolysaccharide-induced inflammation in the rat. *Biosci. Biotechnol. Biochem.* **2006**, *70*, 926–932. [CrossRef]
103. Shiraishi, E.; Iijima, H.; Shinzaki, S.; Nakajima, S.; Inoue, T.; Hiyama, S.; Kawai, S.; Araki, M.; Yamaguchi, T.; Hayashi, Y.; et al. Vitamin K deficiency leads to exacerbation of murine dextran sulfate sodium-induced colitis. *J. Gastroenterol.* **2016**, *51*, 346–356. [CrossRef] [PubMed]
104. Kuwabara, A.; Tanaka, K.; Tsugawa, N.; Nakase, H.; Tsuji, H.; Shide, K.; Kamao, M.; Chiba, T.; Inagaki, N.; Okano, T.; et al. High prevalence of vitamin K and D deficiency and decreased BMD in inflammatory bowel disease. *Osteoporos. Int.* **2009**, *20*, 935–942. [CrossRef] [PubMed]
105. Nakajima, S.; Iijima, H.; Egawa, S.; Shinzaki, S.; Kondo, J.; Inoue, T.; Hayashi, Y.; Ying, J.; Mukai, A.; Akasaka, T.; et al. Association of vitamin K deficiency with bone metabolism and clinical disease activity in inflammatory bowel disease. *Nutrition* **2011**, *27*, 1023–1028. [CrossRef] [PubMed]
106. Schoon, E.J.; Müller, M.C.A.; Vermeer, C.; Schurgers, L.J.; Brummer, R.-J.M.; Stockbrügger, R.W. Low serum and bone vitamin K status in patients with longstanding Crohn's disease: Another pathogenetic factor of osteoporosis in Crohn's disease? *Gut* **2001**, *48*, 473–477. [CrossRef] [PubMed]
107. Ali, T.; Lam, D.; Bronze, M.S.; Humphrey, M.B. Osteoporosis in inflammatory bowel disease. *Am. J. Med.* **2009**, *122*, 599–604. [CrossRef] [PubMed]
108. O'Connor, E.M.; Grealy, G.; McCarthy, J.; Desmond, A.; Craig, O.; Shanahan, F.; Cashman, K.D. Effect of phylloquinone (vitamin K1) supplementation for 12 months on the indices of vitamin K status and bone health in adult patients with Crohn's disease. *Br. J. Nutr.* **2014**, *112*, 1163–1174. [CrossRef]
109. Shishavan, N.G.; Gargari, B.P.; Jafarabadi, M.A.; Kolahi, S.; Haggifar, S.; Noroozi, S. Vitamin K1 supplementation did not alter inflammatory markers and clinical status in patients with rheumatoid arthritis. *Int. J. Vitam. Nutr. Res.* **2019**. [CrossRef]
110. Niepel, D.; Klag, T.; Malek, N.P.; Wehkamp, J. Practical guidance for the management of iron deficiency in patients with inflammatory bowel disease. *Ther. Adv. Gastroenterol.* **2018**, *11*. [CrossRef]
111. Gisbert, J.; Gomollon, F. Common misconceptions in the diagnosis and management of anemia in inflammatory bowel disease. *Am. J. Gastroenterol.* **2008**, *103*, 1299–1307. [CrossRef]
112. Cavallaro, F.; Duca, L.; Pisani, L.F.; Rigolini, R.; Spina, L.; Tontini, G.E.; Munizio, N.; Costa, E.; Cappellini, M.D.; Vecchi, M.; et al. Anti-TNF-mediated modulation of prohepcidin improves iron availability in inflammatory bowel disease, in an IL-6-mediated fashion. *Can. J. Gastroenterol. Hepatol.* **2017**, *2017*, 6843976. [CrossRef] [PubMed]
113. Sobrado, C.W.; Cançado, R.D.; Sobrado, L.F.; Frugis, M.O.; Sobrado, M.F. Treatment of anemia and improvement of quality of life among patients with Crohn's disease: Experience using ferric carboxymaltose *Arq. Gastroenterol.* **2016**, *52*, 255–259. [CrossRef] [PubMed]
114. Dignass, A.U.; Gasche, C.; Bettenworth, D.; Birgegård, G.; Danese, S.; Gisbert, J.P.; Gomollon, F.; Iqbal, T.; Katsanos, K.; Koutroubakis, I.; et al. European consensus on the diagnosis and management of iron deficiency and anaemia in inflammatory bowel diseases. *J. Crohn's Colitis* **2015**, *9*, 211–222. [CrossRef] [PubMed]
115. Bonovas, S.; Fiorino, G.; Allocca, M.; Lytras, T.; Tsantes, A.; Peyrin-Biroulet, L.; Danese, S. Intravenous versus oral iron for the treatment of anemia in inflammatory bowel disease. *Medicine (Baltimore)* **2016**, *95*, e2308 [CrossRef]
116. Lee, T.W.; Kolber, M.R.; Fedorak, R.N.; Van Zanten, S.V. Iron replacement therapy in inflammatory bowel disease patients with iron deficiency anemia: A systematic review and meta-analysis. *J. Crohn's Colitis* **2012**, *6*, 267–275. [CrossRef]
117. Kulnigg, S.; Teischinger, L.; Dejaco, C.; Waldhör, T.; Gasche, C. Rapid recurrence of IBD-associated anemia

and iron deficiency after intravenous iron sucrose and erythropoietin treatment. *Am. J. Gastroenterol.* **2009**, *104*, 1460–1467. [CrossRef]
118. Shankar, A.H.; Prasad, A.S. Zinc and immune function: The biological basis of altered resistance to infection. *Am. J. Clin. Nutr.* **1998**, *68*, 447–463. [CrossRef]
119. Gammoh, N.Z.; Rink, L. Zinc in infection and inflammation. *Nutrients* **2017**, *9*, 624. [CrossRef] [PubMed]
120. Jarosz, M.; Olbert, M.; Wyszogrodzka, G.; Młyniec, K.; Librowski, T. Antioxidant and anti-inflammatory effects of zinc. Zinc-dependent NF-KB signaling. *Inflammopharmacology* **2017**, *25*, 11–24. [CrossRef]
121. Ma, A.; Malynn, B.A. A20: Linking a complex regulator of ubiquitylation to immunity and human disease. *Nat. Rev. Immunol.* **2013**, *12*, 774–785. [CrossRef] [PubMed]
122. Wong, C.P.; Rinaldi, N.A.; Ho, E. Zinc deficiency enhanced inflammatory response by increasing immune cell activation and inducing IL6 promoter demethylation. *Mol. Nutr. Food Res.* **2015**, *59*, 991–999. [CrossRef]
123. Kloubert, V.; Rink, L. Zinc as a micronutrient and its preventive role of oxidative damage in cells. *Food Funct.* **2015**, *6*, 3195–3204. [CrossRef] [PubMed]
124. Mohammadi, E.; Qujeq, D.; Taheri, H.; Hajian-Tilaki, K. Evaluation of serum trace element levels and superoxide dismutase activity in patients with inflammatory bowel disease: Translating basic research into clinical application. *Biol. Trace Elem. Res.* **2017**, *177*, 235–240. [CrossRef] [PubMed]
125. Filippi, J.; Al-Jaouni, R.; Wiroth, J.B.; Hébuterne, X.; Schneider, S.M. Nutritional deficiencies in patients with Crohn's disease in remission. *Inflamm. Bowel Dis.* **2006**, *12*, 185–191. [CrossRef]
126. Lee, H.H.; Prasad, A.S.; Brewer, G.J.; Owyang, C. Zinc absorption in human small intestine. *Am. J. Physiol. Liver Physiol.* **1989**, *256*, G87–G91. [CrossRef] [PubMed]
127. Ananthakrishnan, A.N.; Khalili, H.; Song, M.; Higuchi, L.M.; Richter, J.M.; Chan, A.T. Zinc intake and risk of Crohn's disease and ulcerative colitis: A prospective cohort study. *Int. J. Epidemiol.* **2015**, *44*, 1995–2005. [CrossRef]
128. Siva, S.; Rubin, D.T.; Gulotta, G.; Wroblewski, K.; Pekow, J. Zinc deficiency is associated with poor clinical outcomes in patients with inflammatory bowel disease. *Inflamm. Bowel Dis.* **2017**, *23*, 152–157. [CrossRef]
129. Mulder, T.P.J.; Veer, A.V.D.S.; Verspaget, H.W.; Griffioen, G.; Peña, A.S.; Janssens, A.R.; Lamers, C.B.H.W. Effect of oral zinc supplementation on metallothionein and superoxide dismutase concentrations in patients with inflammatory bowel disease. *J. Gastroenterol. Hepatol.* **1994**, *9*, 472–477. [CrossRef]
130. Kudva, A.K.; Shay, A.E.; Prabhu, K.S. Selenium and inflammatory bowel disease. *Am. J. Physiol. Gastrointest. Liver Physiol.* **2015**, *309*, 71–77. [CrossRef]
131. Barrett, C.W.; Ning, W.; Chen, X.; Smith, J.J.; Washington, M.K.; Hill, K.E.; Coburn, L.A.; Peek, R.M.; Chaturvedi, R.; Wilson, K.T.; et al. Tumor suppressor function of the plasma glutathione peroxidase gpx3 in colitis-associated carcinoma. *Cancer Res.* **2013**, *73*, 1245–1255. [CrossRef] [PubMed]
132. Esworthy, R.S.; Arand, R.; Martin, M.G.; Doroshow, J.H.; Binder, S.W.; Chu, F.F. Mice with combined disruption of Gpx1 and Gpx2 genes have colitis. *Am. J. Physiol. Gastrointest. Liver Physiol.* **2001**, *281*, 848–855. [CrossRef]
133. Esworthy, R.S.; Kim, B.; Larson, G.P.; Yip, M.L.R.; Smith, D.D.; Li, M.; Chu, F. A colitis locus on chromosome 2 impacting the severity of early-onset disease in mice deficient in GPX1 and GPX2. *Inflamm. Bowel Dis.* **2011**, *17*, 1373–1386. [CrossRef] [PubMed]
134. Han, Y.M.; Yoon, H.; Lim, S.; Sung, M.K.; Shin, C.M.; Park, Y.S.; Kim, N.; Lee, D.H.; Kim, J.S. Risk factors for vitamin D, zinc, and selenium deficiencies in Korean patients with inflammatory bowel disease. *Gut Liver* **2017**, *11*, 363–369. [CrossRef] [PubMed]
135. Rannem, T.; Ladefoged, K.; Hylander, E.; Hegnhoj, J.; Jarnum, S. Selenium status in patients with Crohn's disease. *Am. J. Clin. Nutr.* **1992**, *56*, 933–937. [CrossRef] [PubMed]
136. Hinks, L.J.; Inwards, K.D.; Lloyd, B.; Clayton, B. Reduced concentrations of selenium in mild Crohn's disease. *J. Clin. Pathol.* **1988**, *41*, 198–201. [CrossRef] [PubMed]
137. Gentschew, L.; Bishop, K.S.; Han, D.Y.; Morgan, A.R.; Fraser, A.G.; Lam, W.J.; Karunasinghe, N.; Campbell, B.; Ferguson, L.R. Selenium, selenoprotein genes and Crohn's disease in a case-control population from Auckland, New Zealand. *Nutrients* **2012**, *4*, 1247–1259. [CrossRef] [PubMed]
138. Geerlin, B.J.; Badart-Smook, A.; Stockbrugger, R.W.; Brummer, R.-J.M. Comprehensive nutritional status in recently diagnosed patients with inflammatory bowel disease compared with population controls. *Eur. J. Clin. Nutr.* **2000**, *54*, 514–521. [CrossRef]

139. Aguilar-Tablada, T.C.; Navarro-Alarcon, M.; Granados, J.Q.; Sanchez, C.S.; Rufian-Henares, J.A.; Nogueras-Lopez, F. Ulcerative colitis and Crohn's disease are associated with decreased serum selenium concentrations and increased cardiovascular risk. *Nutrients* **2016**, *8*, 780. [CrossRef]
140. Barrett, C.W.; Singh, K.; Motley, A.K.; Lintel, M.K.; Matafonova, E.; Bradley, A.M.; Ning, W.; Poindexter, S.V.; Parang, B.; Reddy, V.K.; et al. Dietary selenium deficiency exacerbates DSS-induced epithelial injury and AOM/DSS-induced tumorigenesis. *PLoS ONE* **2013**, *8*, e67845. [CrossRef]
141. Sun, Z.; Xu, Z.; Wang, D.; Yao, H.; Li, S. Selenium deficiency inhibits differentiation and immune function and imbalances the TH1/TH2 of dendritic cells. *Metabolomics* **2018**, *10*, 759–767. [CrossRef] [PubMed]
142. Benstoem, C.; Goetzenich, A.; Kraemer, S.; Borosch, S.; Manzanares, W.; Hardy, G.; Stoppe, C. Selenium and its supplementation in cardiovascular disease—What do we know? *Nutrients* **2015**, *7*, 3094–3118. [CrossRef] [PubMed]
143. Kaur, R.; Thakur, S.; Rastogi, R.; Kaushal, N. Resolution of cox mediated inflammation by Se supplementation in mouse experimental model of colitis. *PLoS ONE* **2018**, *13*, e0201356. [CrossRef] [PubMed]
144. Gandhi, U.H.; Kaushal, N.; Ravindra, K.C.; Hegde, S.; Nelson, S.M.; Narayan, V.; Vunta, H.; Prabhu, K.S. Selenoprotein-dependent up-regulation of hematopoietic prostaglandin D2 synthase in macrophages is mediated through the activation of peroxisome proliferator-activated receptor (PPAR) gamma. *J. Biol. Chem.* **2011**, *286*, 27471–27482. [CrossRef] [PubMed]
145. Forbes, A.; Escher, J.; Hébuterne, X.; Kłęk, S.; Krznaric, Z.; Schneider, S.; Shamir, R.; Stardelova, K.; Wierdsma, N.; Wiskin, A.E.; et al. ESPEN guideline: Clinical nutrition in inflammatory bowel disease. *Clin. Nutr.* **2017**, *36*, 321–347. [CrossRef] [PubMed]
146. Brignola, C.; Belloli, C.; De Simone, C.; Evangelisti, A.; Parente, R.; Mancini, R.; Iannone, P.; Mocheggiani, E.; Fabris, N.; Morini, M.C.; et al. Zinc supplementation restores plasma concentrations of zinc and thymulin in patients with Crohn's disease. *Aliment. Pharmacol. Ther.* **1993**, *7*, 275–280. [CrossRef] [PubMed]
147. Wegmüller, R.; Tay, F.; Zeder, C.; Brnic, M.; Hurrell, R.F. Zinc absorption by young adults from supplemental zinc citrate is comparable with that from zinc gluconate and higher than from zinc oxide. *J. Nutr.* **2014**, *144*, 132–136. [CrossRef]
148. Jeejeebhoy, K.N. Short bowel syndrome: A nutritional and medical approach. *CMAJ* **2002**, *166*, 1297–1302. [CrossRef]
149. Eiden, K.A. Nutritional considerations in inflammatory bowel disease. *Pract. Gastroenterol.* **2003**, *5*, 33–54.

Permissions

All chapters in this book were first published by MDPI; hereby published with permission under the Creative Commons Attribution License or equivalent. Every chapter published in this book has been scrutinized by our experts. Their significance has been extensively debated. The topics covered herein carry significant findings which will fuel the growth of the discipline. They may even be implemented as practical applications or may be referred to as a beginning point for another development.

The contributors of this book come from diverse backgrounds, making this book a truly international effort. This book will bring forth new frontiers with its revolutionizing research information and detailed analysis of the nascent developments around the world.

We would like to thank all the contributing authors for lending their expertise to make the book truly unique. They have played a crucial role in the development of this book. Without their invaluable contributions this book wouldn't have been possible. They have made vital efforts to compile up to date information on the varied aspects of this subject to make this book a valuable addition to the collection of many professionals and students.

This book was conceptualized with the vision of imparting up-to-date information and advanced data in this field. To ensure the same, a matchless editorial board was set up. Every individual on the board went through rigorous rounds of assessment to prove their worth. After which they invested a large part of their time researching and compiling the most relevant data for our readers.

The editorial board has been involved in producing this book since its inception. They have spent rigorous hours researching and exploring the diverse topics which have resulted in the successful publishing of this book. They have passed on their knowledge of decades through this book. To expedite this challenging task, the publisher supported the team at every step. A small team of assistant editors was also appointed to further simplify the editing procedure and attain best results for the readers.

Apart from the editorial board, the designing team has also invested a significant amount of their time in understanding the subject and creating the most relevant covers. They scrutinized every image to scout for the most suitable representation of the subject and create an appropriate cover for the book.

The publishing team has been an ardent support to the editorial, designing and production team. Their endless efforts to recruit the best for this project, has resulted in the accomplishment of this book. They are a veteran in the field of academics and their pool of knowledge is as vast as their experience in printing. Their expertise and guidance has proved useful at every step. Their uncompromising quality standards have made this book an exceptional effort. Their encouragement from time to time has been an inspiration for everyone.

The publisher and the editorial board hope that this book will prove to be a valuable piece of knowledge for researchers, students, practitioners and scholars across the globe.

List of Contributors

Yun Pan, Ya Liu, Xuanchen Liu and Weiwei Cui
Department of Nutrition and Food Hygiene, School of Public Health, Jilin University, 1163 Xinmin Avenue, Changchun 130021, China

Haizhuo Guo
Department of Radiology, The Second Part of the First Hospital, Jilin University, Changchun 130031, China

Majid Sakhi Jabir
Department of Biotechnology, University of Technology, Baghdad 00964, Iraq

Dong Li
Department of Immunology, College of Basic Medical Sciences, Jilin University, 126 Xinmin Avenue, Changchun 130021, China
Department of Hepatology, The First Hospital, Jilin University, Changchun 130021, China

Yulan Liu and Xiuying Wang
Hubei Collaborative Innovation Center for Animal Nutrition and Feed Safety, Hubei Key Laboratory of Animal Nutrition and Feed Science, Wuhan Polytechnic University,Wuhan 430023, China

Chien-An Andy Hu
Hubei Collaborative Innovation Center for Animal Nutrition and Feed Safety, Hubei Key Laboratory of Animal Nutrition and Feed Science, Wuhan Polytechnic University,Wuhan 430023, China
Department of Biochemistry and Molecular Biology, University of New Mexico School of Medicine, Albuquerque, NM 87131, USA

Krasimira Aleksandrova
Nutrition, Immunity and Metabolism Start-up Lab, Department of Epidemiology, German Institute of Human Nutrition Potsdam-Rehbrücke, Arthur-Scheunert Allee 114-116, 14558 Nuthetal, Germany

Beatriz Romero-Mosquera and Vicent Hernandez
Department of Gastroenterology, Instituto Investigación Sanitaria Galicia Sur, Estrutura Organizativa de Xestión Integrada de Vigo, 36312 Vigo, Spain

Efstathia Papada, Charalampia Amerikanou, Nick Kalogeropoulos, Chara Tzavara and Andriana C. Kaliora
Department of Dietetics and Nutritional Science, School of Health Science and Education, Harokopio University, 17671 Athens, Greece

Alastair Forbes
Norwich Medical School, University of East Anglia, Bob Champion Building, James Watson Road, Norwich NR4 7UQ, UK

Ljilja Torović
Department of Pharmacy, Faculty of Medicine, University of Novi Sad, 21000 Novi Sad, Serbia

John K. Triantafillidis
Inflammatory Bowel Disease Unit, IASO General Hospital, 15562 Athens, Greece

Roger Stanley
Centre for Food Safety and Innovation, Tasmanian Institute of Agriculture, University of Tasmania, Launceston, TAS 7250, Australia

Agampodi Promoda Perera, Ravichandra Vemuri, Sonia Shastri, Benjamin Southam and Rajaraman Eri
School of Health Sciences, College of Health and Medicine, University of Tasmania, Launceston, TAS 7250, Australia

Tanvi Shinde
Centre for Food Safety and Innovation, Tasmanian Institute of Agriculture, University of Tasmania, Launceston, TAS 7250, Australia
School of Health Sciences, College of Health and Medicine, University of Tasmania, Launceston, TAS 7250, Australia

Shakuntla V. Gondalia
Centre for Human Psychopharmacology, Swinburne University of Technology, Hawthorn, VIC 3122, Australia

Avinash V. Karpe and David J. Beale
Land and Water, Commonwealth Scientific and Industrial Research Organization (CSIRO), Ecosciences Precinct, Dutton Park, QLD 4102, Australia

Sing-Chung Li and Wei-Fang Hsu
School of Nutrition and Health Sciences, College of Nutrition, Taipei Medical University, Taipei 11031, Taiwan

Jung-Su Chang
School of Nutrition and Health Sciences, College of Nutrition, Taipei Medical University, Taipei 11031, Taiwan
Graduate Institute of Metabolism and Obesity Sciences, College of Nutrition, Taipei Medical University, Taipei 11031, Taiwan

Chun-Kuang Shih
School of Nutrition and Health Sciences, College of Nutrition, Taipei Medical University, Taipei 11031, Taiwan
School of Food Safety, College of Nutrition, Taipei Medical University, Taipei 11031, Taiwan
Master Program in Food Safety, College of Nutrition, Taipei Medical University, Taipei 11031, Taiwan

Ilse Molendijk and P.W. Jeroen Maljaars
Department of Gastroenterology and Hepatology, Leiden University Medical Center, 2313 ZA Leiden, The Netherlands

Sander van der Marel
Department of Gastroenterology and Hepatology, Haaglanden Medical Center, 2512 VA The Hague, The Netherlands

Fernando Castro
Department of Internal Medicine, School of Medicine, Federal University of Rio de Janeiro, 21941-913 Rio de Janeiro, Brazil

Heitor S. P. de Souza
Department of Internal Medicine, School of Medicine, Federal University of Rio de Janeiro, 21941-913 Rio de Janeiro, Brazil
Department of Internal Medicine, D'Or Institute for Research and Education (IDOR), 22281-100 Rio de Janeiro, Brazil

Scott N. Schoeman and Amanda Lim
IBD Service, Department of Gastroenterology and Hepatology, The Queen Elizabeth Hospital, 28Woodville Road, Woodville 5011, Australia

Robert Venning Bryant and Samuel Paul Costello
IBD Service, Department of Gastroenterology and Hepatology, The Queen Elizabeth Hospital, 28Woodville Road, Woodville 5011, Australia
School of Medicine, Faculty of Health Sciences, University of Adelaide, Adelaide 5000, Australia

Christopher G. Schultz and Francis Dylan Bartholomeusz
Department of Nuclear Medicine, PET and Bone Densitometry, Royal Adelaide Hospital, Port Road, Adelaide 5000, Australia

Soong Ooi and Charlotte Goess
IBD Service, Department of Gastroenterology and Hepatology, Royal Adelaide Hospital, Port Road, Adelaide 5000, Australia

Jane Mary Andrews
School of Medicine, Faculty of Health Sciences, University of Adelaide, Adelaide 5000, Australia
IBD Service, Department of Gastroenterology and Hepatology, Royal Adelaide Hospital, Port Road, Adelaide 5000, Australia

Andrew D. Vincent
Freemasons Foundation Centre for Men's Health, School of Medicine, University of Adelaide, North Terrace, Adelaide 5000, Australia

Simon P.L. Travis
Translational Gastroenterology Unit, John Radcliffe Hospital, Headley Way, Headington, Oxford OX3 9DU, UK

Nicole Green, Talya Miller, David Suskind and Dale Lee
Department of Pediatric Gastroenterology and Hepatology, Seattle Children's Hospital, Seattle, WA 98105, USA

Pedro López-Muñoz
Inflammatory Bowel Disease Unit, Gastroenterology Department, La Fe University and Polytechnic Hospital, 46026 Valencia, Spain

Esteban Sáez-González and Beatriz Mateos
Inflammatory Bowel Disease Unit, Gastroenterology Department, La Fe University and Polytechnic Hospital, 46026 Valencia, Spain
Inflammatory Bowel Disease Research Group, Medical Research Institute Hospital La Fe (IIS La Fe), 46026 Valencia, Spain

Marisa Iborra, Inés Moret, Pilar Nos and Belén Beltrán
Inflammatory Bowel Disease Unit, Gastroenterology Department, La Fe University and Polytechnic Hospital, 46026 Valencia, Spain
Inflammatory Bowel Disease Research Group, Medical Research Institute Hospital La Fe (IIS La Fe), 46026 Valencia, Spain
Biomedical Research Network Center for Liver and Digestive Diseases (CIBEREHD), 28029 Madrid, Spain

Ammar Hassanzadeh Keshteli, Karen L. Madsen and Levinus A. Dieleman
Department of Medicine, University of Alberta, Edmonton, AB T6G 2P5, Canada
Centre of Excellence for Gastrointestinal Inflammation and Immunity Research (CEGIIR), Edmonton, AB T6G 2X8, Canada

Fernando Rizzello, Elisabetta Giovanardi, Veronica Imbesi, Marco Salice and Paolo Gionchetti
Department of Medical and Surgical Sciences, University of Bologna, Via Massarenti 9, 40138 Bologna, Italy

Enzo Spisni
Department of Biological, Geological and Environmental Sciences, University of Bologna, Via Selmi 3, 40126 Bologna, Italy

Maria Chiara Valerii
Department of Medical and Surgical Sciences, University of Bologna, Via Massarenti 9, 40138 Bologna, Italy
Department of Biological, Geological and Environmental Sciences, University of Bologna, Via Selmi 3, 40126 Bologna, Italy

Patrizia Alvisi
Pediatric Unit, Maggiore Hospital, Largo Bartolo Nigrisoli, 2, 40133 Bologna, Italy

Helena Rolandsdotter and Yigael Finkel
Department of Clinical Science and Education, Södersjukhuset, Karolinska Institutet, 11883 Stockholm, Sweden
Department of Gastroenterology, Sachs' Children and Youth Hospital, Södersjukhuset, 11883 Stockholm, Sweden

Kerstin Jönsson-Videsäter
Clinical Immunology and Transfusion Medicine, Karolinska University Hospital, 14157 Huddinge, Sweden
Department of Medicine, Huddinge, Karolinska Institutet, 14157 Huddinge, Sweden

Ulrika L. Fagerberg
Department of Women's and Children's Health, Karolinska Institutet, 17177 Stockholm, Sweden
Center for Clinical Research, Västmanland Hospital, Uppsala University, 72189 Västerås, Sweden

Michael Eberhardson
Department of Gastroenterology, Karolinska University Hospital, 17177 Stockholm, Sweden
Department of Medicine Solna, Karolinska Institutet, 17176 Stockholm, Sweden

Kyle Kilby
Faculty of Medicine, Dalhousie University, 1459 Oxford Street, Halifax, NS B3J 4R2, Canada

Holly Mathias
School of Health and Human Performance, Dalhousie University, 6230 South Street, Halifax, NS B3H 1T8, Canada

Lindsay Boisvenue
Seaway Valley Community Health Care, 353 Pitt Street, Cornwall, ON K6J 3R1, Canada

Courtney Heisler and Jennifer L. Jones
Nova Scotia Collaborative Inflammatory Bowel Disease Program, Division of Digestive Care and Endoscopy, QEII Health Science Centre, Room 932, Victoria Building, 1276 South Park Street, Halifax, NS B3H 2Y9, Canada

Index